Manual Therapy

Jean-Pierre Barral • Alain Croibier

BARRAL PRODUCTIONS

Manual Therapy for the Cranial Nerves

Manual Therapy for the Peripheral Nerves

Manual Therapy for the Prostate

From Manual Evaluation to General Diagnosis

Visceral Vascular Manipulation

New Manual Articular Approach; Upper Extremity

New Manual Articular Approach; Lower Extremity

Manual Thermal Evaluation

Understanding the Messages of Your Body

Understanding the Messages of Your Joints

Your source for quality educational materials.

com

New Manual Articular Approach; Lower Extremity

Project Managers: Dawn Langnes, Vicki McCabe
Translator: Annabel Mackenzie
Editors: Gail Wetzler, Deb Delmar, Fred von Kamecke
Production Artists: Jennifer Prater, Jeri Monastero
Illustrations and Photographs: Totem Studio (Pierre-Francoise Couderc)

New Manual Articular Approach; Lower Extremity

Jean-Pierre Barral

Osteopathe DO (UK)
Member of the Registre des Ostéopathes de France
Diplomed from the European School of Osteopathy of Maidstone (UK)
Faculty of Medicine of Paris – North, Department of Manual Medicine and Osteopathy

Alain Croibier

Osteopathe DO, MRO (F)
Member of the Registre des Ostéopathes de France
Member of the Academie d'Osteopathie de France
Lecturer in visceral manipulation and osteopathic diagnosis at the osteopathic college, A.T. Still Academy, Lyon, France

BARRAL PRODUCTIONS

PALM BEACH GARDENS, FLORIDA

First published 2011

LCCN: 2016933693

ISBN-13: 978-0-9860262-8-7

Barral Productions
11211 Prosperity Farms Road, Suite D-325
Palm Beach Gardens, Florida 33410 USA
561.622.3761

BARRAL PRODUCTIONS
Your source for quality educational materials.

www.Barralinstitute.com

Printed in USA

Contents

Introduction

Patients often use their ingenuity to direct therapists to where they think their problem lies. They determine that all care and attention should be focused precisely where they experience pain.

The practitioner has a choice to make. Either he focuses locally on symptoms, an action that runs contrary to osteopathic principle, or he takes a comprehensive approach to the problem.

General listening allows the hand to be attracted to the major tissue tension. *Local listening* refines the evaluation.

A joint in pain and dysfunction can have a local or a remote cause. Knee pain can result from a sprain. On the other hand, the sprain can occur because of a dysfunctional genital system, whose repercussions land at the knee, by way of the myofascial or neural systems. The source of the trouble might be an adhesion at the cecum, creating mechanical conflict for the adjacent ovary and obturator nerve.

Over time, local consequences that occur from a more general imbalance become the primary dysfunctions. Thus the local knee problem must be treated, as well. In answer, the therapist might might treat the capsule, retinacula, and saphenous nerve together with the genicular arteries.

We can always ask why such injuries and problems occurred. Was it a last straw, like the drop of water that overfills the vase, or simply the result of a forceful or maladapted movement?

There are diehards who believe that nothing happens by chance; that all events are preordained as part of some vast program. While it has certainly been our experience that dysfunctions tend to arise over time, this is not always true.

The bottom line is, whether or not the cause of the problem originates beyond the joint itself, the pain is real, and sooner or later, it interferes with proper function. Joint pain gradually causes stiffness, edema, circulatory deficiency, the beginnings of osteoarthritis, and eventually postural changes.

Our objective as therapists is to address the source of the trouble.

1
General Introduction

Review and generalities

1

The first book in the New Manual Articular Approach series is devoted to the upper extremity. For readers unfamiliar with this earlier book, we will review the essential elements of what constitute the "novelty" of our manipulative approach. For a more complete description, we invite you to consult the opening chapters of *New Manual Articular Approach; Upper Extremity.*

This volume expands on our systemic approach to joints and their biomechanics. We explain why it seems necessary to step back from reductionist biomechanics and how our practice has led us to envisage a more clinically anchored model that integrates mechanical aspects and biological principles.

We examine the lower extremity in terms of its role in overall body stability as well as evolutionary adaptations it has made in terms of vertical stance and bipedal locomotion.

1.1 BRIEF OVERVIEW OF THE NEW MANUAL APPROACH

1.1.1 Beyond structure and function

This book presents both a fresh concept and a range of new technique possibilities. Together they amount to a very different approach to manual joint treatment that is far from abiding by the classic division between function and structure. Our techniques are based on results achieved with a wide range of patients in clinical practice with patient safety in mind.

This work was originally formatted as a collection of clinical tips developed chiefly by senior author Jean-Pierre Barral. Since then, the authors have refined techniques together. This has come as a function of clinical cases encountered over many years of daily practice.

After we grouped these techniques together, they lacked certain cohesion. This desire for unity prompted us to take a good look at the fundamentals of joint function and reconsider some of our basic premises.

In the end we mapped out our manipulations in reference to an enlarged biomechanical framework that is more in line with a systems approach, in which parts are joined together in a web of relationships.

This strategy proves very useful when dealing with acute or complex pain and whenever classic techniques are not working, are difficult, or are impossible to perform.

1.1.2 Our perspective

We envision a joint as being made up of several subsystems whose interactions create an intricate complex. By complex we do not mean complicated. Edgar Morin (2005) defined complexus as "that which is chained together," like an aggregate of parts in an entanglement of interlacing branches, organized much as we picture a neurological plexus.

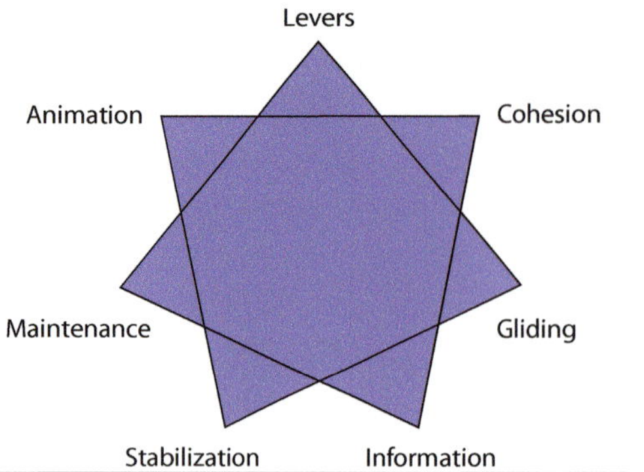

Fig. 1.1 The seven joint subsystems.

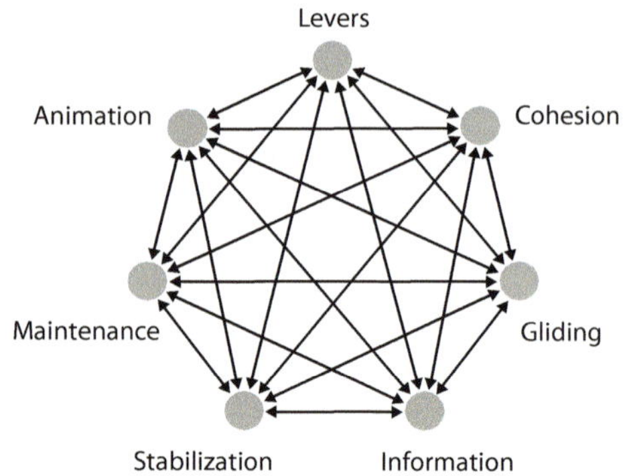

Fig. 1.2 Joint subsystem interactions.

We distinguish seven basic subsystems that work in combination to support function (Fig. 1.1).

1.1.3 The system interactions

From the systems perspective, good joint function is inseparable from the sound working order of each subsystem, along with the seamless interaction and communication between the subsystems (Fig. 1.2). Further, a joint can be conceptualized as an "organ complex" dedicated to movement. This function also relies on proper cooperation and communication between each component part.

1.1.4 Interactions outside the system

From a holistic perspective, the human being is an aggregate of systems that operates in exchange with each other and with the environment. The joint system is part of this grand totality, constantly interacting with other dimensions of the individual. It is subjected to the functioning of many parts of the body such as visceral, vascular, nervous, and psychoemotional elements. Moreover, it continually compensates for and adapts to internal and external conditions.

A tremendous range of interactions occurs. While some interactions are quite apparent, others are less obvious, but they all influence joint system function to varying degrees.

1.2 THE SYSTEMS APPROACH

To gain a new perspective about any therapeutic course of action in the field of joint work, it is helpful to first review some essentials of the systems approach.

The systemic approach is an interdisciplinary field that originated in the mid-1970s. Sometimes referred to as systems analysis, it is a way of studying objects in their complexity. It attempts to understand how systems influence each other within a whole. This methodology can be applied to the domain of physics, human beings, and even society. A systems way of understanding can be viewed as a language, a state of mind, or even a philosophy. Systems analysis has applications and tangible benefits for a great number of disciplines ranging from ecology and biology to the study of human culture. This line of thinking is especially well-suited to the osteopathic approach in general and to joints in particular.

1.2.1 Definitions

The systems approach rests on the notion of system. A system can be defined as a group of elements that interacts with sufficient strength to form a whole that cannot be described by considering its elements separately.

Joël De Rosnay defined a system as "a group of elements in dynamic interaction organized toward a common end state."

The theory describes two systems:

- closed systems with very little external environmental exchange;
- open systems that exchange matter, energy, and information with their environment.

From this perspective, living organisms as well as their cells and some organ groups can be defined as open systems to the extent that they interact with their environment.

1.2.2 Principles

Ludwig von Bertalanffy was an Austrian-born biologist known as one of the pioneers of general systems theory. Every open system operates under three structural and functional principles:

- the principle of totality;
- the principle of homeostasis;
- the principle of equifinality.

These three principles give the system autonomy, independent of time or initial conditions, something whose state is determined solely by parameters of the system (Von Bertalanffy 1973).

Principle of totality: interactions

A system is a whole that is more than the sum of its parts and is not reducible to its parts. It is not possible to understand the function of a system by simply deducing the function of each component. If the whole is greater than the sum of its parts, it is due to the interplay of elements—exchanges from inside the system and interactions between these elements and the exterior context of the system.

One cannot predict the behavior of the whole merely through the detailed knowledge of it parts. From a certain level of complexity, new properties can appear in a system. These are called emergent properties. In any systemic intervention, the focus shifts to the interaction of the parts rather than their behavior taken separately.

Principle of homeostasis: regulations

An open system has regulatory mechanisms that allow it to remain stable in all circumstances, even when its environment changes. Constant regulation permits the system to survive and maintain itself. The regulator mechanisms function by way of feedback loops that operate in relationship to internal or external factors. Feedback mechanisms are usually implicit in joint systems.

Feedback loops can be positive or negative.

Negative feedback cancels the action of internal or external factors and can alter the balance of a system. Because system balance and stability depend on these feedback mechanisms, they are termed stabilizers.

Positive feedback accentuates the effect of disruptive factors and tends to destabilize the system to the point it achieves a new position of equilibrium. The effects of such mechanisms are cumulative. In the extreme they can have a snowball effect that expands indefinitely, generating the explosion of blockages in the system. The dynamics of change rest on positive feedback.

Circular causality is a notion that derives from the feedback concept. Feedback responses sometimes make it difficult to distinguish between cause and effect in a phenomenon at the heart of a system. In fact, it becomes a meaningless question. Better to consider such a loop in its global dynamic. If one hopes to observe it in order to study it, it is preferable not to open or sever it.

Such a systemic approach is operational in any therapy that makes use of a structure's capacity to regulate itself. This sometimes involves activating transformative possibilities in unblocking a system or cutting certain circular causality loops. Isn't this exactly what we strive to do in osteopathy?

Circular causality in osteopathy

We are quite familiar with this type of feedback loop in osteopathy. These are invariable instances where an effect has a retroactive outcome on its cause. This becomes an effect in itself. In some pathologies it can be next to impossible to determine the true origin of the problem.

A common example of this quandary is a somatic vertebral dysfunction that irritates the laterovertebral sympathetic chain, causing organ dysfunction. The irritated organ, in turn, sends nociceptive messages through the already dysfunctional vertebral segments. The result is an exacerbation of vertebral muscle spasms, an aggravation of the vertebral segment irritation. The sympathetic chain then sends more efferent messages that increase organ irritation, and so it continues.

Principle of equifinality: adaptability

Equifinality is the capacity of a system to reach a given end state from different initial conditions and by many potential means. A system is deemed equifinal when "the same end state can be reached from different initial states and by alternate paths" (Von Bertalanffy 1973). The organism may not be able to rely on past structural hierarchies to resolve a given problem. Rather, corrective action comes from informational exchange among the interconnected and interdependent component parts.

1.3 HUMAN MECHANICS

1.3.1 How this works in practice

This new manipulative approach can be a little disconcerting for osteopaths who remain "osteocentric" in their view of joint manipulations. It is not our intention to question classic manipulations. We have learned them and use several on a daily basis. Far be it from us to deny our origins. We simply wish to expand our concept of joint dysfunction, moving beyond notions of simple "mechanical disturbances." Such an approach limits itself to axes and planes of movement that quickly find their conceptual and operational limits.

Opening our mind to other parameters has allowed a different vision of joint physiology to emerge. This revamping enables us to better help our patients find solutions or improve their conditions, especially in cases that respond poorly to classic manual treatment.

1.3.2 Biomechanics

There are many ways to look at joint biomechanics. They range from the most abstract of mathematical configurations to the most concrete of biological phenomenon. Any understanding of human mechanics vacillates between two camps: (1) notions of the mechanical and the physical; and (2) principles of life and physiology. The two propositions are worlds apart. They are put further at odds in everyday reality, especially as they apply to the static and moving body. Nervous, muscular, and vascular regulations all complicate any exact functional joint study.

The mechanical level

The mechanical aspect concerns all studies focusing on vectors, angles, load forces, and geometrical figures. Results are expressed in numbers, graphs, and mathematical calculations that are conceptually closer to engineering than to osteopathy.

According to Ficat et al. (1987), while the encoding of physiology is perhaps a laudable ambition, it has the hidden agenda of turning biology into an exact science in the face of uncertainty and multiple unknown factors inherent to all things human. Even if these more or less abstract physical data lend biomechanics a "scientific" character, one must not overestimate their value. Such findings can never be more than approximations, serving only as guidelines. It certainly is wrong to dismiss them entirely, but it is equally unjustified to give them much credence in terms of designing our manipulations.

The biological level

Human biomechanics requires us to take

into account the structural and functional complexity of all soft tissue and joint components; this includes their reciprocal interactions together with their muscular, nervous, and vascular connections. The musculoskeletal system is strictly subordinate to all organic functions operating in close relationship with the central nervous system. The motor function escapes to absolute automatism, and confers to Man his physical freedom and autonomy.

1.3.3 Necessary clinical biomechanics

Reductionism

In the view of Dr. Adalbert I. Kapandji (1987), most biomechanical data and models must be put in perspective. Such science, often technically inspired, is fundamentally reductionist. Beware! He believes it is important to differentiate clearly between clinical biomechanics and industrial mechanics, and to dispense with the acquired reflexes of thinking in overly rigid, mechanical terms.

In an article on the biomechanical "spud," Kapandji emphasized the basic difference between industrial and living mechanics. Living biomechanics operate in four dimensions, in which time does not have the same value as it does in industrial mechanics. Furthermore, mechanical play is omnipresent in the living joint, whereas it is to be challenged in industrial joints. Planes and axes of movement are materialized and fixed in industrial mechanics but are far from being so in living motion.

The dimension of time

Kapandji also imagined biomechanics as a four-dimensional space where the "the time dimension" counts for double.

In general terms, time is naturally involved in movement. Standard kinematics describes motion as a relationship between space and time.

While all motion requires time, time is twice as involved in living structures because living beings are born, transform, and evolve. Growth and renewal are continuous until an irreversible degenerative tendency takes the upper hand (Fig. 1.3).

According to Kapandji, man by definition can only be observed at a given moment of his existence. In this way, biomechanics are

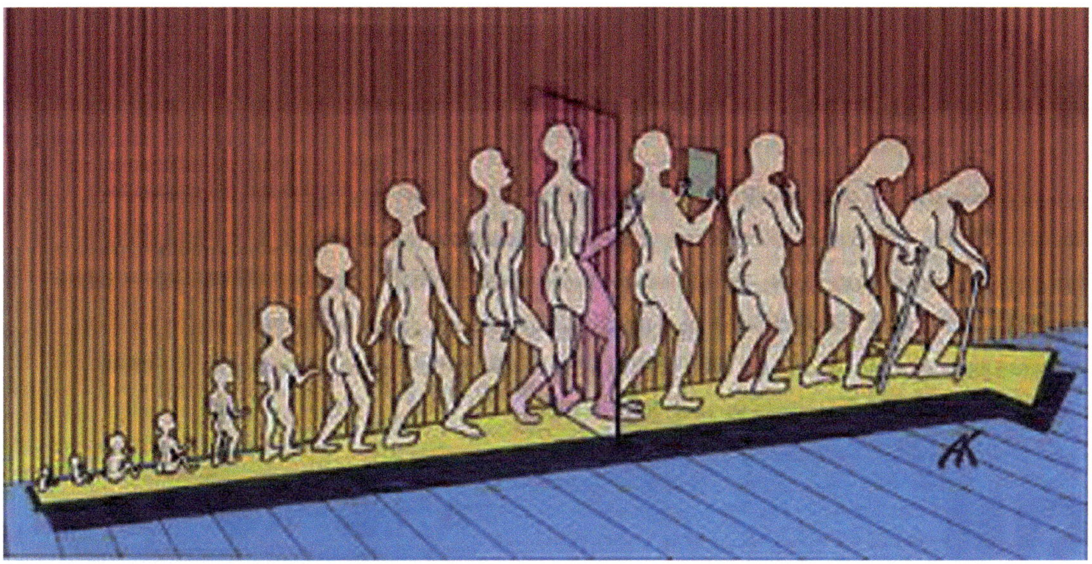

Fig. 1.3 Life's walking belt. (A. Kapandji. 2011, What is biomechanics? Sauramps edition.)

radically distinct from standard mechanics. Man is to be viewed as the "temporal section" of a four-dimensional entity. His status is the combination of mechanical constraints he undergoes and his growth and deterioration potential.

Negentropy

Behind this somewhat barbaric-sounding term lies one of life's basic mechanisms. The terms negentropy, or negative entropy, refer to the organizing factor that counterbalances a system's natural gradual decline into disorder, which is defined as entropy.

The effects of temporal evolution are seen in the constant remodeling of every part of the living mechanism. The capacity for dynamic structural change differentiates biomechanics from industrial mechanics.

Living systems possess homeostasis. Homeostasis (from homeo, the same, and stasis, standing still) is defined as the capacity of a system to maintain itself in a constant state in terms of form and internal conditions, despite external disturbances. A system that finds itself in a state of complete stable equilibrium has, in principle, exhausted all possible exchanges with its environment. This represents the state of "death" of the system. All closed systems end up this way sooner or later; it is the physical principle called entropy. Through homeostasis the living world counters degradation linked to the "arrow of time." By this process living systems fight to reverse entropy.

System wear and tear

Even if all living beings could provisionally reverse entropy, they would still never return to their original state. The tendency is to evolve toward a slightly different condition that comes as close as possible to their initial state. There is always a certain inherent wearing down of the system.

Wear is the enemy of industrial mechanics. But life constantly rebuilds all biomechanical parts. Our bones, muscles, and joints are never the same way twice. We transform and we repair. Over the course of a lifetime, any deterioration of parts is compensated for by their reconstitution.

System evolution

From the initial cell, the living being develops and builds itself by self-duplication. Plasticity confers yet another distinctive feature to living mechanical structures: adaptation. Connective tissue studies suggest that life forces adapt body parts to environmental conditions. Life responds to mechanical tensions, which allows the system to adjust to environmental variations.

Repetitive strain can cause certain mechanical structures to strengthen their efforts against environmental changes. This happens, for example, when tissue becomes fibrotic or when joints form bone spurs or lay down extra bone in an attempt to adapt to new conditions. Inversely, lack of mechanical demand, such as during bed rest, causes significant demineralization in bones that are no longer required to be as solid and rigid.

Therapeutic interests

Through the march of time, the living mechanism can: (1) maintain its shape and combat wear and tear, all the while continuing to function; and (2) conserve relative stability without excluding some margin of evolution and adaptation.

At any given moment, an individual's mechanical condition is determined by mechanical stresses it undergoes and its capacity for growth and regeneration. By supporting forces of growth and maintenance, manual therapy can also influence the conditions of joint function.

1.3.4 The use of mechanical play

Kapandji highlighted another functional difference between industrial and living articulations. In industrial joints, wear and tear is proportional to mechanical play. Lack of mechanical play is important in industrial joints because it can cause damage. By contrast, Kapandji considers that some degree of play is necessary in living joints. Whereas parts are able to be perfectly adjusted in industrial mechanics, this is never the case in the living mechanics.

Kapandji identified three basic factors that generate mechanical joint play:

- tendency of joint axis to evolve;
- irregularity of joint surfaces;
- reciprocal joint surfaces conformation (complementary conformation).

The tendency of joint axes to evolve

Axes are fixed and often materialized in industrial mechanics. In biomechanics, axes are not so tangible; they tend to evolve as instantaneous axes. Consequently, artificial joint production is a tricky process. It is necessary to think biomechanically in order to construct prosthetic parts whose axes are neither materialized nor fixed. In addition, the axes of these joints are almost never perpendicular to each other (orthogonal). They are usually oblique and do not correspond to the orthonormal planes that regularly serve as anatomical reference. Standard planes and axes were a creation of early anatomists, drawn in the Cartesian spirit from the frontal, transversal, and sagittal planes of the dissection table.

This is why Kapandji speaks of a biomechanical "spud," because nothing biomechanical is perpendicular like it is in industrial construction. A potato has neither a defined shape nor a clear axis, and it rolls in an inconsistent fashion. As a result, the axis of movement follows along imaginary lines.

Beware all conceptual joint comparisons to mechanical models. While such schemes provide some initial understanding and allow us to visualize a given movement, they ought not to confine our thinking. This is particularly true at the foot, an extraordinarily complex and fascinating ensemble that is too often reduced to mechanical caricatures, such as the heterokinetic toggle joint, lever, or torsion bar. The reality is much more subtle and far less distorted.

Joint surface irregularity

The second aspect of "spud" mechanics, which graces it with the very qualities that industrial engineers search to eliminate, concerns generally accepted ideas about joint surfaces. For example, the femoral head is commonly described as a ball that fits into the socket of the hip bone. The true picture is more nuanced.

In terms of form, even the most regular joint surfaces are far from being perfect geometric figures. Spherical surfaces that form enarthroses, such as the femoral head, are not the ideal spheres we imagine.

As for congruence, most joints fit together with some mechanical play included in their construction. Far from being harmful to function, an element of play is favorable to lubrication and joint shock absorption.

Reciprocally conforming joint surfaces have a complementary structural arrangement. This is a process of osseous rounding off, which fine-tunes our genetically predetermined fabrication.

Research by Rudolf Fick (1911) contributes greatly to our understanding of this process. His experiments looked at what happens when two epiphyses come into contact. One takes on a convex shape while the other becomes concave as it molds to the first. Analysis shows that movement generates form, and that musculotendinous junctions (lever arms) determine the location of concave and convex surfaces. Joint surfaces are simultaneously constructed and refined thanks to automatic movements, beginning with voluntary gesture in utero and continuing through joint usage.

Here we find yet another fundamental characteristic of biomechanics: the indivisible link between form and movement. A prefabricated form delineates movement, but movement then defines and refines the form.

1.3.5 An approach geared toward a joint system

In view of the above, it only makes sense to abandon any purely mechanical approach to human joints. One way to reframe the proposition is to view the joint as the happy result of an extraordinary set of circumstances.

Putting the joint in its proper context

Movement as a system can be organized into several levels:

- Level one includes the anatomical components of the joint unit, which consists of all the classic elements: bone, cartilage, capsule, synovial membrane, synovial fluid, meniscus, labrum, ligaments, and short monoarticular muscles.
- The second level arranges diverse joint systems into a sort of supersystem that can be designated as an articular chain or articular segment. Here we find fascia, aponeuroses, long muscles, and generally all manner of polyarticular components that mechanically strengthen and unite various joint units. The spine and limbs are in this category.
- A third level, the locomotive apparatus, is an integral part of the individual. One can conceive of it as a megasystem, encompassing all the subunits. This apparatus permits a person to act at will in his environment through individual decisions and neuromotor possibilities. This apparatus interacts with numerous other systems, such as the circulatory, that are central to both function and maintenance. It is at this level that psychopostural and posturoemotional effects show up as postural responses to emotional stimuli.

Each level is self-regulating, a property necessary to the conservation of a constant or stable state. In fact, each level exercises control over not just itself but also adjacent categories of organization. As a result, the base level is subject to the most regulation. Whenever we wish to act on an element situated low on the organizational pyramid, it can be useful to identify local regulatory dysfunctions at organizational levels higher up.

Protection requirement

Any movement of living tissue must respect the so-called "noble" structures, which provide nutrition and nerve supply to mobilizing segments. One can only move on the condition that these anatomical elements are not imperiled.

It is imperative to protect neurovascular structures, as they are "hidden" elements of joint load specification. Accordingly, certain actions are simply forbidden in the mechanical joint program. When neurovascular tissues become dysfunctional, mechanoreceptors located within these structures, called interoceptors, detect stimuli that can disturb local proprioception and joint play.

Future outlook

Regrettably, biomechanics are all too often presented from the perspective of pure and hard mechanics, something akin to Newtonian physics. Divested of its true biological nature, biomechanics can even be reduced to an industrial mechanical caricature, drawn up as a sequence of equations or a string of vectors. Some basic understanding of biomechanics is indispensable, but it cannot explain everything.

A citation from Professor Jean Castaing, in the preface to a book by Jean Giraudet (1976), summarizes well the mindset required of an osteopath seeking to understand human mechanics:

"It is important that mechanics not shield life away. The adventure of the body is difficult and problematic to summarize or reduce to an abstract schematic. No matter how complex and sophisticated the model, a machine is still only subject to mechanical, biomechanical, or cybernetic laws."

Life forces are omnipresent and an integral

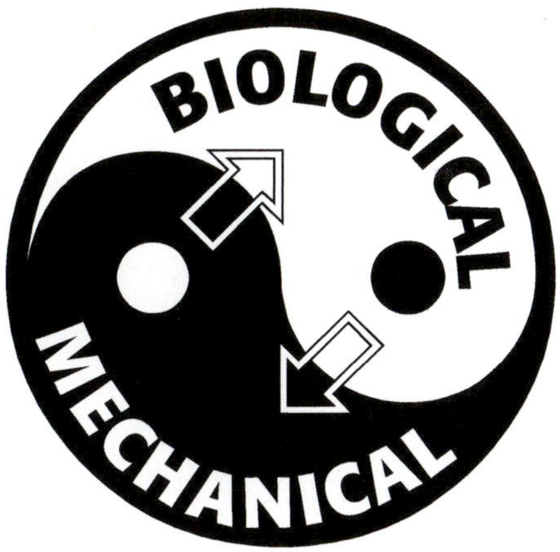

Fig. 1.4 Biomechanical consubstantiality.

part of our new approach to joint treatment. Ficat et al. (1987) describe it this way: "The mechanical and the biological are consubstantial, essentially two expressions of the same discipline, as interpenetrated and inseparable as the yin and yang of Chinese philosophy" (Fig. 1.4).

Example of systemic interaction

We are generally conditioned by our knowledge and preconceived ideas. In order to progress we must sometimes reconsider the way we see things and cast aside conventional wisdom. For example, when we think of a bone as something solid, it is because biomechanics and histomechanics have shown us numerous properties of spongy and cortical bone. Having been inundated with masses of numerical data concerning resistance anisotropy, or even Young's Modulus model of different osseous tissues, we have built up a picture of bone rigidity in terms of these elements alone.

By and large a bone's structural resistance is attributed to the strength of cortical bone and the trabecular layout of the spongy component that strengthens the cortical layer. It is well-known that lines of force materialize the various tensions that are applied to a given bone segment. Nevertheless, the structure of spongy and cortical bone represents no more than the skeleton of the mineral framework of dry bone. It can make us forget the soft parts of bone that fill the intertrabecular spaces of living bone.

- Soft bone has a lining of fatty and hematopoietic components.
- Vessels provide nutrients to osseous tissues and are able to balance anabolism and catabolism through their exchanges.

Living bone is more appropriately visualized as a pressurized solid organ insofar as its vasculomedullary contents exert pressure in the range of 20 mm of mercury against the lining of the inner cavity, the endosteum.

This vasculomedullary turgescence is called the turgor effect, something we are familiar with in the visceral system (Fig. 1.5). Studies show that this force, even if it remains modest compared to the intrinsic resistance of the boney tissue, augments increased trabecular resistance and bone elasticity. The turgor effect, being of vascular origin, is even designated as a form of hydraulic reinforcement. By augmenting the

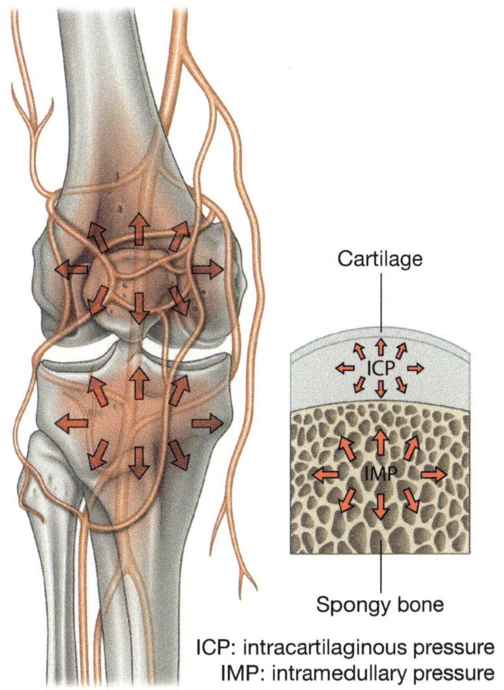

Fig. 1.5 Interosseous vasculomedullary forces.

rigidity of spongy bone as well as reinforcing cortical bone, turgor effectively strengthens the entire bone (Liebschner et al. 2005).

Hydraulic reinforcement is particularly significant in the long bones of the lower extremities that are permanently "inflated" by the prevailing blood pressure within the epiphyses. This force enables the end of the bone to better cushion cartilage stress while, at the same time, strengthening the epiphysis. Vascular architecture is very distinctive at the hip, where venous capacity is six to eight times greater than arterial capacity (Ficat et al. 1987). In addition to their metabolic function, circulatory forces at the hip joint have a physical influence on the mechanical qualities of subchondral bone and play a role in cartilage protection.

Through this simple example we can see how vascular structure together with circulator function bring a biological note into the mechanical domain that is generally seen as belonging to skeletal elements alone.

The lower extremity; key to stability

2

Commonly studied for its role in walking and locomotion, the lower extremity is key to stability in humans. The bipedal human being cannot carry out even ordinary weight transfer and displacement without satisfying stability requirements. Stability of the lower extremity is rarely static. Rather, true steadiness occurs at the heart of movement.

2.1 STABILITY: A DIFFICULT CONCEPT TO DEFINE

Joint problems are largely subordinate to stability, which in and of itself is a multifaceted concept. Each of us has assumptions and references as to what constitutes a stable or unstable joint.

Working clinically with our hands allows us to measure suppleness or stiffness, tissue retraction or laxity. From a theoretical standpoint, however, stability cannot be conceived of piecemeal. In the broader view, several aspects and components should be considered.

2.1.1 Physical considerations: stability and balance

Stability of a solid can be defined as "the resistance opposed anytime a solid wants to move away from a position of balance" (Giraudet 1976). All factors that help a solid to conserve its equilibrium constitute stability. Stability is linked to balance in the sense

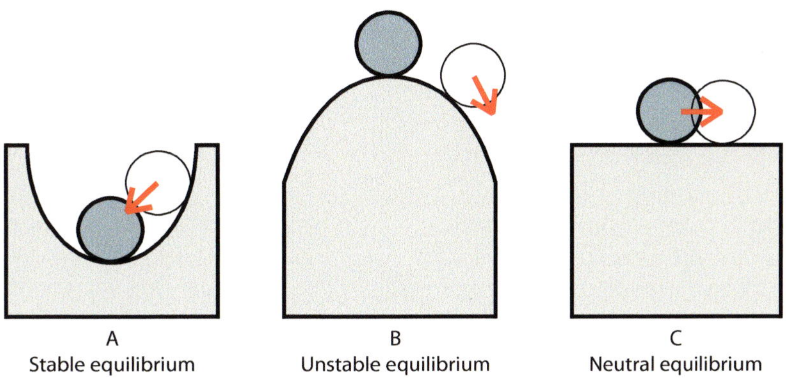

A: A body is in stable equilibrium, if after undergoing a displacement, it tends to return to its initial position.
B: A body is in unstable equilibrium, if after undergoing a displacement, it tends to continue along its course.
C: A body is in neutral equilibrium, if after a displacement, it retains its new position.

Fig. 2.1 The three types of equilibrium.

that physics distinguishes three types of equilibrium of a solid—instable, stable, and neutral (Fig 2.1).

- A body is in unstable equilibrium if it tends to continue movement after being slightly displaced.
- A body is in stable equilibrium if it tends to return to the initial position following displacement.
- A body is in neutral equilibrium when it retains its new position following slight displacement.

2.1.2 Clinical considerations

Where joints are concerned, notions of stability are at once contradictory, complementary, and inseparable from mobility. In simplified terms, the stronger one joint component is, the weaker another joint component may be. This tenet leads to a basic clinical principle that defines joint stability in terms of the anatomical relationship between the joint surfaces of adjacent bones.

The concept of joint stability is not as absolute as it might appear, in that stability indexes are only based on clinical observations. Medicine and surgery are gradually coming around to the idea that essential stability exists in reference to instability when it comes to joint pathology or trauma.

Stability turns out to be a multifaceted notion that can be variously explained depending on context. Clinically, the concept of stability rests on criteria such as degrees of coaptation, cohesion, congruence, and the presence or absence of contact between joint surfaces (Fig. 2.2).

- In a normal joint, congruence and cohesion are preserved.
- In a lax or hypermobile joint, joint play is exaggerated. Cohesion is diminished, but congruence is maintained.
- In a subluxed joint, there is partial contact between joint surfaces with a loss of congruence.
- In a dislocated joint, there is loss of contact between joint surfaces.

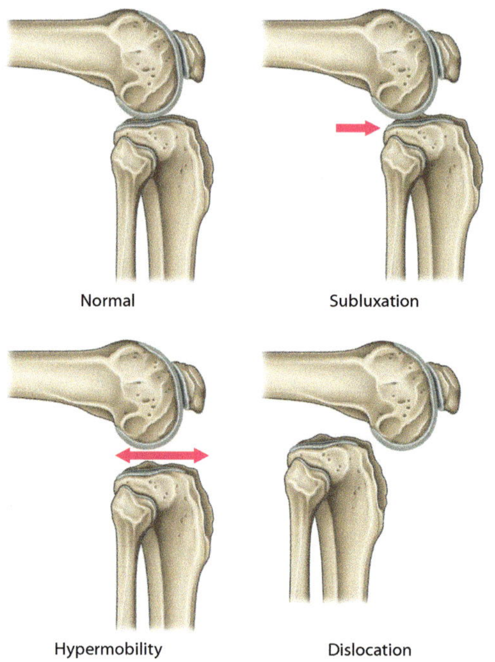

Fig. 2.2 Clinical considerations concerning joint stability.

2.1.3 Energetic considerations

From a perspective closer to physics, joint stability can be envisioned as the energetic potential brought to bear on the joint by the anatomical structural components that guarantee joint play. In other words, joint stability is subject to the quantity of external energy required to destabilize a given articulation. The amount of energy is equal to the work necessary to bring the system to its point of instability.

Take for example a marble in stable equilibrium. The work required to dislodge it from a pit depends on the depth of the hole. One can easily understand that the deeper the hole, the higher the displacement and the greater the effort required to create movement (Fig. 2.3).

The same principle applies to a joint. Stability exists in proportion to the amount of energy required to destabilize the unit. The external effort required must be greater or equal to the sum of anatomical and physio-

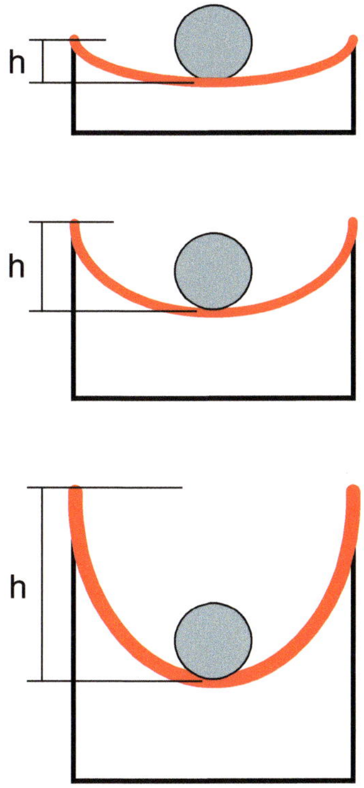

Fig. 2.3 Energy and stability. The height increases from the top to the bottom drawing. "h" depicts the depth of the "well" of potential energy available for the marble. The energy required to destabilize the marble increases with the depth of the well.

logical factors involved in joint stability.

In practical terms, the amount of energy is difficult to quantify. Orthopedic tests to determine ligament rupture, sprain, abnormal movement, or joint laxity all involve degrees of energy applied in precise directions to bring the joint close to destabilization.

2.1.4 Stability: a systemic necessity

Conservation

A system's primary imperative is its own conservation. It strives to remain in a constant state geared toward optimal function. Otherwise, functional systems sooner or later find themselves in a state of imbalance. Various constraints maintain steady conditions for relative stability within which imbalances naturally exist.

Joint integrity

From this perspective a joint is a system that preserves itself in spite of movement. Several factors determine joint stability.

Articular and periarticular structures are configured to resist destabilizing forces.

- They possess both the resistance and the viscoelasticity required to reestablish balance should any major destabilization occur.
- Ligaments are passive viscoelastic structures.
- Muscles are dynamic viscoelastic organs.

All together these properties function in keeping with joint kinematics, permitting full bone movement while providing adequate protection to all joint sectors. Viscoelasticity equals passive stretch (properties).

The concept of visceral articulation has been developed at length in the Visceral Manipulation books (Barral & Mercier, 1984).

Levels of stability

In chapter one we described the components of the movement system according to three levels of organization:

- joint unity;
- the articular chain or articulated segment;
- the locomotive apparatus on which the entire body balances.

Each level is self-regulatory in the service of maintaining a constant or stable state. While autoregulation takes various forms, the abiding rule is the preservation of joint integrity.

The joint makes every effort to avoid actions that can dislocate, deteriorate, or damage it. This is achieved either by defense mechanisms or by the elimination of certain movement components. Each level has implicit specifications for carrying out movement. These blueprints must respect the integrity of the constituent parts involved in the action. Structures adapt as a function of movement, but their stability is both the precondition and the absolute necessity of movement.

Stabilizing elements are of particular importance at the lower extremities. They operate in two ways:

- They provide a stable base of support essential to all body displacement.
- They are the home base for balance mechanisms essential to the biped.

In sum, the entire lower extremity, spinal equilibrium, and all static and dynamic movement possibilities are influenced by the state of joint balance and joint stability. With this in mind, we will examine how individual levels participate in the stability of the human structure.

2.2 JOINT UNIT STABILITY

Joint stability is the result of many closely linked mechanisms: joint geometry; passive, restricting elements (capsuloligamentous tissues); dynamic stabilizers; and intra-articular pressures and forces.

Stability goes hand-in-hand with two different conditions: static stability and dynamic stability. Bones are the main elements of static stability. Capsuloligamentous structures are involved in both static and dynamic stability. Muscles are the major players in dynamic stability.

Depending on the configuration of their articulating surfaces, joints present two very different arrangements. The surfaces of the hip joint fit well together; this results in excellent osseous and static stability. While a meniscus cushions the boney arrangement of the knee, joint stability is essentially dynamic; it relies on an effective musculoligamentous configuration along with extraordinary proprioception. At the ankle, boney stability is not strong; here, again, dynamic stability is of prime importance.

Structural factors: joint geometry

According to Dufour and Pillu (2006), boney stability depends on several factors:

- Stability relies on concordance between surface curves; the closer the radius, the less glide there is.
- Congruence refers to the connecting of joint surfaces; it is sometimes enhanced by an interposed fibrocartilage.
- The angular relationships of neighboring bones determine the way force is transmitted. Joints are more stable when this transmission occurs along one and the same axis.
- Stability is affected by irregularity of the joint line. For example, a broken line lends more stability to a joint.
- Weight plays a role in bringing joint parts together and thus exerts a stabilizing force.

Passive and active factors: dynamic interactions

Capsuloligamentous structures are more than just mechanical strongholds protecting the body from joint subluxation. They provide vital sensory information for the control of movement. They participate in the regulation of involuntary muscular activity (neuromuscular control) necessary to joint stability. Musculotendinous function itself generates joint stability.

Intra-articular pressures

Joint stress is generally studied in reference to osseous constraint. According to Wolff's law, osseous structures adapt according to the lines of force transmitted from bone to bone. But joint pressure is something entirely different.

Intra-articular pressure results from capsuloligamentous forces, synovial fluid pressure, and compression or traction stress applied to a given joint segment.

The capsuloligamentous sleeve is a viscoelastic tube containing a watertight fluid-filled sac made up of synovial membrane and synovial fluid. Two types of constraints operate alternately in the joints of the lower extremity:

- compression constraint when the foot is supported on the ground;
- traction constraint when the foot lifts off.

What results is perpetual intra-articular pressure variation. The capsuloligamentous system and synovial fluid continuously adapt as a pair to these pressure changes. A healthy joint relies on dynamic equilibrium between fluid volume and the elasticity of the passive viscoelastic structures that form the capsuloligamentous unit.

An increase in synovial fluid sometimes upsets this balance. Other times, altered ligamentous elasticity causes rapidly visible changes. This complementary relationship between passive viscoelastic structures and synovial fluid volume generates joint cohesion.

Synovial fluid: laminar cohesion

Laminar cohesion represents the bond strength of a fluid. This force usually acts within a substance. When water, for example, meets the earth or sand, it acts like a paste. It links particles of earth or grains of sand, thereby forming capillary bridges that tend to bring the grains closer together. This attraction is called capillary cohesion.

This type of force can act between two surfaces where intervening fluid opposes their separation. The process involves viscosity and fluid volume, and it affects local pressure conditions. Synovial fluid plays this role notably when the inferior limb hangs freely. Capillary cohesion created by synovial fluid counters separation of the joint surfaces of the knee.

There is an optimal fluid level at which cohesion force is maximal. Insufficient fluid causes inadequate laminal cohesion force. The synovial membrane can adjust volume by either secreting or absorbing joint fluid.

Good joint cohesion requires that intra-articular pressures not vary to any great degree. The capsuloligamentous sleeve regulates pressure within joints. If it is too elastic, peripheral retention becomes insufficient, intra-articular pressure weakens, and cohesion force can be affected. If the sleeve is not elastic enough, fluid volume becomes depleted; here again, the force of cohesion can diminish.

Synovial fluid and capsuloligamentous tissues work in combination to generate cohesion and resist joint dislocation. It is noteworthy that fluid film is doubled at the knee in the peripheral part of the articulation because of the interposed meniscus. Laminar cohesion is strengthened as a result.

2.3 STABILITY OF THE ARTICULAR CHAIN

In a traditional orthopedic analysis, joint stability is evaluated in terms of displacement. The tests need to reveal the ligamentous state of the joint between the two adjacent bones. In pathology, ligament rupture translates into abnormal movements, which in turn generate instability.

Sound physiological stability is generally attributed to the integrity of various ligaments attached to a particular joint. For example, joint ligaments are tensed when the lower extremity is in extension; this occurs in standing. Joints are under relative pre-stress, lending stability to the entire articular chain.

Ligamentous sensory perception

Ligaments are central to stability, but they do not carry out their role solely in the way we often imagine. Before acting as the last strongholds against subluxation, ligaments are first and foremost dynamic strain gauges. They constantly register joint deformations during mobility. Information coming from ligaments induces the body to adapt muscle postures that best and most efficiently serve joint stability.

Over the past 25 years, numerous experiments have shown that muscle activity contributes greatly to joint stability in terms of both articular movements and dynamic stability. Ligaments help to regulate muscle function. Rich in mechanoreceptors, the information they deliver influences muscle tone and stabilizing activity.

As such, many of the muscles involved in this phenomenon are muscles whose attachments bridge several joints. These polyarticular muscles stabilize and animate articular chains and reinforce the interdependence of several units within a particular chain. For example, there are long muscles of the foot that affect as many as four or five different joint units.

It is clear that information provided by the ligamentous mechanoreceptors and issued from various joint units plays a central role in adjusting the tone and contractions of these muscles.

Ligaments and joint communication with the rest of the body

Loss of balance

When muscle protection is insufficient, ligaments are the next in line to help the body avoid a loss of balance. Ligaments themselves only become the ultimate recourse of stabilization when the proprioceptive feedback loop fails. Physiologically, ligaments should never find themselves in such a situation. This default situation indicates that the ligaments are unable to play their proprioceptive role correctly; they lose normal muscle protection as a result. Keep this in mind whenever a joint tends toward instability and repetitive sprain.

Dysfunctional ligaments

Proprioception deficits are a result of deafferentation. Deafferentation is the interruption of the afferent connection of nerve cells. This happens when animals demonstrate their spontaneity of locomotion.

A good deal has been written about proprioceptive deficits resulting from interrupted peripheral mechanoreceptors, especially with regard to diminished function of the knee. Studies have shown that restored proprioception can improve functional knee stability, depending on the condition of the joint.

Experiments show that ligaments are far removed from the "all or nothing" proposition to which they are too often reduced. The simplified view of ligaments as either intact and functional or ruptured and incompetent is far from clinical reality. In practice, ligaments suffer a range of dysfunction and injury that can diminish their informational function. This proprioceptive loss is what disturbs normal neuromotor feedback and impairs full recovery.

Injury to the ligament not only causes mechanical instability but also leads to a functional deficit in the form of diminished proprioception of the knee joint. Functional recovery is often incomplete even after arthroscopic anterior cruciate ligament reconstruction. Some patients with a clinically satisfactory repair and good ligament tension continue to complain of a feeling of instability and giving way, although the knee does not sublux on clinical testing.

Factors that may play a role could be proprioceptive elements, as the intact anterior cruciate ligament has been shown to have significant receptors. Proprioception is an important component of functional knee stability.

A collection of seemingly minor sprains, quick turns of the foot, or putting the foot down wrong during gait can deprive ligaments of elasticity. Diminished proprioception has significant implications for stability in terms of the joint involved as well as the entire articular chain.

We are always surprised to find that small fixations are not only detectible by trained hands but that releasing them can have spectacular results for functional joint recovery. Furthermore, it is astonishing to realize that standard neurophysiological and imaging examinations fail to reveal what the educated and trained hand can detect.

Ligamentous fixations are often concentrated at areas of boney or fibrocartilage attachment. These locations yield the best results. It is advisable to treat them in all joint dysfunctions.

2.4 CORPORAL STABILITY

2.4.1 The "solid" human

Earlier in the chapter we described the stability of a solid strictly in terms of physical considerations. Needless to say, the human body is well understood to be neither solid nor rigid. Nevertheless, it is customary to calculate a theoretical center of gravity as well as a line of gravity around which, like any solid, an individual finds equilibrium.

Center of gravity

The center of gravity of a geometric volume is perceived easily, even intuitively. It is quite another story for irregular figures and solids. The distribution of the human body mass is asymmetrical. Body segments are articulated and their relationships changeable. The center of mass displaces to the largest and heaviest extremity.

The center of gravity varies from one individual to another; it depends on body shape, morphological type, age, and sex. A person's center of gravity shifts as the result of:

- changes in position: standing, sitting, crouching, rolling like a ball;
- changes in position of limb segments: arms in the air, doing the splits;
- activity and movement: walking, running, sports;
- weight bearing, etc.

When a person stands erect with arms at the sides, palms forward in the anatomical position (which is rarely the case), the center of mass is entirely situated in the pelvis, in front of the second sacral segment.

Line of gravity and the static body

With a subject standing in the anatomical position, one can define a line of gravity, also referred to as the central line of gravity, as an imaginary vertical line passing through the center of gravity.

According to Giraudet (1976), this line classically:

- passes in front of the external auditory canal;
- grazes the concavity of the cervical spine;
- cuts along the 10th dorsal vertebra;
- skims the posterior border of the fifth lumbar vertebra;
- passes slightly behind the coxofemoral joint (under tension of the ischiofemoral ligament);
- passes slightly anterior of the knee joint (with the posterior and lateral ligaments tensed);
- arrives at the ankle on the midtarsal joint (Chopart's joint).

In the anatomical position of reference, the line of gravity is the vertical line that passes through the center of gravity, which is found in the lesser pelvis facing the second sacral segment.

Support polygon

The base of support or support polygon is a surface where all points of contact land either on the inside or on the perimeter. The surface cannot be concave.

2.4.2 Bipedal and quadrupedal stability

Stability conditions

If we apply the preceding notion to animal or human stability, it is evident that the number and position of an animal's paws help to determine stability. The basic premise is that stability exists in relation to the surface that we have defined as a "support polygon." An animal or human body is deemed stable only if its center of gravity is located above the polygon (Fig. 2.4).

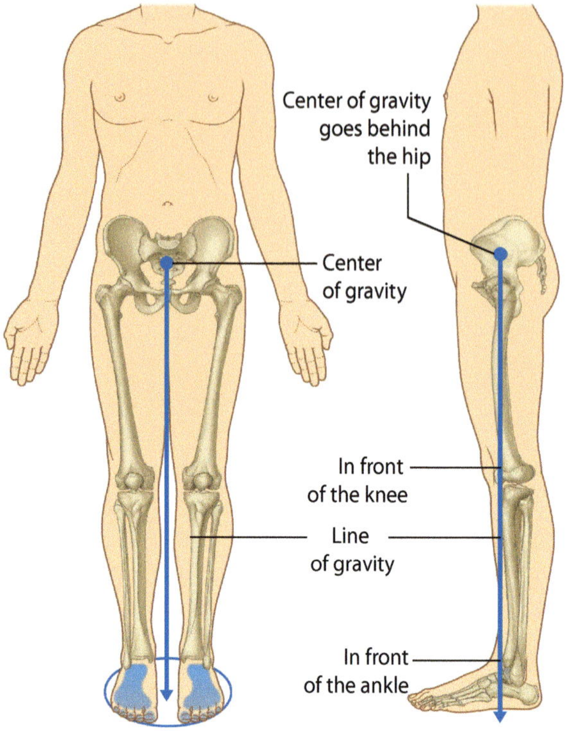

Fig. 2.4 Gravity line and polygon support.

Balance

A person's stability rests on two factors:

- the degree to which the line of gravity reconciles with the geometric center of the support polygon;
- the size of the support polygon.

The stability of an object is inversely proportional to the height of its center of gravity. An object whose center of mass is located very low and near the support polygon is more stable than one whose center of gravity is higher up.

In the acquisition of erect vertical posture, the human body lost a good deal of stability when compared to quadrupeds. The bipedal body is comparable to a line of gravity that remains in balance as long as the line remains within the base of support. A relatively high center of gravity combined with a reduced support base creates less stable conditions, even instability.

2.4.3 Problems linked to bipedalism

Preamble

In approaching the adaptations required by bipedalism, it is useful to be clear from the start that it is not our intention to pick up on debates centered on the whys and wherefores of evolution, notably between the followers of Jean Baptiste Lamarck and Charles Darwin. Neither do we promote the anthropocentrism favored by certain scientific circles. Accordingly, we emphasize that bipedalism is not the preserve of man alone. Most birds are bipedal, their tail often serving as a third foot as it does for most primates.

While some species walk on two legs for a short time or for a few meters, Homo sapiens are the only extant species of the primate family who permanently walk on their two feet, heels touching the ground.

Most scientists accept the current evolutionary model that suggests men evolved from primate simians (apes). This approach would seem to place man at the top of the pyramid of living being. Contrarily, there are anthropologists who defend the theory of initial bipedalism. Based on embryological elements and comparative anatomy, they contend that the human form is not the outcome but rather a starting point to once and future lineages of the animal world.

We keep out of such discussions. Our approach is limited to the specifics of the lower extremity and adaptations required by bipedalism, without regard to any evolutionary view.

Problems of bipedalism

We have seen that standing erect on the lower extremities and maintaining positioning with a high center of gravity poses stability problems not imposed on quadrupeds. In erect posture the center of gravity is more than one meter from the ground. The head rises to at least 1.60 meters, while the foot surface contact with the ground is limited to the support polygon.

Elements of bipedalism

Osteoarticular modifications have been well studied by anthropologists and anatomists. Comparisons between homologous skeletal elements permit a better understanding of the biological significance of human structures.

Neuromotor adaptations facilitate sophisticated neurological coordination. The very nature of the mechanisms that control our balance remains poorly understood. A long apprenticeship on the subject and a certain maturity on the part of the nervous system are required for study. We know that even after acquiring coordination skills, balance control remains vulnerable. To be persuaded of this, just try having a few drinks.

2.4.4 Modifications linked to bipedalism

Osteoarticular adaptations

Many changes to the human model can be identified (Cyrille Cazeau 2006):

- The pelvis is now broad and short. There is enlargement of the iliac wings, while the symphysis pubis has shortened to form a "bowl."
- The lower limbs switched from the transversal stage to the parasaggital erect stage, so they are very mobile in the sagittal plane.
- There is significant elongation of the femur accompanied by a decentering and reinforcement of the femoral neck; the general axis of the shaft is oblique below and medially.
- The tibia is bound with the fibula. There is no rotation at the knee and ankle and only weak inversion of the foot.
- A semirigid longitudinal and transversal arch permits walking on the soles of the feet (plantigrade walking).

Adaptations of the foot

The foot is usually our only contact with the ground. It has at least three functions:

- Being in direct contact with the ground that supports it, the foot is first and foremost a sensory organ. It provides a substantial part of the information we receive about the exact nature of the ground underfoot and our position in space.
- The foot is also an organ of support. It must carry the weight of the body, sometimes even much more, without collapsing. It must be strong without being too rigid.
- The foot is also an organ of movement. It must adapt itself to uneven terrain and propel us forward.

The foot gives us our sense of space and how to move in it. The foot provides sensory information, supports load, maintains balance, and provides for locomotion all at the same time. It must conjugate sensitivity, force, skill, and agility.

Neuromotor adaptations

Gravity

The force of gravity is familiar to us, as it keeps our feet on the ground. It is one of the four basic forces of nature along with electromagnetic force and the weak and strong nuclear forces. This natural attraction acts on all masses and constitutes what some have called the "glue of the cosmos."

Gravity gives weight to physical objects. It concentrates, densifies, and attracts all that is subject to it toward the center of the earth. Gravitational force penetrates the human body, impregnating all tissues and influencing each cell. As such, gravity is a cosmic organizing principle of the human structure.

Harisson H. Fryette (1983) described gravity as an "inexorable factor" that places a constant load on all support structures of human organism. According to Fryette, this force is also what kills our patients, as the weight of gravity can mechanically disrupt health. But it can also release curative forces, which is how we put it to use in osteopathy.

Gravity is a basic parameter that presides over both health disruption of mechanical origin and the release of curative forces that we attempt to do in osteopathy.

The struggle against gravity

Gravitational load requires that internal forces be in place to oppose structural collapse. Upright stance implies the meeting of two forces: gravity and the ceaseless implementation of automatic activity.

Ernst Michael Kranich (2006) expressed this state vividly when he said, "Erect stance is a constant protest against the forces that would pull us down." And, "What confers the seal of humanity on the body is its erect posture."

The distinctive feature of mankind is his relationship to gravity. Indeed, even when animals stand on two legs they never achieve the same degree of victory over gravity that characterizes human posture (Fig. 2.5).

Constant surveillance

The struggle for balance when standing or walking is perpetual (Fig. 2.6). In the end, the achievement depends very little on static and geometric conditions of each of the joints that compose the articular chains of the body.

Somatosensory information is integrated at the cerebellum together with labyrinthic input. The lower extremities represent two articulated chains that act constantly to remedy disruptions in equilibrium and reestablish better balance.

The motor program uses the lower extremities to keep its balance in two ways:

- Muscle vigilance modulates activity, allowing small degrees of anterior, posterior, and lateral sway. In this way muscles maintain the line of gravity within the base of support and in line with that of the mobility axis of the joints of the rear foot.

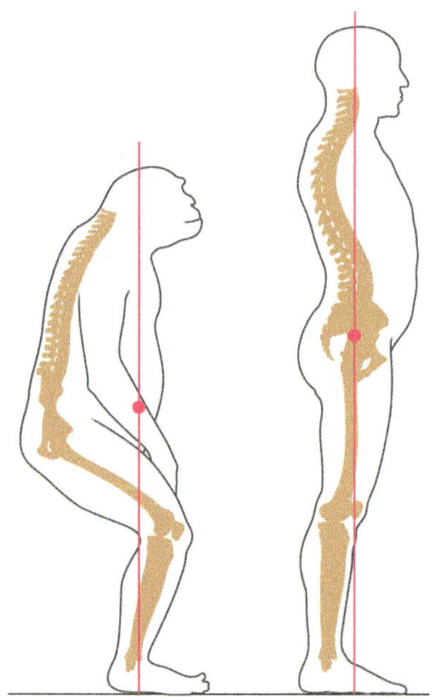

Fig. 2.5 Animal biped and human posture.

- Adaptations occur at the level of the support base itself. Adjacent imbalances are rectified mainly by moving or widening to bring the base back under the line of gravity.

2.4.5 Bipedal balance sheet

Advantages

Man essentially owes his characteristics to the vertical appearance of his body.

- The axis of the trunk almost coincides with the line of gravity.
- By remaining close to the gravitational axis, various parts of the body are distributed in a more balanced way.
- The weight of the viscera is supported in part by the pelvis and no longer hangs from the vertebral column.
- The upper extremities are free from the constraints of locomotion, making them available for other purposes, such as prehension and the evolution of the hand. Orthopedic surgeons Jean Bénichou and Marc Libotte (2002) view the biped as static heresy, because the foot is fraught with trouble; nevertheless, this represents a liberating option.
- The migration of the foramen magnum toward the base of the cranium permits a precise and economical centering of the head on the neck.
- Due to the proximity of the head to the body and the line of gravity, the work of the cervical muscles is diminished.

It is also classically acknowledged that bipedalism saves energy in the standing position, and walking upright is linked to brain development.

Inconveniences

Upright trunk posture requires a good many musculoskeletal adaptations. It is conventionally accepted that this process may have caused mechanical weak points such as the lumbosacral junction or the thoracic inlet, which are subject to strong tensions and sometimes operate under duress.

The human hand has long been considered the great beneficiary of bipedalism. Some authors view it as the distinctive char-

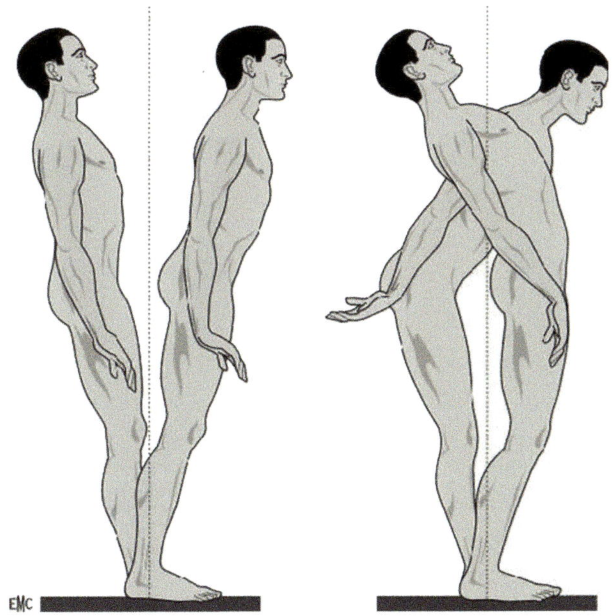

Fig. 2.6 Rebalancing strategies. Strategy of the ankle (left) and the hip (right). (A.M. Eber, M. Collart. 2002. "Balance disorders and posture." EMC Neurology 17-005-E-10: 1-11. Paris: Elsevier Masson. All rights reserved.)

acteristic of man. It is easy to forget that the human foot was markedly differentiated and specialized in the course of bipedalism. In place of the classic "liberation of the hand," some authors prefer to emphasize "the enslavement of the foot" (G. Richards 1986).

Summary

Gravity places a constant and permanent load on the support structures of the organism. Like all living beings, humans are in a perpetual struggle against gravitational stress.

Certainly the stability of erect stance is a tribute to mechanical factors that govern static joint function within each of the corporal chains. But this is not enough. Dynamic factors come into play, controlling movement and stability as well as adjusting and regaining balance. Let us keep in mind that psychoemotional factors can alter a person's posture considerably.

Two-legged locomotion compels human beings to work constantly on their proprioceptive sense in the struggle and dynamic adaptation to gravity's perpetual pull. A sense of body position, posture, balance, and motion maintains the body's center of gravity in line with the support polygon. Precise ligamentous, tendinous, and muscular information is integrated at central neurological circuits. The brain's balance strategies then guide coordinated muscle and joint activity.

2
The Hip

Functional anatomy

3

3.1 ANATOMICAL REVIEW

Here are a few characteristics to help the reader understand the hip joint.

3.1.1 Joint surfaces

Femoral head (Fig. 3.1A-C)

- The femoral head forms two-thirds of a full sphere, about 4–5 cm in diameter.
- It is smaller than the humeral head. While its surface area is larger and rounder, the femoral head forms just two-thirds of a sphere in contrast to the nearly hemispheric form of the humeral head.
- The semilunar acetabular surface and the acetabular labrum cover two-thirds of the femoral head.
- The femoral head is covered with articular cartilage except anteriorly, where strong ligaments are required.
- It comes in contact with the roof of the acetabulum, where 50% or more of the entire weight of the upper body is supported by the femur during activity.
- It is directed cranially, anteriorly, and medially.
- The fovea capitis is a pit on the head of the femur where the round ligament inserts. It is situated a little below and

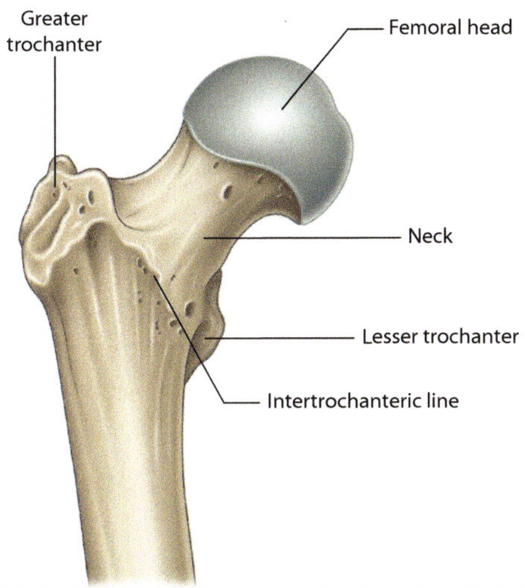

Fig. 3.1A Femoral head (anterior view).

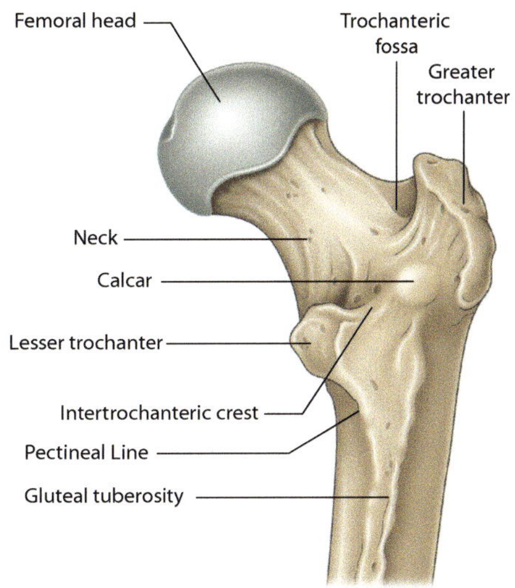

Fig. 3.1B Femoral head (posterior view).

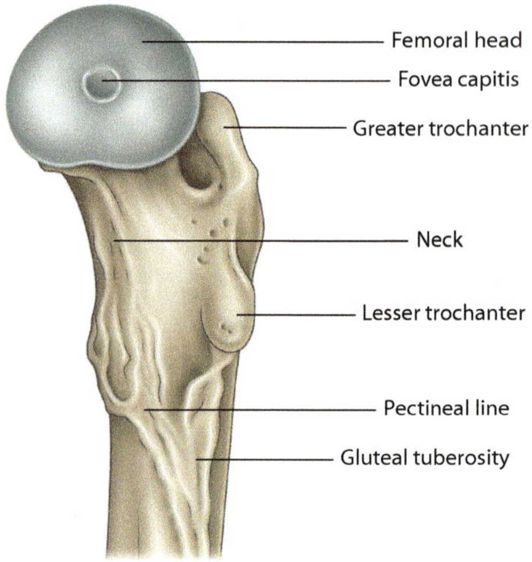

Fig. 3.1C Femoral head (medial view).

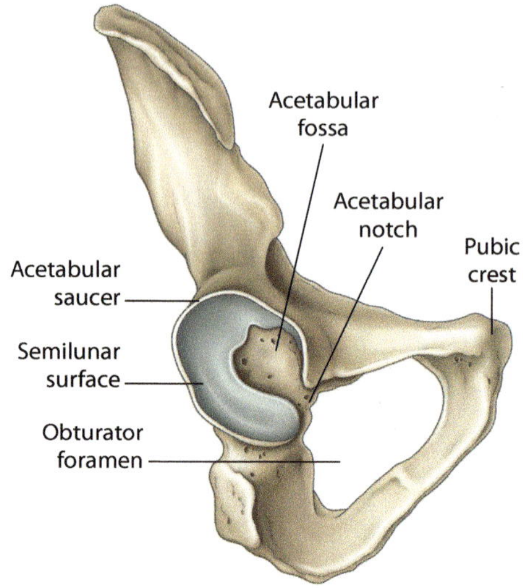

Fig. 3.2 Acetabulum.

behind the center of the femoral head.

- The round ligament is ensheathed in synovial membrane. The artery of the femoral head enters through it.
- The thickness of the femoral cartilage diminishes from the center toward the periphery and is more developed at its anterior cranial part.
- The extracapsular part of the femur narrows to form the neck, which is wider posteriorly.

Deeply situated, the hip is not very accessible to the hand; hence it is mainly treated through the surrounding soft tissues.

Acetabulum (Fig. 3.2)

- Three once-distinct bones fuse to form the acetabulum: the ilium, ischium, and pubis.
- The hip bone, as it is known collectively, forms an open crest-like structure, wider at the top and bottom than at the center.
- It is bounded by the acetabular rim to which the labrum attaches.
- The coxofemoral angle is more open in humans than in animals.

Acetabular labrum or cotyloid labrum

- This ring of fibrocartilage runs around the bony rim of the acetabulum. The transverse acetabular ligament is a fibrous continuation of the labrum, whose peripheral surface attaches to the capsule.
- The labrum increases the depth of the acetabulum to better suit the head of the femur in the formation of the hip joint.
- The articular surface is covered by cartilage whose thickness increases from the center toward the periphery.
- The labrum increases the joint surface by as much as 25%.
- It faces obliquely downward and forward, like the femoral head.
- It constitutes a semirigid intermediary zone between the bones of the joint and the capsule.

Transverse acetabular ligament (Fig. 3.3)

- It straddles the inferior limit of the acetabulum and merges with the two ends of the semilunar labrum.
- It blends superior medially with one of three roots of the round ligament of the femoral head.

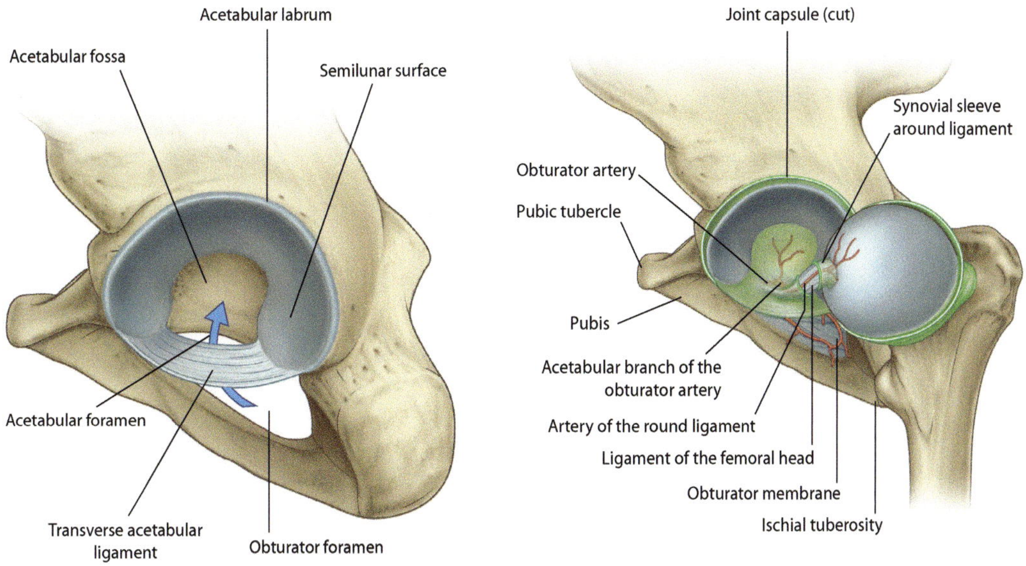

Fig. 3.3 Transverse acetabular ligament.

- It bridges the ischiopubic notch to transform the notch into a passageway.
- It exchanges fibers with the external obturator membrane.

3.1.2 Capsules and ligaments (Fig. 3.4)

The capsule enveloping the hip joint is tough, strong, and flexible. It comprises an outer fibrous layer and an inner synovial membrane.

Proximally the fibrous capsule attaches to the acetabulum at the outer margins of the labrum where the transverse acetabular ligament connects. Distally the fibrous capsule attaches anteriorly to the intertrochanteric line and to the root of the greater trochanter. Posteriorly it encloses the neck of the femur. The capsule is reinforced by circular fibers that form a collar around the femoral neck, known as the zona orbicularis.

The capsule fibers are strengthened by the:

- iliofemoral ligament, in the shape of an inverted Y;
- pupofemoral ligament;
- ischiofemoral ligament.

The ligament of the head of the femur is weak and of little importance in terms of strengthening the hip joint. This intra-articular band attaches to the acetabular notch and to the transverse acetabular ligament. Its narrow end implants at a pit in the femoral head (fovea capitis).

3.1.3 Muscles and movements

The movements that can occur at the hip joint are flexion-extension, abduction-adduction, medial and lateral rotation, and circumduction. Trunk biomechanics also come into play at the hip.

Muscles that act on the hip joint can be grouped by function:

- flexors: iliopsoas, sartorius, tensor fasciae latae, rectus femoris, pectineus, adductor longus, adductor brevis, adductor magnus (anterior part), and gracilis;
- adductors: adductor longus, adductor brevis, adductor magnus, gracilis, pectineus, and obturator externus;
- lateral rotators: obturator externus, obturator internus, gemellus, piriformis, quadratus femoris, and gluteus maximus;
- extensors: semitendinosus, semimembranosus, biceps femoris (long head), adductor magnus (posterior part),

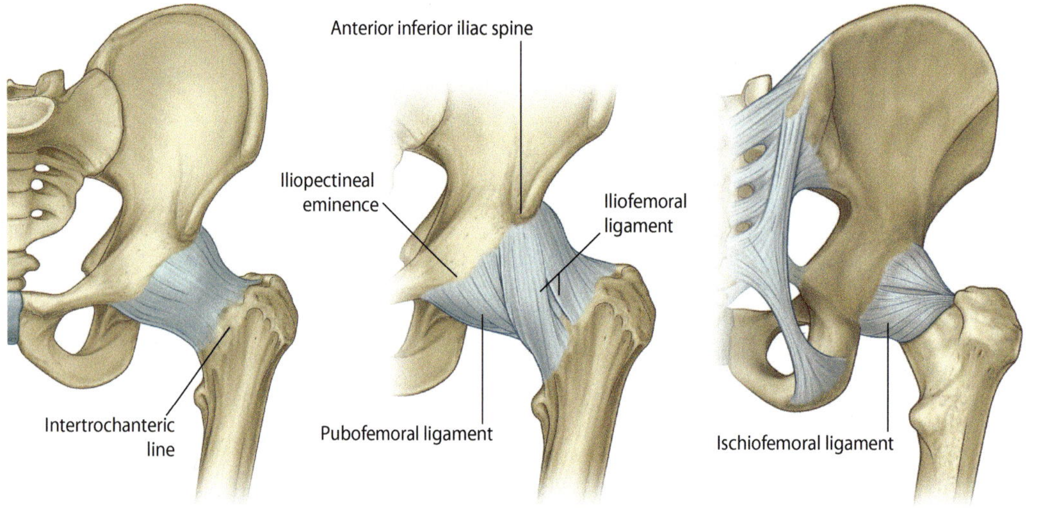

Fig. 3.4 Capsule and ligaments of the hip.

and gluteus maximus;
- abductors: gluteus medius, gluteus minimus, and tensor fasciae latae;
- medial rotators: gluteus medius, gluteus minimus (anterior part), and tensor fasciae latae.

3.1.4 Vascularization (Fig. 3.5)

The femoral head is well vascularized by peri- and intraosseous anastomoses that provide arteries that include the:
- femoral (medial and lateral circumflex femoral arteries);
- superior gluteal;
- inferior gluteal;
- obturator (for the ligament of the femoral head), a division of the internal iliac artery.

Thanks to microcirculation, venous capacity is six to eight times greater than arterial capacity. The adductors play a role in sweeping along venous circulation. The anterior and posterior venous systems are joined by numerous anastomoses. While the hip has a tremendous blood supply, circulation is vulnerable to intraosseous pressures.

3.1.5 Innervation (Fig. 3.6)

The hip joint is supplied by nerves that include the:
- sciatic;
- femoral;
- obturator;
- femoral cutaneous;
- posterior cutaneous;
- lateral cutaneous.

3.2 JOINT PHYSIOLOGY

3.2.1 General considerations

The hip forms the connection between the femur and the pelvic girdle. While the hip and shoulder are analogous to ball-and-socket joints, the shoulder is oriented toward mobility, whereas the hip and pelvis are geared to strength and stability. The hip is soundly made and well planted for weight bearing. A powerful muscle system reinforces good joint congruence. The hip joint is designed to combine stability and movement.

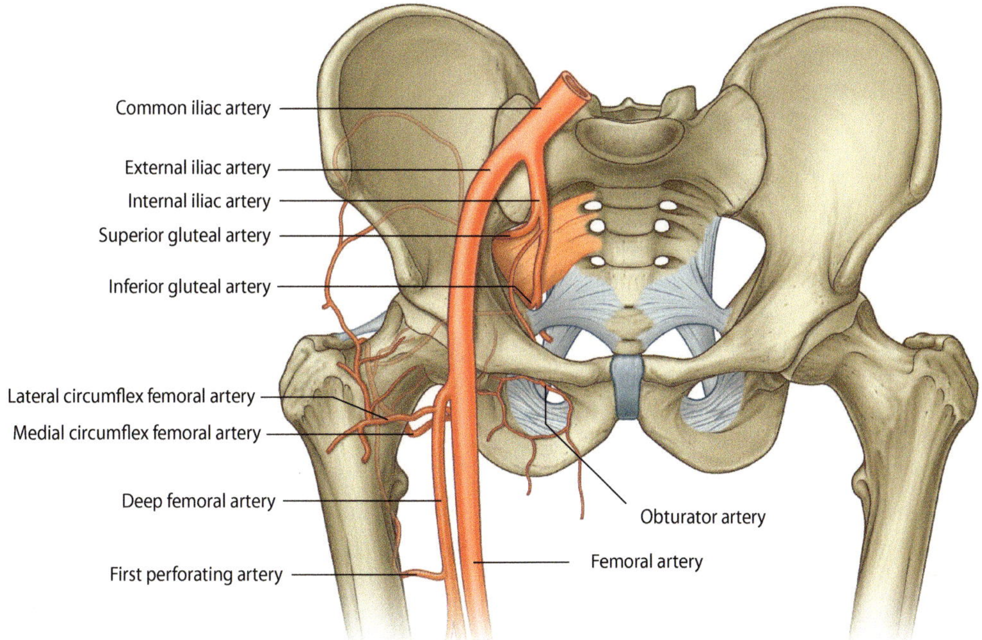

Fig. 3.5 General view of vascularization of the hip.

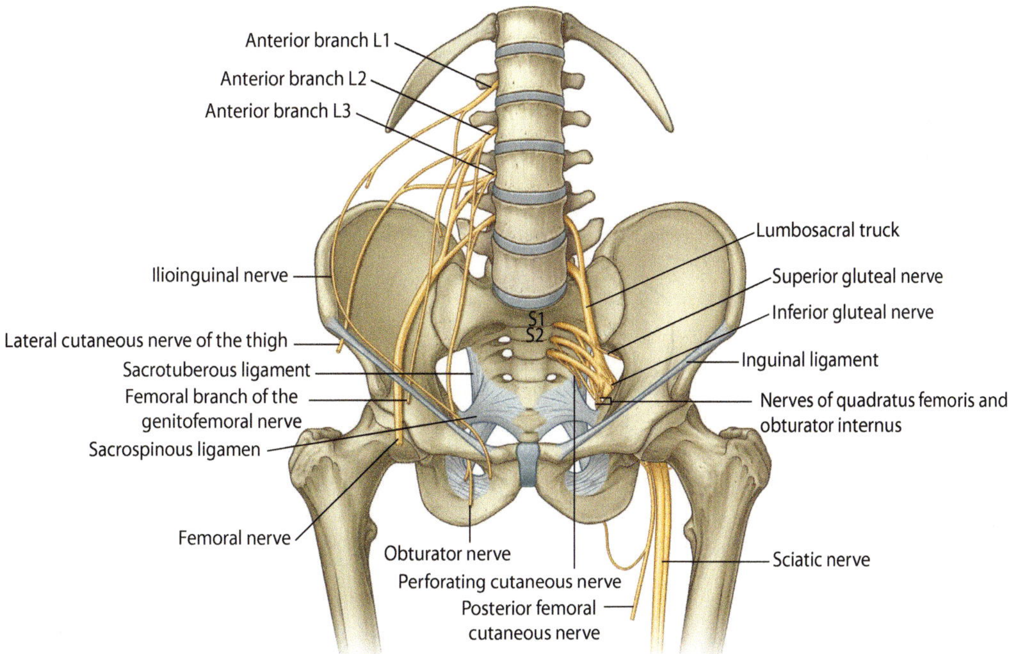

Fig. 3.6 General view of the innervation of the hip.

Mechanical imperative

Like all joints, the hip has specific requirements. Hip imperatives center on the following characteristics:

- The hip must be stable. It must support the weight of the upper body in both static and dynamic posture.
- The hip must be dynamic. Movement must be possible in all directions, accommodating for walking, running, crouching, jumping, and sitting.
- The hip must be static. Loads are transmitted through the trunk and hip to the lower extremities.

Kneecap on three axes

The joint type that responds best to these contradictory imperatives is the spheroid model, a multiaxial ball-and-socket joint. The patella is a mechanical example of this type of joint, as it is somewhat like a large ball well-fitted in a spherical cavity.

The hip moves in three planes around three axes of rotation. The combination of these movements allows the hip to circumduct freely. The hip is surrounded by powerful muscles that provide movement, strength, and stability.

Double stability

Hip stabilization is provided by a support system that is both passive and active.

Passive system of stabilization

Components:

- The fitting of the femoral head as it sits in the acetabulum;
- A joint vacuum that improves surface adherence thanks to null or negative joint pressure;
- The joint capsule, whose annular ligament is a key structure for hip stability in distraction;
- Joint ligaments that wind up tightly when the hip is fully extended;
- The ligament of the femoral head that secures the head of the femur to the three bones that form the acetabulum.

Active system of stabilization

Muscles of the hip, together with the force of gravity, create axial compression and thus mechanical stability. Certain muscles act as active ligaments. We can have an effect on the coxofemoral joint through these muscles.

3.2.2 Hip stabilizing factors

Osteocartilaginous components

Osseous elements

The femoral neck angle stabilizes the hip considerably.

In the frontal plane, the angle of inclination is where the axis of the shaft meets the long axis of the neck. It is formed at about 120°–125°. Coxa valga is a congenital deformity in which the angle opens to as much as 140°. The increased angle commonly results in shortening of the adductor muscles, causing them to overpower hip abductors. This is why adduction is a position of instability, whereas abduction makes the hip more secure.

In the horizontal plane, the angle of declination can be defined as the angle formed where the bicondylar plane meets the plane running through the center of the neck and femoral head. If this angle passes behind the center of the femoral head, the anterior part of the head of the femur is no longer covered by the acetabulum. The neck angle increases, causing anteversion of the femoral neck. In this instance, an angle of 20° will cause the head to be exposed to pathological dislocation. Conversely, retroversion of the femoral neck stabilizes the joint, as occurs in medial hip rotation.

Luxating positions

The most stable position for the hip joint is quadrupedia. Being on all fours offers the best congruence, but instability can easily arise in other situations:

- In positions combining hip flexion, adduction, and medial rotation, the femoral head has a tendency to slip posteriorly.
- In positions of extension, adduction, and lateral rotation, the femoral head has a tendency to slip anteriorly.

Nevertheless, the hip remains stable during the course of everyday activity. Dislocations tend to happen only in trauma involving high-level force.

Articular factors

Joint coupling

The relationship between joint stability and mobility is determined by the value of its interlocking pairs. Joint congruence is the measurement of two joint surfaces as they relate to one another. The better the fit, the greater the stability. By contrast, a weaker fit favors mobility.

The ball-and-socket hip joint is the most stable joint in the body. Congruence approaches 50%, representing the highest level in the animal kingdom (Adalbert Ibrahim Kapandji 2011). A ring of cartilage runs around the cup-shaped acetabulum and deepens the cavity so the femur fits beyond its circumference.

The deformable cartilaginous labrum is an ingenious way of increasing joint congruence without sacrificing range of motion. Increased socket depth allows more than half of the head of the femur to fit within the acetabulum. This interlocking fibrous coupling (Kapandji 2009) effectively increases hip strength.

Congruence

The femoral and acetabular joint surfaces are not entirely congruent. Maximum contact between joint surfaces occurs in the close-packed position: flexion, abduction, and internal rotation.

While not perfectly congruent, the acetabulum and femur fit together so well that it is difficult for the femoral head to slip out of place. We will see that congruence changes under the effect of weight bearing. Acetabular deformability is discussed further in chapter 8.

Negative pressure

When the coxofemoral joint is unloaded, intracapsular pressure is subatmospheric. This feature is common to most large joints and is a major cohesive factor. Negative pressure depends on the integrity of the capsuloligamentous system.

Weber brothers' experiments

The Weber brothers performed an interesting experiment to show the key role played by atmospheric pressure. Ligaments and muscles were first detached from the limbs of a cadaver. The lower limbs were left to hang free. It was observed that the head of the femur did not leave the acetabulum.

The next step was to bore a small hole in the wall of the acetabulum, whereupon the head of the femur was driven away at once by the atmospheric air. The head of the femur was then replaced in the acetabulum. When the small hole was plugged with a finger, the lower limb stayed in place; when the finger was removed, it fell out again.

Joint suction

Intracapsular pressure is lower than atmospheric pressure. The suction effect is substantial between 30° and 90° of flexion; in this position joint pressure is minimal.

According to Hall, the suction effect alone is able to resist traction forces up to 18.25 kg, and thus provide stability (Raymond Paul Ficat and Christian Ficat 1987). Suction force is what causes the snapping noise known as "Larrey kiss" during hip dislocation.

While opening a joint during arthrotomy, surgeons sometimes report hearing an audible sucking noise, the sound of sudden air intake.

Larrey was a surgeon of the empire, specialized in amputation on the battle fields. He described the noise made by the joint suction of the hip when he was disarticulating the hip joint. This noise was named "Larrey kiss" by the surgeons after him and is well known in the surgical world in France.

Muscle factors

Muscular orientation

Muscles are essential to hip stability. They are grouped according to orientation:

- Muscles parallel to the neck of the femur. Muscles that run closely to the femoral neck keep the femoral head in the acetabulum. These are mainly the pelvitrochanteric group: piriformis, obturatur externus, obturator internus, superior and inferior gemella, and quadratus femoris. The gluteus minimus and gluteus maximus combined draw the hip bones together so powerfully that they are sometimes called the hip appenders.
- Muscles parallel to the shaft of the femur. The longitudinal muscles have a tendency to cause superior hip luxation, where the femoral head can slip above the acetabulum when the hip is everted. This type of instability is characterized by a shallow acetabulum of the type found in cogenital hip dysplasia. Destabilizing muscle action diminishes with abduction to the point where muscles become coadaptors in full hip abduction.

Muscle constraint

Movement is controlled according to muscle group:

- Muscles running longitudinally near the femoral shaft put tension on the superior pole of the femoral head. Enduring hypertonicity or spasm can cause expulsive coxarthrosis (ventral instability) to develop.
- Muscles lying transversally near the femoral head push the head of the femur toward the acetabular fossa. This muscle tension tends to promote protrusive coxathroses.

3.2.3 Hip equilibrium

Stability in the sagittal plane

Bipedal footing

The central line of gravity passes slightly behind the geometric center of the femoral head. Remaining close to the center of rotation, it has a very short lever action on the joint and does not generate much constraint. In a subject whose central line of gravity passes behind the center of the joint, balance is maintained by the passive elastic force of the capsule and the anterior ligaments, particularly the iliofemoral ligament.

In addition, the iliacus muscle works in a state of continuous static and eccentric contraction. A part of this muscle known as the lesser or accessory iliacus plays a stabilizing role through its connection with the coxofemoral joint capsule. We refer to this muscle in the practical section of this book.

In subjects whose central line of gravity passes behind the joint center, hip balance is mostly assured by the passive elastic force of the posterior muscle group known as the gluteals.

Unipodal footing

In the course of walking, the central line of gravity passes continually behind and in front of the center of the femoral head. Accordingly, the hip alternates between flexion and extension.

When the hip is in extension, the central line of gravity momentarily exerts a force favoring extension of the hip and retroversion of the pelvis. Balance is provided by the passive elastic force of the iliofemoral ligament and the active eccentric action of the hip flexor muscles, particularly iliacus.

When the hip is in flexion, the central

line of gravity momentarily exerts a force that favors hip flexion and pelvic anterversion. Equilibrium is achieved by the active eccentric work of the hip extensors.

In both cases, the leverage exerted by gravitational forces remains low.

Stability in the frontal plane

Bipodal support

The central line of gravity falls in the midsagittal plane. A passive elastic force exerted by the abductor and adductor muscles is enough to maintain balance. Movement restraints are feeble, as only half the weight of the body lands on each hip.

Unipodal support

The central line of gravity moves in the frontal plane. It translates from the weight-bearing side to rest over the support polygon that is reduced to the surface contact of the supporting foot. To avoid the weight of the pelvis collapsing on the femoral head and the hip, massive contraction of the abductor muscle occurs.

Gluteus medius, gluteus minimus, tensor fasciae latae, and gluteus maximus are the main muscles that stabilize the hip by counterbalancing the weight of the body. Considerable leverage is brought to bear by these offsetting muscle forces. The resulting load on the hips is equivalent to many times the weight of the body, as we shall see.

Stability in the transverse plane

Pelvic and hip rotations are involved in walking. When the advancing limb swings in relation to the weight-bearing limb, the pelvis twists around the vertical axis on the head of the femur of the bearing limb. The pelvis rotates medially on the femoral head of the bearing limb. At the same time, the femoral head of the swinging limb rotates laterally. This double action creates a virtual torsion of the pelvis involving the medial rotator muscle of the bearing hip and the lateral rotators of the swaying hip. The level of constraint generated by balance requirements remains low in this plane.

3.2.4 The hip joint under tension

Bearing stress

Hip stress is elevated during walking. In monopodal support, the hip is vulnerable to imbalance in the frontal plane. The so-called balance of Pauwels (1935) calculates compression forces to which joint surfaces are subject. In unipodal support, the hip remains horizontal despite the momentum of the body weight tipping toward the supporting limb. Abductorial forces act strongly to counterbalance this tendency.

The equilibrium system can be likened to a weight scale in which the femur is the vertical pivot and the hip the balance beam. The two arms of the beam are unequal in length; the arm on which the abductor muscles act is about three times smaller than the beam supporting the weight of the body. Thus the abductor muscles must produce forces equal to three times the weight of the body to equilibrate the hip when it is supported on one leg. With each step, the femoral head receives forces equivalent to at least four times the body weight.

The importance of angles

Hip angles are important in that they affect lever arm length. For example, an increase in the angle of the femoral neck shaft can raise stress on the femur from four to as much as six times the body weight.

Dynamic forces

The hip is submitted to two types of force: muscle force and weight force, with its echo in the reverberating forces coming up from the ground. While muscle actions improve coxofemoral coaption and joint balance, they also increase joint stress.

These dynamics are not limited to static conditions. In everyday activities, such as walking, running, or jumping, muscle forces join with movement, giving rise to dynamic forces of intensity beyond theoretical calculation. Dynamic forces are at play in motor impulse and acceleration.

Measurement values

Theoretical calculations describe forces applied to the hip in order of magnitude. To illustrate, here are some values expressed in reference to body weight:
- In bipodal support, the applied force is in the range of 1/3–1/2 times times body weight.
- In monopodal support, force is on the order of 2 ½–4 times body weight.
- Normal walking imposes a maximum of 5–6 times body weight for less than 1/10 of a second.
- Brisk walking involves 6–7½ times times body weight for just under 1/10 of a second.
- Walking 10% up ramp exerts about 5 times body weight.
- Walking 10% down ramp exerts about 6 times body weight.

In terms of load coefficients, it is easy to see that each kilo of extra weight can be a real burden on the hip.

3.2.5 Pressure on the femoral head

Thrust on the femoral head: a triple demand (Fig. 3.7)

In dismantling hip prostheses, Ficat et al. (1987) demonstrated that the sum of forces acting on the hip involves threefold pressure to the femoral head:
- from back to front (protrusion);
- from up to down (varisation);
- from front to back (retroversion).

These pulls tend to put a strain on prosthetics and/or bones and sometimes even deform them.

Weak zone

Cartilage plays a central role in hip constraint. Their forces determine the critical hip zone situated on:
- the head of the femur, midway between the superior pole and the anterior surface;
- the superior internal surface of the acetabulum.

Maximal demands converge at the critical area. Localized osteoarthritis or osteonecrosis can arise in this zone. Experiential data shows that high pressure is a probable cause in these afflictions.

Biomechanical hip balance

Ficat et al. (1987) emphasized that biomechanical hip equilibrium is a sum of balances:
- between muscles that cause or inhibit movement;
- between the forces of muscle and weight;
- between structure and function.

The profound and constant interactions that stabilize the structure and function of the hip are good illustrations of the fusion of the mechanical and the biological, a concept that we spoke of in the opening chapter. Ficat et al. add that "their interdependence is so closely woven, their collusion so intimate that it is sometimes difficult to discern the effect from the cause."

Coxofemoral hyperpressure syndrome

This fragile anatomophysiological balance can be disrupted by multiple factors that Ficat et al. (1987) grouped together under four headings:
- Higher than normal forces of coaption create true coxofemoral hyperpressure in absolute value. Often these stresses surpass hip resistance in a hip that is considered normal in all other respects. High pressure can arise from diverse causes: abnormally tense muscle chains

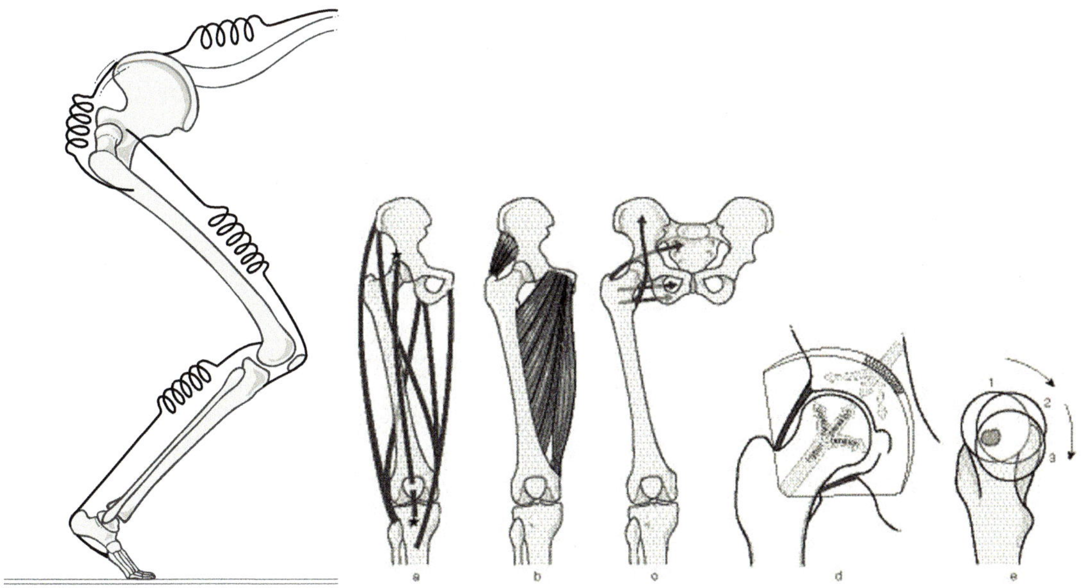

Fig. 3.7 Pressure on the hip. (Ficat et al 1987. Mechanical pathology of the hip. Paris: Masson.)

or capsuloligamentous cuffs and, of course, being overweight.

- Bones that present structural anomalies lead to poor distribution of forces, displacement of the resulting load, and/or diminution of load-bearing surfaces. While forces of coaption and coxofemoral pressure can be normal, hyperpressure is relative. For example, these consequences arise in cases of dysplasia or postural disorders.
- Structures present reduced resistance. This shortfall can occur at any point along the trochanter-acetabulum axis (joint cartilage, spongy bone, subchondral, or growth plate in the infant). The defect can affect the slant of the femur, the tilt of the acetabulum, or both. Here again it can amount to relative high pressure, where the hip load is absolutely normal.
- Functional demand made of the hip can exceed these adaptation and resistance capacities. This happens to the body that is overweight or is subjected to sporting excess, to overtaxing amateur or professional sports, or to trauma and its aftermath.

In practice, we often encounter a combination of these factors.

Consequences of loss of balance

Any one of the four factors can be enough by itself to create diverse pathological situations. For Ficat et al. (1987), the coxofemoral hyperpressure phenomenon is without a doubt, in absolute or relative terms, the dominant factor in all mechanical hip pathologies.

Loss of equilibrium has two outcomes:

- If the hip has good adaptation potential, only minor malfunctions occur. These can be compensated for and result in fairly simple, generally nonpathogenic anomalies.
- If the tolerance threshold is overcome, major malfunctions can result. These can be the basis of a great variety of osteoarticular problems:
  - degenerative (arthritis or osteonecrosis);
  - malformations (protrusion, retroversion, variation);
  - traumatic (femoral head or acetabulum fracture).

It is imperative that permanent equilibrium be maintained between all parts of the hip in order that the enumerated factors remain within normal range.

3.2.6 Cartilaginous protection

Necessary protection

Coxofemoral joint cartilage lives and works between the hammer and the anvil. Over the course of a lifetime enormous locomotive strain is exerted, accumulated, and sometimes stored up in the hip. Each step can be sheer torture for the cartilage. Kapandji (2009) considered that "walking is nothing but a succession of avoided and controlled falls." This everyday activity generates vibration and shock waves that contribute to the stresses described above.

A weight-bearing joint is very weak; as a consequence, the unitary pressures bearing down on cartilage are tremendous. In addition, they fall on the critical zone. Taken together, these parameters seem reason enough to expect joint cartilage resistance of the femoral head and acetabulum to break down rapidly. If the joint is functioning well, however, this does not happen. What then makes the "good adaptation potential" that Ficat et al. describe?

We will see that, thanks to certain devices, constraint by itself does not always get the better of cartilage. Several mechanisms converge to protect cartilage.

Pressure alterations

An imperative

As explained in the first volume of this series, *New Manual Articular Approach; Upper Extremity*, cartilage is reliant on pressure to ensure proper exchange with synovial fluid. Cartilage function and survival have the same requirement. Alternating phases of load and discharge are essential to cartilage maintenance and to its exchanges with capsulosynovial structures.

True joint unloading

In order for cartilage to exchange nutrients with synovial fluid effectively, intra-articular pressure must change radically. At the lower extremity, alternating phases of weight bearing as well as swinging back and forth while walking supposedly offer ideal conditions. Unfortunately, this is not always the case.

When we consider compression stress on the hip, we often think first of body weight. While obesity can certainly generate or exacerbate coxarthrosis, this factor is not really important except when the lower extremity is under load.

It is generally forgotten that a rise in intra-articular pressure during load discharge can be just as harmful for the joint. Increased pressure on the unloaded hip has nothing to do with body weight. Rather, it is more often attributed to deficient elasticity in the musculoligamentous system. Shortening, fibrosity, or spasm of these structures can become significant factors in arthrosis. For example, musculoligamentous tensions can put exaggerated pressure on the superior pole of the femur, or it can cause the femoral head to protrude in the acetabulum.

An accumulation of compressive stress can also drive cartilage wear. Periarticular tissue tension can create major circulatory disturbance that reinforces the lesional chain.

Cushioning strategies

Many cushioning conveniences are distributed through the lower extremity and trunk to absorb impacts and vibrations engendered by locomotion. Shock absorption is a collective function that can be conceptualized as a sports team. If just one player fails to play correctly, the whole enterprise is compromised. We revisit the various levels of joint cushioning in the chapter concerning the foot (see "Shock absorbers" in chapter 21).

At the hip, shock absorption is crucial to

the preservation of joint cartilage. The joint does not have to submit to the crush of ascending and descending forces that would rapidly flatten the femoral heads, because it has at least three available shock-absorbing strategies: flexion, pelvic tilt, and the gemellus-obturator hammock.

Work in flexion

Most theoretical hip strain studies are done with the joint in extension. Yet in real life the hip and knee operate in concert to accomplish flexion. Flexion movements are controlled by the biarticular thigh muscles, a powerful means of cushioning femoral head stress (Fig. 3.8). This happens, for example, when landing a jump.

Cantilevered pelvis

Lumbopelvic shock absorbers also serve to dampen hip stress. The lumbopelvic forward pitch acts like a shock absorber.

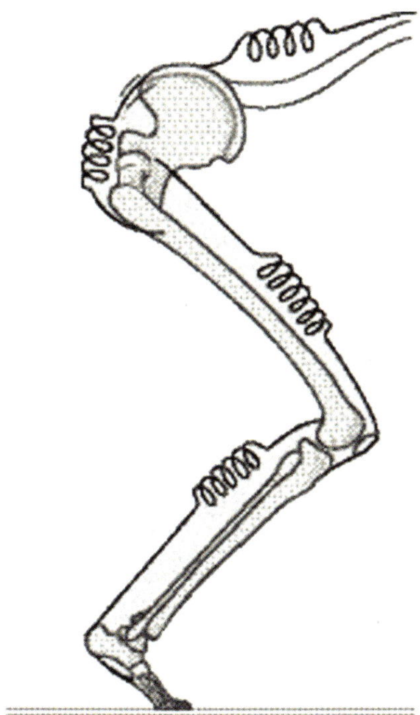

Fig. 3.8 Shock-absorbing flexors. (Ficat et al 1987. Mechanical pathology of the hip. Paris: Masson.)

According to Paul Klein and Peter Sommerfeld (2008), this system is passively supported by extrinsic pelvic ligaments such as sacrotuberous and sacrospinous. Hip flexor and pelvic floor muscles actively complete this cantilevered position.

In this arrangement, muscles of the pelvic floor can be likened to a safety net or trampoline that limits organ descent.

The hip, a joint suspended

Gemellus-obturator hammock

Boris Dolto (1967) envisaged the obturator externus, obturator internus, and gemellus as a single muscle. He said the unit is simply divided by the obturator membrane and essentially forms a single connective tissue muscular band. This muscle arrangement lies in a slightly upward direction, "ascending from the ischiopubic area toward the lesser trochanter."

Dolto compared the system to a hammock stretched between two trees. The "gemellus-obturator hammock" concept (Fig. 3.9) makes it easy to see how this set of muscles contributes to preserving and economizing the cartilage of the femoral head. It operates like a suspension sling that supports and cushions gravitational stress.

It is interesting to note that the activity of this muscle group "relieves" femoral heads of constraint. This runs counter to classic biomechanical theory that links muscle activity to increased joint cushioning. According to Dolto (1967), "If these shock absorbers give way, become atrophied, or lose their tone or passive stretch, the pelvis collapses on the coxofemoral cartilage, which, bereft of its protectors, wears away and degenerates into debilitating arthritis."

In the service of the obturator membrane

Twenty years of dissection experience has led us to conclude that the gemellus-

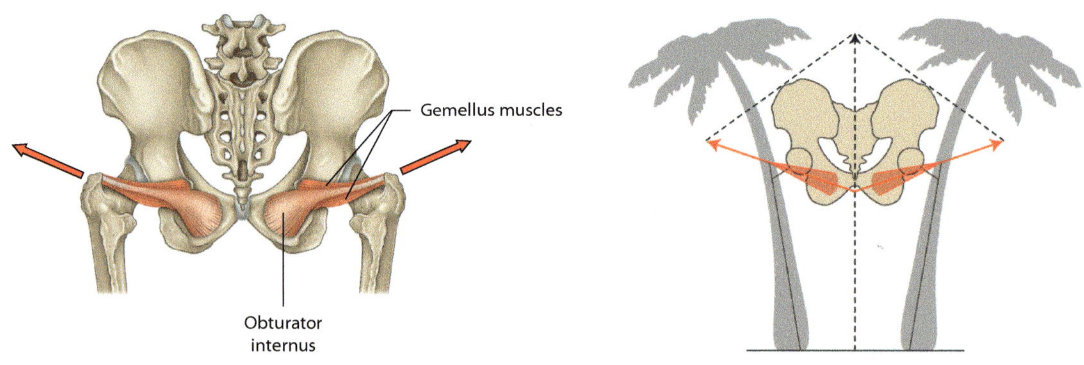

Fig. 3.9 Dolto's gemellus-obturator hammock. (Michel Dufour and Michel Pilu 2006.)

obturator hammock cushioning system is subservient to the obturator membrane (Alain Croibier 1991). We have been able to demonstrate the anatomical and functional relationships that exist between the obturator membranes and the coxofemoral joint. The transverse acetabular ligament and the subpubic band are not uninterrupted in their adherence to the bone. An anatomical continuum exists between the round ligament, the transverse acetabular ligament, and the subpubic band or external obturator membrane. Mobilizing the lower extremity in a way that puts the round ligament on tension also alters the tensions of the subpubic band. These changes reverberate to the internal obturator membrane, creating a reciprocal tension system. When one element tenses, the other relaxes.

We think that this variable tension system likely plays a proprioceptive role for the obturator muscles. This arrangement becomes activated as a function of hip position. The shock absorber that constitutes the gemellus-obturator would seem regulable as a function of information supplied by the obturator membranes.

Interdependence with the visceral column

Moreover, available tension on the obturator internus membrane is able to deform, diminishing abdominal pressures bearing down on the pelvic visceral contents. This observation prompted us to compare the obturator membrane to an active abdominal pressure outlet—or even a trampoline—that is nevertheless dependent on hip mechanics. Coxofemoral shock absorption and pelvic viscera cushioning appears to be effectively linked. This partly explains how mechanical bladder problems can affect the coxofemoral joint and vice versa.

Elements of diagnosis

4

4.1 HIP ANGLES

4.1.1 Definitions

Coxometry

Hip angle measurement is a standard part of hip imaging. Some of the angles are important to know, for they can help in understanding hip mechanics. They allow us to see how certain anatomical hip changes can increase stress at a dizzying rate on load-bearing surfaces and lever arms. Angles convey the structural component of hip pathologies that result from irregular bone formation (Fig. 4.1 and Table 4.1).

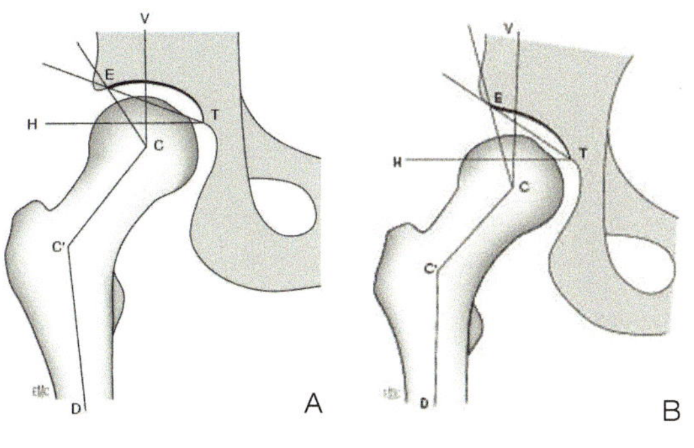

Fig. 4.1 A = normal; B = dysplasia. (C. Le Breton, P. M'Bappé, J. Korzec, J. M. Bigot, M. F. Carette, A. Sobotka. 2002. "Imagery of the normal and pathological hip." EMC Medical radiology and imagery: Musculoskeletal–Neurological–Maxillofacial 30-450-A-10: 1–28. 2002 Paris: Elsevier Masson. All rights reserved.)

Table 4.1 Fundamental hip angle values

Angles	Normal hip	Dysplastic hip
CE or VCE	≥ 25°	≤ 20°
AOA	≤ 10°	≥ 12°
CDA	120°–135°	≥ 140°
VAC	≥ 25°	≤ 25°
Femoral anteversion	7°–15°	> 20°–25°
Acetabular anteversion	20°–25°	> 25°
CE=	angle of Wiberg	
VCE=	external coverage angle of the femoral head	
AOA=	acetabular obliquity angle	
CDA=	cervicodyaphysary angle	
VCA=	anterior coverage angle of the femoral head	

(C. Le Breton, P. M'Bappé, J. Korzec, J. M. Bigot, M. F. Carette, A. Sobotka. 2002. "Imagery of the normal and pathological hip." EMC Medical radiology and imagery: Musculoskeletal–Neurological–Maxillofacial 30-450-A-10: 1–28. 2002 Paris: Elsevier Masson. All rights reserved.)

Frontal plane

Three angles are generally measured in the frontal plane:

1. Obliquity of the femoral neck. The cervicodiaphysary angle, also called the angle of inclination, is formed by the axis of the femoral neck and the axis of the femoral shaft. Its average value is in the neighborhood of 130°. Normal values should be less than or equal to 135°. The angle evolves throughout life, having a value of about 150° in newborns and 120° in the elderly (Fig. 4.2). Changes to this angle show up in Pauwel's considerations of sheer stress, compressive stress, tensile force, and torque mechanics.

2. Opening of the femoral head angle (of Wiberg). This is the measure of the angle formed by:
   - a vertical line drawn through the center of the femoral head;
   - a line drawn from the outer edge of the acetabulum to the center of the femoral head.

Normal values should be greater than 125°. The average value is 30°. A decreased angle implies insufficient femoral coverage and a diminished weight-bearing surface that is increasing unit stress on the joint cartilage.

3. Acetabular angle. This angle is formed by:
   - a horizontal line;
   - a line extending from medial to lateral edges of the acetabulum.

The normal value is 10°.

Horizontal plane

Two angles are generally measured in the horizontal plane:

1. Angle of femoral anteversion. This angle is formed by:
   - the axis of the femoral neck;
   - the axis of the femoral condyle at the knee.

At birth the angle is in the order of 35°. It decreases to 15° after age 10. The average adult value is 12°. Normal range is between 10° and 15°. Pathological increase is any angle above 20°.

2. Angle of acetabular anteversion. This angle is formed by:
   - a tangent line to the anterior and posterior acetabular borders;
   - a frontal or sagittal plane of reference.

Anteversion measured with a densitometer (a device registering degrees of darkness found in film negatives) values angles in the sagittal plane at about 15° plus or minus 3°

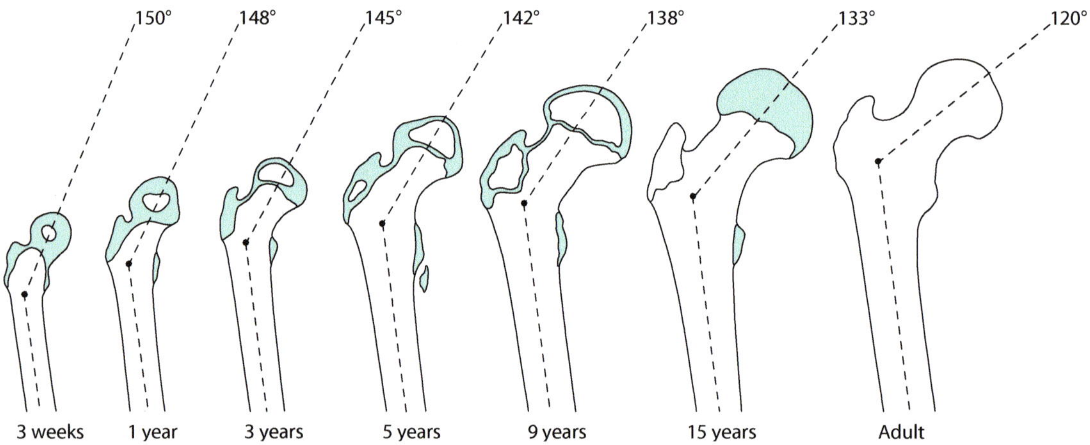

Fig. 4.2 Evolution of the cervico-diasyphary angle as a function of age. (G. Kalifa, A. E. Millischer-Bellaiche, M. Lahutte. 2007. "Cosa vara." EMC Medical radiology and imagery: Musculoskeletal – Neurological –Maxillofacial 31- 143-A-10: 1–6. 2010 Paris: Elsevier Masson.)

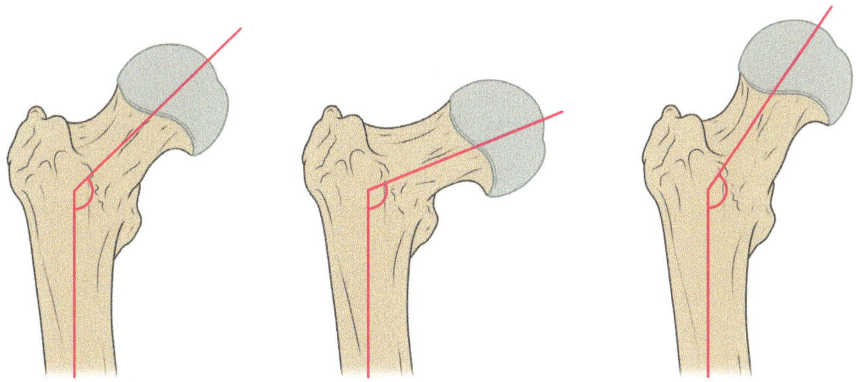

Fig. 4.3 Hip deformities.

in men and 20° plus or minus 3° in women. Kapandji and Castaing found the angle to be on the order of 30°–40° in the frontal plane.

4.1.2 Hip deformities (Fig. 4.3)

Coxa vara

Coxa vara is a deformity of the hip whereby the angle between the neck of the femur and the shaft is reduced. This orientation may be congenital or acquired in the aftermath of epiphysiolysis, rickets, or trauma.

Coxa valga

This deformity is the inverse of coxa vara. The angle between the head and neck of the femur and its shaft (cephalocervico-diaphysary) is increased, producing a straighter bone. When it is unilateral, leg length disparity results.

Coxa antetorsa

The axis of the femoral neck is exaggerated toward the front and can cause hip dysplasia.

Coxa retrotorsa

This is the inverse of the above. The axis of the neck of the femur is oriented toward the back.

Coxa adducta and coxa flexa

This is similar to coxa vara, in which the femoral neck becomes more horizontal. Clinically, the lower extremity is found to be in medial rotation and adduction.

Coxa magna

Latin for large hip, this broadening of the head and neck of the femur causes:

- acute transitory synovitis of the hip;
- acute epiphysitis of the hip;
- irritable hip;
- a cold in the hip (more on this later).

Coxa plana

Coxa plana is a deformity in which the head of the femur becomes flattened like a beret and subluxes. The femoral neck is shortened and thickened. Coxa plana is synonymous with juvenile osteochondritis.

4.2 DIFFERENTIAL EXAMINATION OF ROTATIONS AND TORSIONS OF THE LOWER EXTREMITY

4.2.1 Rotator test

The classic osteopathic hip test evaluates the comparative range and quality of movement by mobilizing both hips simultaneously in medial and lateral rotation. Due to the great number of lateral hip rotators it is easy enough to find limited medial rotation in the unbalanced or pathological hip.

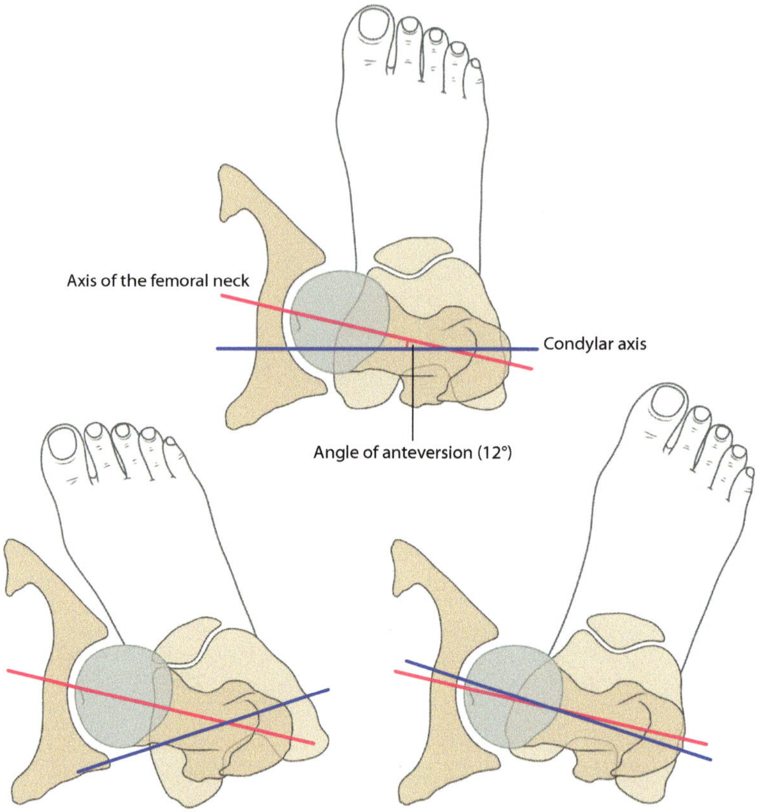

Fig. 4.4 Foot position and anteversion angle of the femoral neck.

4.2.2 Deceptive first glance

Be careful not to extrapolate. This test cannot be replaced by simply observing the position of a patient's feet resting on the table. Such visual inspection leads to improper deductions. This is a classic mistake. A foot resting on its lateral edge does not necessarily imply lateral rotation of the hip any more than toes pointing inward indicate medial hip rotation (Fig. 4.4).

4.2.3 Rotation is not torsion

Innumerable and frequent skeletal torsions of the lower extremity can induce particular foot positions and create the impression that the lower limb is in rotation. As Fabrice Duparc (2009) reminds us, rotation is a movement, whereas torsion is the twisting of an object (Fig. 4.5). For the inferior limb, torsions can land in the long bones of the tibia and femur. These bones tend toward inverse rotation.

As a rule, femoral torsion is medial. This corresponds to anteversion of the femoral neck, where the distal femur rotates inward in relation to the proximal shaft. Tibial torsion is normally lateral. The distal tibia rotates toward the outside of the body in relation to the proximal epiphyses. Torsion of the bones of the lower limb evolves in the course of growth and development, and it changes again in adulthood (Fig. 4.6).

The two long bones of the lower limb have opposite torsion patterns. The reciprocal movement of the bones creates femoral tibial rotation between the two segments.

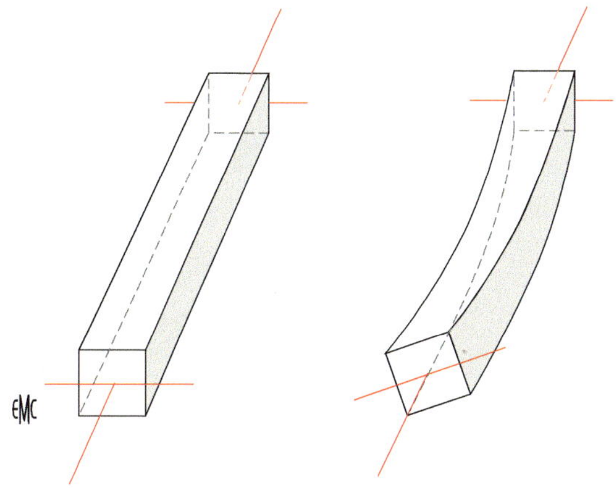

Fig. 4.5 Torsion within a solid. (F. Duparc. 2009. "Skeletal torsion problems of the adult lower limb." EMC Locomotor system 15-322-A-10: 1–12. 2009 Paris: Elsevier Masson. All rights reserved.)

4.2.4 Clinical application

In his excellent article written for The medical surgical encyclopedia, Duparc provides clinical applications of what he refers to as global morphotype torsions of the lower limb. These tests can be used in common practice to differentiate dysfunctions of the hip from problems belonging to interosseous constraints with the entailing deformities. Here is how Duparc evaluates skeletal torsions of the lower limb:

In standing position (Fig. 4.7)

Observing the patient while walking allows you to observe the angle of the foot in relation to the line of displacement of the body. In standing position, two postures are useful and easy to compare: standing with feet together and standing with the knees facing forward (patella at the zenith). The angle between the sagittal axis of the knee and the axis of the foot gives information regarding tibial torsion.

- Standing with feet together, knee orientation (patellar strabismus) displays tibial torsion (TT).
- Standing with the knees facing straight on, the axis of the feet displays tibial torsion (TT).

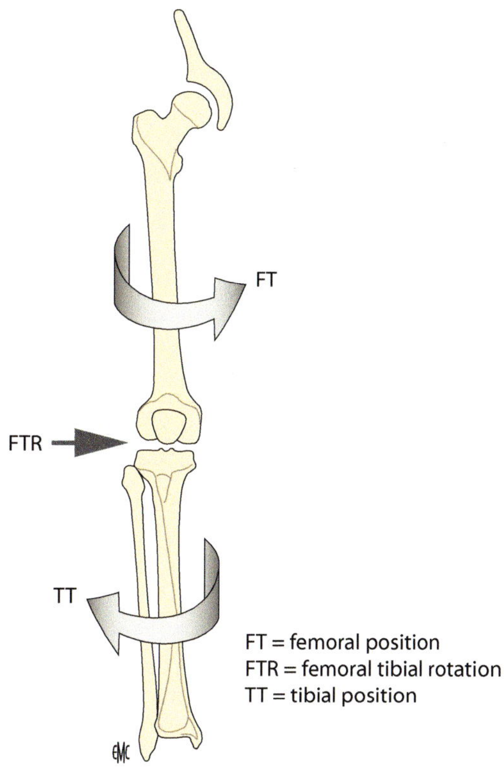

Fig. 4.6 Long Bone torsions. The two long bones of the lower limb have opposite torsion patterns. The reciprocal movement of the bones creates femoral tibial rotation (FTR) between the two segments. FT: femoral position; TT: tibial position (F. Duparc. 2009. "Skeletal torsion problems of the adult lower limb." EMC Locomotor system 15-322-A-10: 1–12. 2009 Paris: Elsevier Masson. All rights reserved.)

In sitting position (Fig. 4.8)

The patient sits at the edge of the exam table. Observe how the tibial condyles contact the edge of the table. The vertical axis of the leg acts like a compass in revealing degrees of femoral torsion. This same angle between the two skeletal extremities of the leg can also be evaluated from the posterior view. The patient stands on the contralateral foot. The knee under examination is flexed to 90° and supported on a stool or lowered table. Measure the angle between the horizontal support axis and the distal bimalleolar axis.

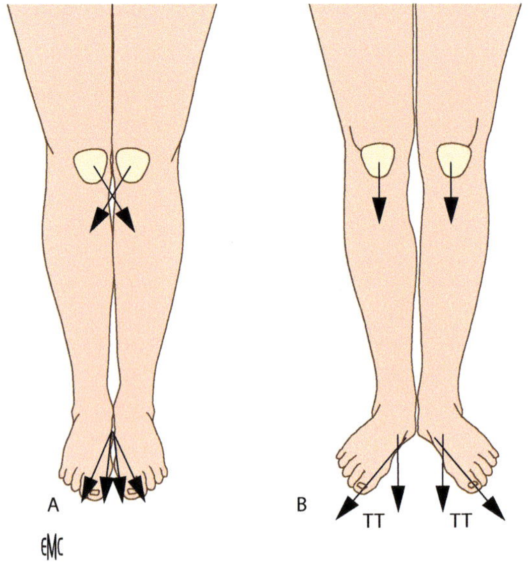

Fig. 4.7 Standing evaluation. A) Standing with feet together: knee orientation (patellar strabismus) displays tibial torsion. B) Standing with the knees facing straight on the axis of the feet: displays tibial torsion (TT). (F. Duparc. 2009. "Torsion problems of the adult lower extremity skeleton." EMC Locomotor system 15-322-A-10: 1–12. 2009 Paris: Elsevier Masson. All rights reserved.)

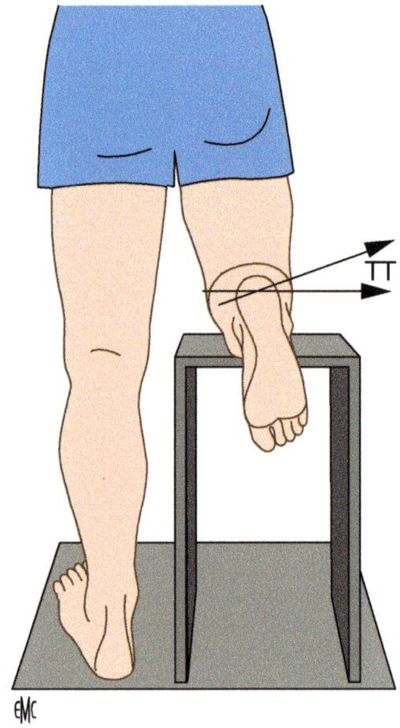

Fig. 4.8 Evaluation on table or stool. The axis of the upper end of the tibia is considered to be parallel to the stool. The angle between this plane and the bimalleolar axis reveals tibial torsion (TT). (F. Duparc. 2009. "Torsion problems of the adult lower extremity skeleton." EMC Locomotor system 15-322-1-10: 1–12. 2009 Paris: Elsevier Masson. All rights reserved.)

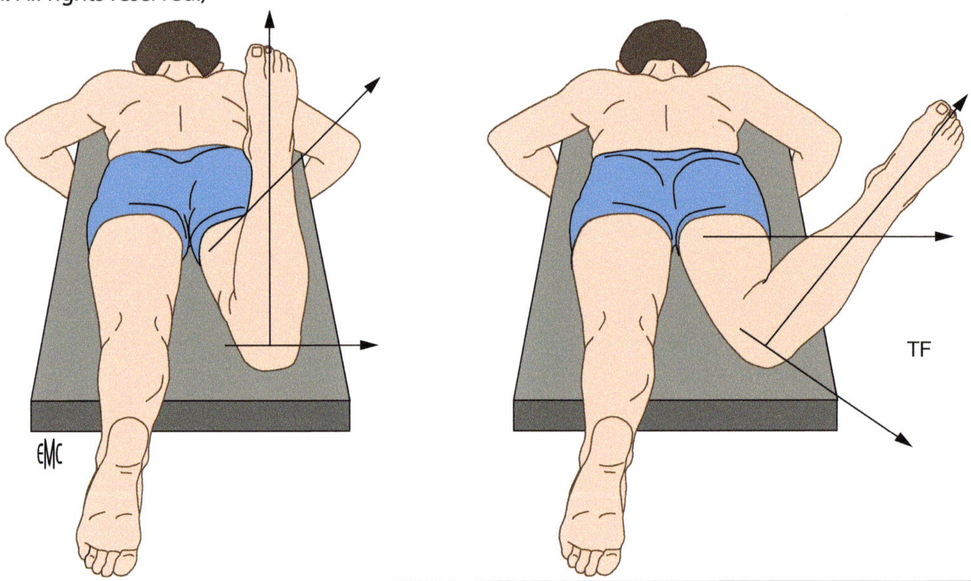

Fig. 4.9 Evaluation in procubitus. In prone position during medial rotation of the hip, the axis of the upper end of the femur is considered to be horizontal and parallel to the plane of the table. The leg axis is perpendicular to the axis of the lower end of the femur, and acts like a compass in the measuring of femoral torsion (FT). (F. Duparc. 2009. "Torsion problems of the adult lower extremity skeleton." EMC Locomotor system 15-322-A-10: 1–12. 2009 Paris: Elsevier Masson. All rights reserved.)

The axis of the upper end of the tibia is considered to be parallel to the stool. The angle between this plane and the bimalleolar axis reveals tibial torsion (TT).

In procubitus (Fig. 4.9)

It is possible to measure the angle between the axis of the leg in medial rotation of the hip and the vertical line. Place the axis of the upper end of the femur so that it is horizontal and parallel to the table. The leg is raised perpendicularly to the inferior end of the femur. In medial rotation of the hip, the leg serves as a compass, giving the measure of femoral torsion.

These simple clinical measures are a way to screen for morphological torsional abnormalities. While this evaluation is a little imprecise, it provides valuable diagnostic guidance. Medical imaging tests are warranted when deformities appear to be clinically significant.

In prone position during medial rotation of the hip, the axis of the upper end of the femur is considered to be horizontal and parallel to the plane of the table. The leg axis is perpendicular to the axis of the lower end of the femur and acts like a compass in the measuring of femoral torsion (FT).

4.3 MANUAL EXPLORATION OF THE GREATER TROCHANTER

Palpation of the hip itself is difficult because of the depth at which the hip lies in the tissues. On the other hand, the greater trochanter is fairly accessible and a key zone for hip manipulations because so many muscles attach to it (Fig. 4.10). Most play an important role in distributing intra-articular coxofemoral pressures on:

- the superior facet–piriformis;
- the lateral facet–gluteus medius, medially, and gluteus minimus, laterally;
- the medial surface–obturator externus and obturator internus, whose tendon is shared with the two gemelli;
- the posterior facet–quadratus femoris.

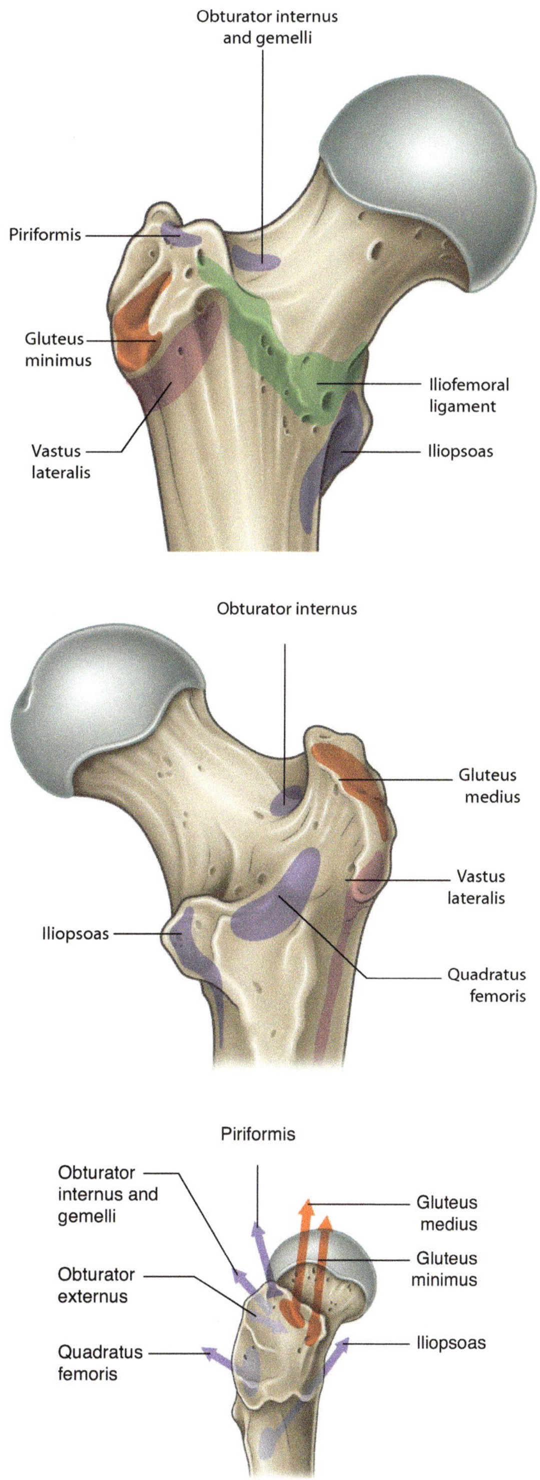

Fig. 4.10 Overview of insertions on the greater trochanter.

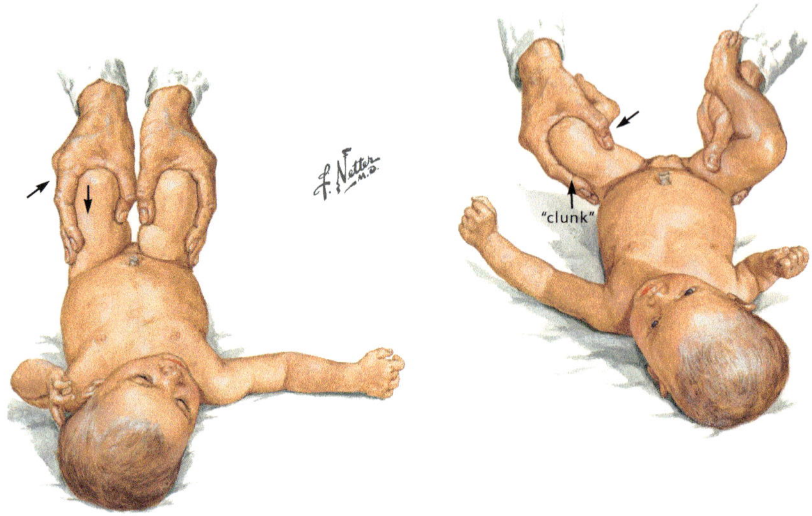

Fig. 4.11 Ortolani test and Barlow maneuver. (After Netter's Orthopaedics, 2nd edition, p.388, Walter Greene. With permission of the editor.)

It is important to be familiar with these insertions in order to refine contact when manipulating the muscles of the hip.

4.4 COMMON HIP PROBLEMS

4.4.1 Developmental dysplasia

Definition of dysplasia

The word dysplasia comes from the Greek dys, meaning bad or difficult, and plasis, meaning formation. It is the abnormal development of tissues such as cartilage, capsule, and ligaments.

Forms of dysplasia at the hip

- Hypoplasia of the epiphysis of the femoral head
- Acetabular dysplasia
- Superior lateral migration of the head of the femur
- Labral irregularities
- Capsular ligament laxity

Tests

Ortolani's test (Fig. 4.11)

The examiner flexes the hips of a supine infant to 90° and then gently abducts the legs. A positive sign is a distinctive "clunk" when the femoral head relocates anterior of the hip socket. The hips can be positioned in an abduction harness, or the infant can wear double diapers to remedy simpler cases.

Barlow's test

The hip can be dislocated easily if the adducted hip can be popped out of its socket using gentle posterior pressure through the knee.

Galeazzi's sign (Fig. 4.12)

This sign is used after the neonatal period, anywhere from two weeks to three months. When both feet are placed firmly on the table, the knees are found not to be level. A unilateral dislocation appears as a shortened thigh on the affected side. There is also limited abduction, which is quite obvious in bilateral testing.

> **Pediatric approach**
>
> In pediatric osteopathy for babies, we recommend that you work systematically on all the muscles of the hip, knee, and foot in combination with cranial and neural manipulations. Pay special attention to the rectus femoris, gluteals, and pelvitrochanteric muscles.

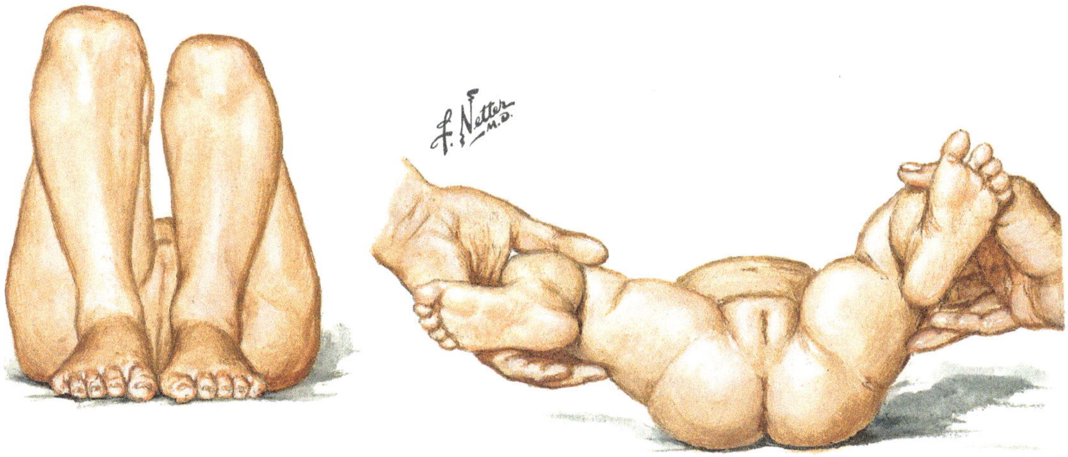

Fig. 4.12 Galeazzi's sign. (After Netter's Orthopaedics, 2nd edition, p. 389, Walter Greene. With permission of the editor.)

4.4.2 Avascular necrosis of the femoral head

This type of necrosis is usually due to displacement fracture of the femoral neck, and it can sometimes occur with hip dislocation. Nevertheless, we have come across several cases of avascular necrosis in patients who simply landed on their heel doing nothing more dramatic than missing a step. It seems in these cases that the problem likely lies with rupture to the ligament of the femoral head. The artery that nourishes the femur runs in the ligament and is damaged accordingly. Necrosis from interrupted blood supply to the bone can take place over a few months or up to two to three years.

Clinical presentation

Pain resides deep in the folds of the groin, especially on weight bearing. Joint range of motion is diminished, particularly medial and lateral rotation. Be alert for contralateral problems, as they are not uncommon.

Predispositions and risk factors

- Alcoholism due to the abuse of wine
- Corticosteroid use
- Osteoporosis
- Trauma (femoral neck fracture, dislocation)
- Tumors, benign or malignant

Test

The test is performed in decubitus with hip flexed to 90°. Exert compression with both hands along the femoral axis in combination with rotations. The test is positive when the patient feels sharp pain. In our clinic we tend to see less involved situations, so-called cases of "a minima," in which pain tends to be muted and difficult to elicit. Alarming pain generally sends the patient for medical workup and referral to a rheumatologist.

Osteopathic considerations

Osteopathy is not indicated for vascular necrosis of the femoral head. Surgery is generally the best option.

Coxarthrosis

The hip is particularly susceptible to osteoarthritis. This condition generally appears after age 60, but it can afflict younger people who endure trauma or microtrauma.

Radiographic signs

Degenerative osteoarthritis of the hip shows up as reduced joint space at the ball–and–socket, with loss of cartilage and subchondral cystic changes. The femoral head is no longer in its normal axis; it is usually displaced cranially or craniolaterally (expulsive coxarthrosis). More rarely, the femur is displaced medially together with acetabular protrusion (protrusive coxarthrosis). The femoral head and the roof of the acetabulum are sclerosed. Osteophytes appear on the acetabulum, particularly the lateral part.

Etiology

- Congenital malformations
- Trauma and microtrauma, local and distant
- Vascular problems
- Heredity
- Malposition in utero

4.4.3 Irritable hip

We have treated approximately 20 cases of irritable hip. The exact cause of this acute condition is unknown. Infants experience hip pain and functional impairment together with a mild fever, which is what unsettles parents the most. The condition is short-lived, however, and pain usually passes within two weeks.

X-ray sometimes reveals enlargement of the head of the femur, giving rise to the term coxa magna. Osteopathy is not indicated for this condition. Check to see if this transient synovitis appeared after pharyngitis, vaccination, or simply a too-long walk. Some parents forget the osteochondral fragility of small children, and they take them on extended walks. If a child consults with hip pain, think to explore the lymphatic ganglions in the groin crease and behind the knee. A child has little purely mechanical reason for hip pain, and it is best to remain vigilant.

The legion of Latin denominations for hip problems proves how common they are and have always been. This would support the recommendation of visiting an osteopath before and after childbirth. Given that a malposition in utero can deform the cranium (plagiocephalia), malposition can also have consequences for the rest of the body, including the hip. Gentle, low-amplitude movements can alter congenital predispositions to disease. In our clinic we teach parents to perform gentle treatment.

4.5 APPROACHES TO HIP PAIN

Acute or chronic pain is the most common reason for hip consultation. When acute pain appears for no apparent reason, ask for an X-ray. Here are the chief causes of hip pain.

4.5.1 Sudden acute pain

Meshed fractures are fractures in which fragments are nestled one inside the other at the fracture line. We have seen patients consult with a slight limp that turned out to be a fracture.

Other common causes of sudden acute pain are:

- cartilage compression (landing hard on the feet);
- phlebitis, veinitis;
- tumors, benign or malignant;
- sprain (rare);
- neuralgia (femoral, lumbar plexus), often secondary;
- muscle tear (psoas, adductors, hamstrings);
- general arterial disorders as well as problems with the artery of the ligament of the femoral head (arteriopathy).

4.5.2 Chronic pain

- Coxarthrosis
- Compensation for the knee or foot
- Muscle fibrosis
- Arteriovenous insufficiency
- Osteoporosis
- Lumbosacral neuralgia compensated at the hip

4.5.3 Referred pain: the visceral hip

Signs and symptoms

As a rule, hip pain of visceral origin provokes pain with passive and active flexion. But this type of pain does not limit range of motion. Be aware that active movement is often more painful than passive movement, because muscle contractions raise intra-articular pressure.

If you encounter firm resistance that worsens pain during passive mobilization, you might well be looking at degenerative arthritis. When this type of arthritis is due to long-standing visceral dysfunction, the patient has more often than not suffered episodic pain for a considerable length of time.

Elements involved

Pain is referred to the hip by the subcostal (12th intercostal) femoral, ilioinguinal, and iliohypogastric nerves. From a neurological perspective, the renal plexus is often involved as well. This is especially true when the kidneys, ureters, intestines, bladder, and ovaries are part of the picture. Hip and flank pain commonly accompany kidney or ureter pyelonephritis or kidney stones in the urinary tract. In women, hip pain of pelvic origin generally points to the ovaries. In men, the same pain can indicate fairly advanced prostate disease.

Pain laterality

Right hip

- Cecum
- Iliocecal junction
- Right ovary
- Right kidney and ureter

Left hip

- Sigmoid
- Left ovary
- Left kidney and ureter

Hip pain linked to the bladder usually involves the ureterovesical junction or bladder fixations connected with the soft tissues of the obturator foramen.

5 Treatment of the active stabilizers

In our approach we tend to view the muscles grouped around the hip as analogous to remote ligaments. Nevertheless, some muscles exert direct influence over the coxofemoral joint proper.

- The rectus femoris has three tendons that stabilize the femoral head anteriorly. Its reflected tendon attaches directly to the iliofemoral ligament.
- The gluteus minimis contributes fibers that directly reinforce the capsule.
- The iliopsoas has a femoral attachment that holds the femoral head in the acetabulum.
- The obturators internus and externus exert an upward force on the pelvis toward the femur (Dolto's gemellus-obturator hammock). The obturator externus passes the infra-acetabular groove and spirals posteriorly to the femoral neck to contact the joint capsule.
- The tensor fasciae latae and the iliotibial tract contribute as a pair to coxofemoral and femorotibial joint cohesion.

All of these muscles help to maintain the trunk in the erect posture and act as restraint straps around the coxofemoral joint.

What interests us is not pure muscle function but rather the effects of muscle action on periarticular elements, particularly intra-articular pressures. In order to follow muscle orientation, our maneuvers must be superb and precise.

Beyond the labrum, the reflected tendon of rectus femoris attaches to the anterior fibrous capsule. This connection allows us to treat the capsule by way of the muscle. In addition, capsuloligamentous manipulations benefit the labrum and vice versa.

5.1 GLUTEUS MAXIMUS (FIG. 5.1)

5.1.1 Review

Origin: Gluteus maximus is the strongest muscle in the human body. It has a deep and superficial origin.

The superficial part arises from:

- the lateral lip of the iliac crest;
- the posterior superior iliac spine;
- the thoracolumbar fascia;
- the sacrum and coccyx.

The deep part arises from:

- the posterior gluteal line of the inner upper llium;
- the sacrotuberous ligament;
- the fascia covering the gluteus medius (gluteal aponeurosis).

Direction

- Caudal and lateral

Termination

- Iliotibial tract
- Femur, gluteal tuberosity

Vascularization

- Superior gluteal artery
- Inferior gluteal artery

Useful relationships: The gluteus maximus covers the sciatic notches over the emergence of the sciatic nerve. Our sacral plexus and sciatic nerve techniques are performed through the gluteus maximus. It also covers the pelvitrochanteric muscles.

Actions

- Statically:
  - It is a cushion for sitting and protects the sciatic nerve from compression.
  - It is a posterior caudal tensor of the fascia lata.
  - It strengthens the anal sphincter.
  - It is one of the muscles stabilizing the trunk in upright posture.
- Dynamically:
  - It is a hip extensor.
  - It is a lateral rotator.
  - It is both an abductor and an adductor, depending on fiber direction.
  - It works when we climb stairs.

Erect posture has evolved at the expense of the hamstrings, which have become increasingly fibrous over the course of time.

5.1.2 Techniques

In decubitus (Fig. 5.2)

The patient flexes the leg of the involved hip. You position yourself either on the same side or across the body from the involved hip. Use the fingers of your distal hand to grasp the femur as near to the gluteal tuberosity as possible. Place your proximal fingers

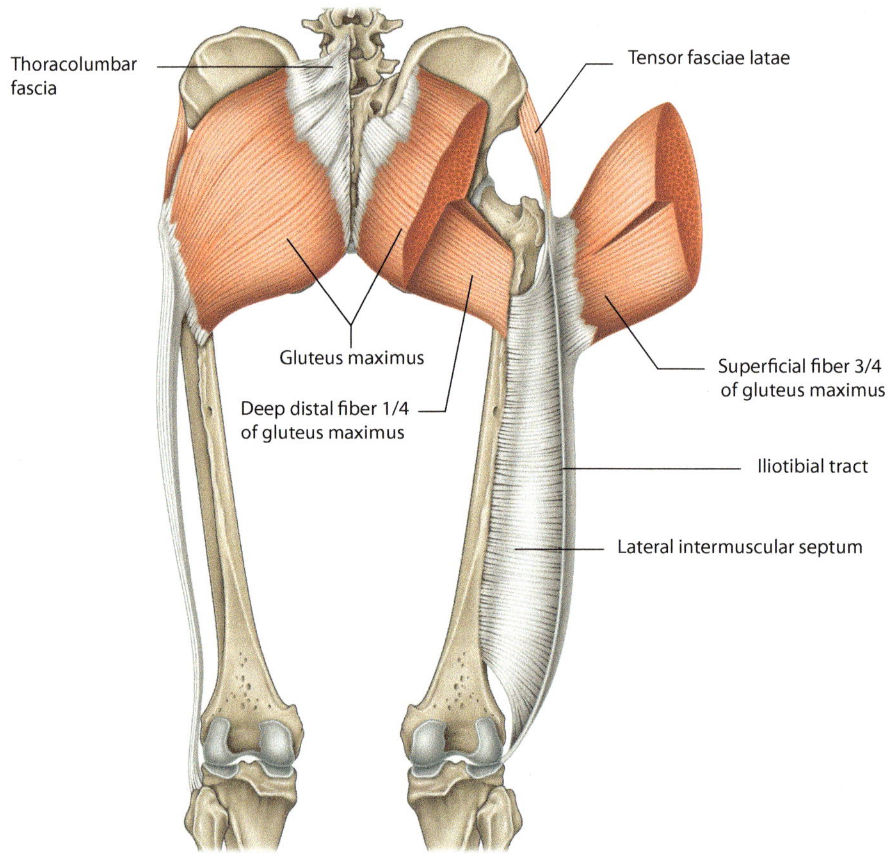

Fig. 5.1 Gluteus maximus.

either on the iliac crest and the posterior superior iliac spine or on the sacrococcygeal region.

Ask the patient to adduct his leg starting from a position of abduction. Accompany the movement, drawing the femur into medial rotation and adduction. Ask more flexible patients to begin with their foot outside the straight leg to increase musculotendinous tension.

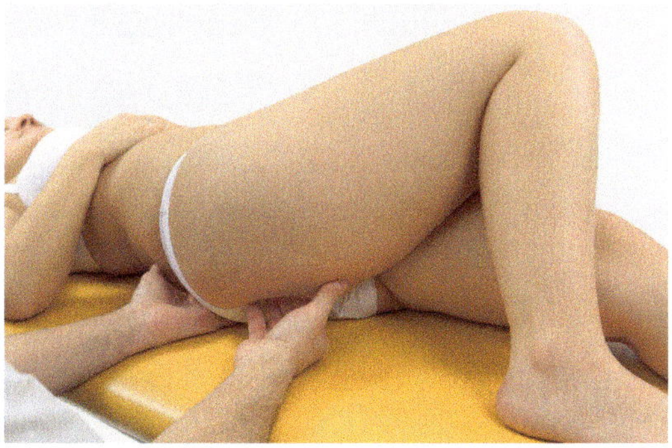

Fig. 5.2 Gluteus maximus in decubitus.

In lateral decubitus (Fig. 5.3)

The patient lies on the side opposite the treatment hip. You place your thumb as close to the gluteal tuberosity of the femur as possible. Position the fingers of your other hand on the posterior superior iliac spine. Ask the patient to flex the hip and accompany the movement while simultaneously drawing the femur into medial rotation.

Gluteus maximus–fascia lata junction (Fig. 5.4)

This maneuver benefits both the hip and the knee, because the fascia lata attaches to the tibia under its reinforced band, the iliotibial tract. The patient lies on the side opposite the hip in question, leg extended. You position yourself three-quarters behind the patient. Place both thumbs behind the greater trochanter, on the musculofascial junction.

Ask the patient to extend his leg as far as possible, as if trying to make it grow longer.

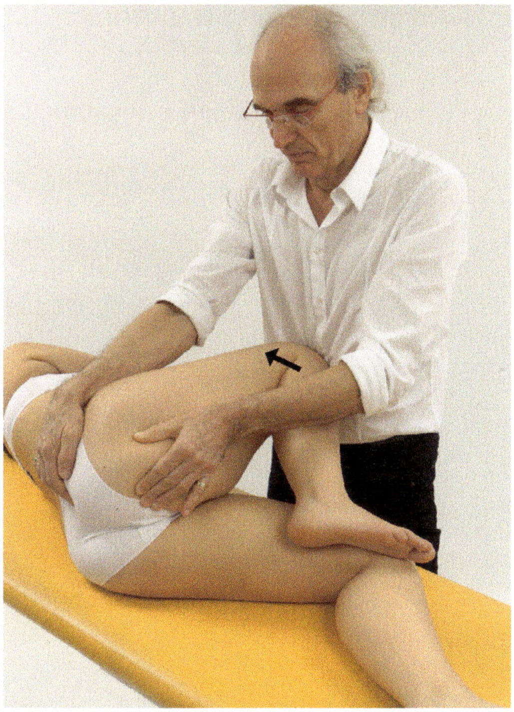

Fig. 5.3 Gluteus maximus in lateral decubitus.

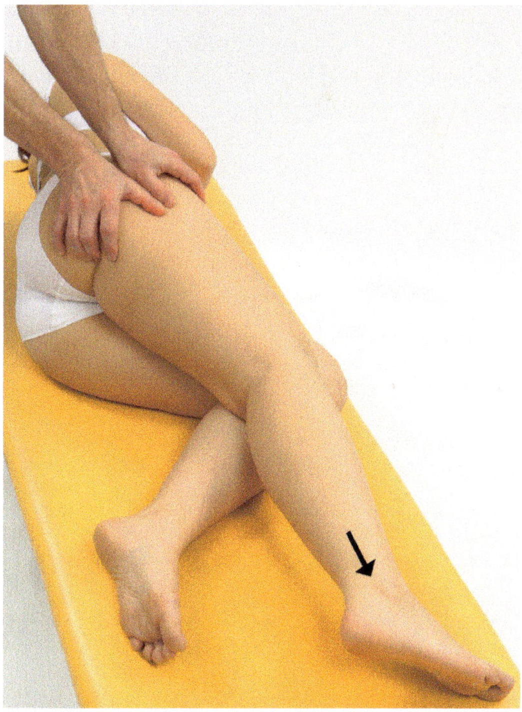

Fig. 5.4 Gluteus maximus–fascia lata junction.

Simultaneously stretch the gluteus maximus–fascia lata junction distally, adding a little medial rotation.

5.2 GLUTEUS MEDIUS (FIG. 5.5)

Gluteus medius is important to hip stability and intra-articular pressures.

5.2.1 Review

Origin

- Outer surface of the iliac wing, between the posterior and middle gluteal lines
- Gluteal aponeurosis

Direction

- Caudal and lateral

Termination

- Lateral surface of the proximal greater trochanter

A serous bursa separates the muscle tendon from the surface of the trochanter over which it glides. The trochanteric bursa pads the bone.

Innervation

- Superior gluteal nerve (L4–L5)

Vascularization

- Superior gluteal artery

Important relationships

The lower part of the muscle is partially covered by the gluteus maximus. The gluteus medius, in turn, covers the gluteus minimus and the coxofemoral joint. It relates to tensor fasciae latae and piriformis, parallel to its posterior border.

Actions

The action differs according to static or dynamic function.

- Statically:
  - It stabilizes the pelvis laterally.
  - It supports the body on one leg during gait.
- Dynamically:
  - The anterior part flexes the hip and internally rotates the thigh.
  - The posterior part extends the hip and internally rotates the thigh.
  - Both parts of the muscle together abduct the hip.

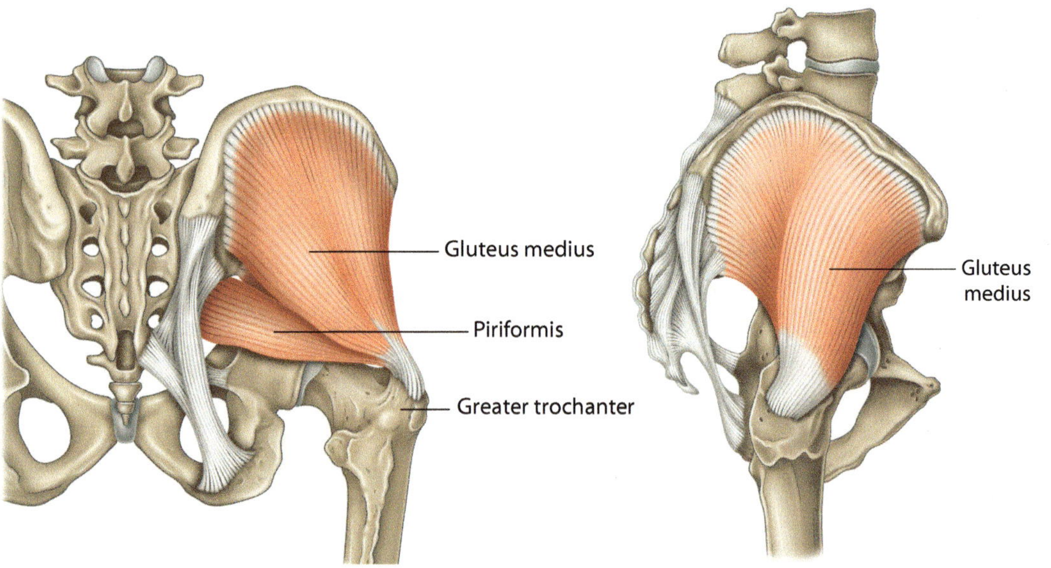

Fig. 5.5 Gluteus medius.

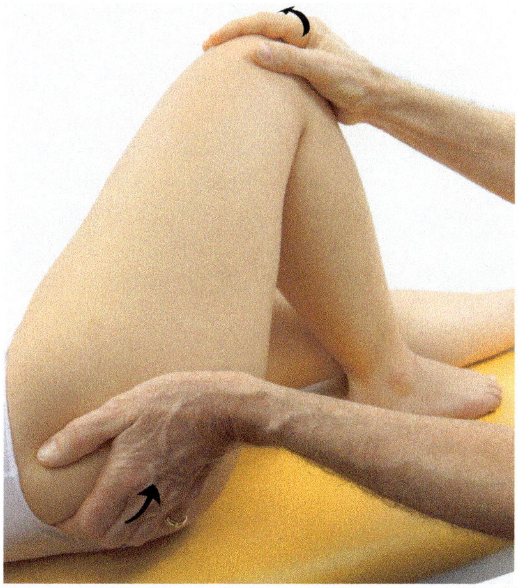

Fig. 5.6 Gluteus medius in decubitus (first method).

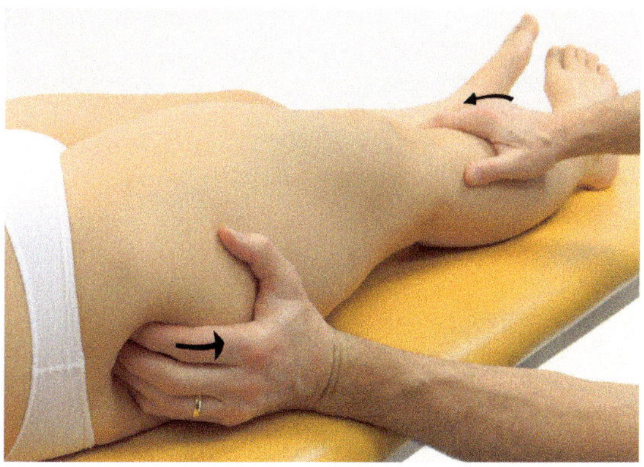

Fig. 5.7 Gluteus medius in decubitus (second method).

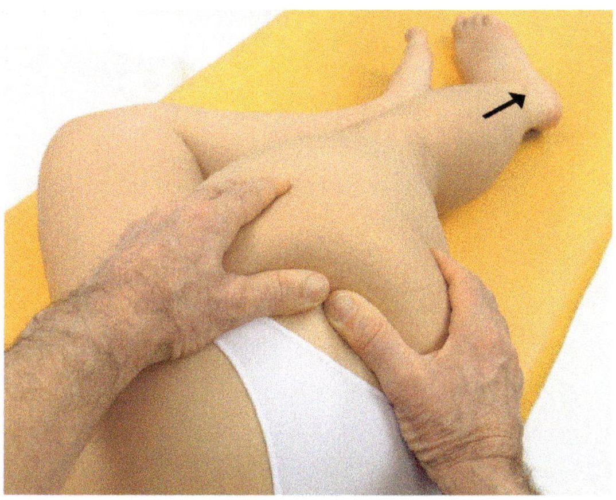

Fig. 5.8 Gluteus medius in lateral decubitus.

- The muscle is important to long-distance walkers and dancers.

5.2.2 Techniques

The patient lies on the table, leg flexed or extended.

In decubitus, leg flexed—first method (Fig. 5.6)

Place your fingers side by side on the cranial facet of the greater trochanter. For especially robust or heavy patients, place both hands under the trochanter. Ask the patient to laterally rotate and abduct the hip to engage the anterior fibers.

To treat the anterior fibers, accompany the movement while tractioning the greater trochanter distally and laterally. To treat the posterior fibers, rotate the leg medially together with adduction of the hip. You can progressively amplify the effect by accompanying the movement.

In decubitus, leg extended—second method (Fig. 5.7)

The patient lies on the table, leg extended in slight medial rotation. With your fingers on the trochanter, traction the muscle caudally and laterally. Ask the patient to simultaneously rotate the leg outwardly.

In lateral decubitus (Fig. 5.8)

The patient lies on the side opposite the treatment. Place your thumbs side by side or place several fingers on the superior facet of the greater trochanter. Exert pressure with your thumbs if you are positioned above the hip. Exert traction if you are standing distally and using your fingers. Draw distally and laterally to affect anterior fibers. Draw distally and medially to affect posterior fibers.

This same maneuver can be used to stretch the gluteus minimus. At the end of the movement, ask the patient to elongate his leg by pushing the foot distally.

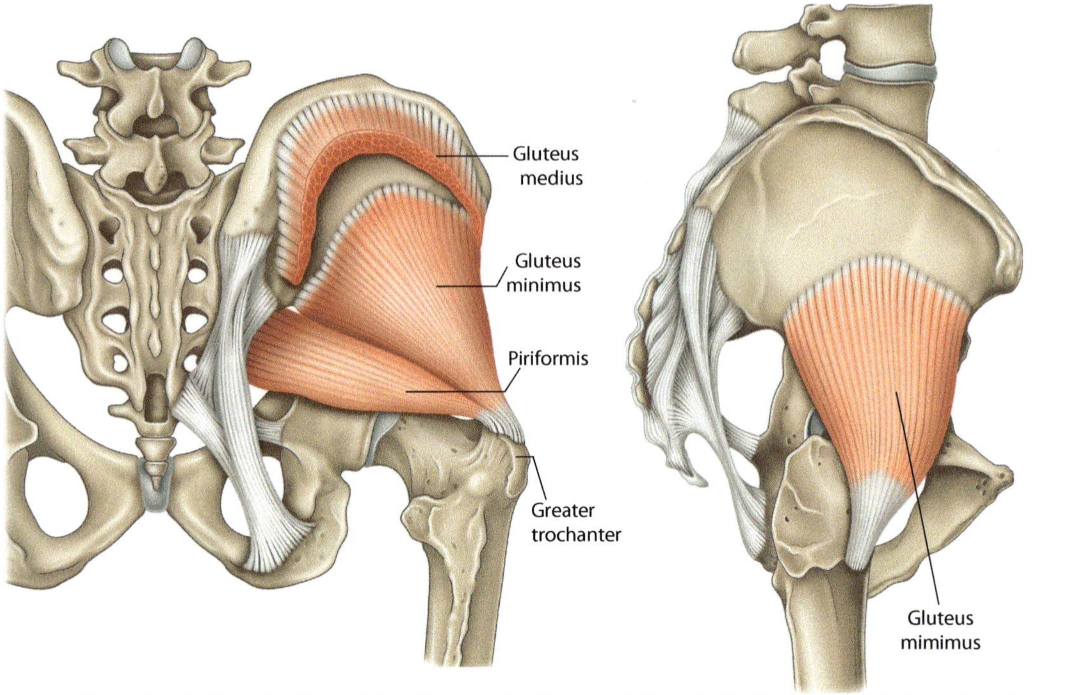

Fig. 5.9 Gluteus minimus.

5.3 GLUTEUS MINIMUS (FIG. 5.9)

This muscle is of special interest due to its intimate relationship to the joint capsule by way of the iliofemoral ligament.

5.3.1 Review

Origin

- Outer surface of ilium between the anterior and inferior gluteal lines

Direction

- Caudal and lateral

Termination

- Greater trochanter, superior facet

Innervation

- Superior gluteal nerve (L4–L5)

Vascularization

- Superior gluteal artery

Actions

- Statically:
  - It has the same function as the gluteus medius.
  - It is a hip stabilizer.
  - It is called into action to support the body standing on one leg.
- Dynamically:
  - It flexes and abducts the thigh.
  - Anterior fibers are medial rotators.
  - Posterior fibers are lateral rotators.

Important relationships

- Exchanges fibers with the iliofemoral ligament
- Is part of the deep muscle group of the hip along with the:
  - piriformis;
  - obturator internus;
  - gemelli;
  - quadratus femoris;
  - adductor magnus.

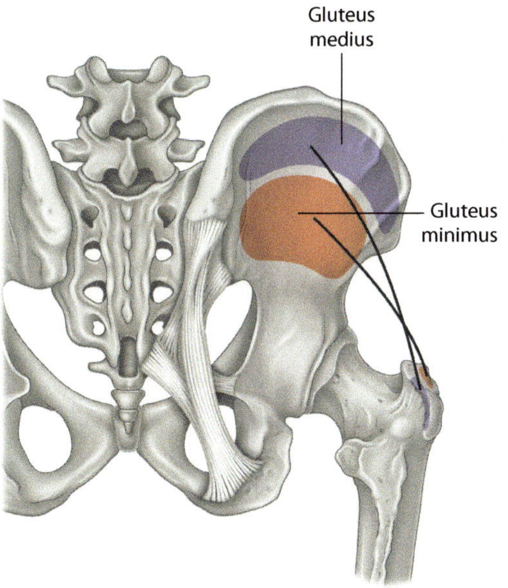

Fig. 5.9 Gluteus minimus.

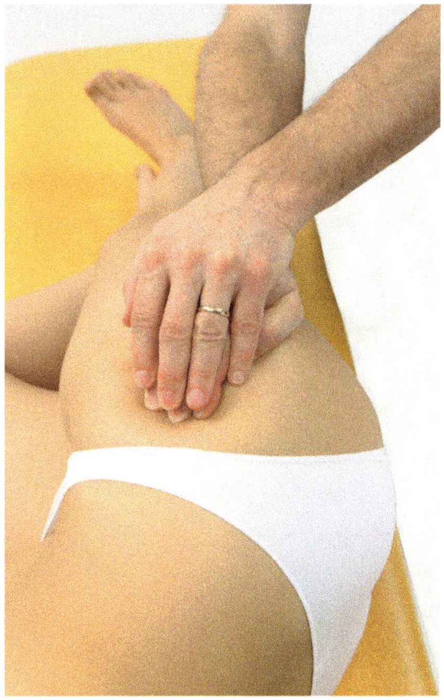

Fig. 5.10 Gluteus minimus in lateral decubitus.

5.3.2 Techniques

The smallest of the gluteal muscles is treated the same way as the gluteus medius, with a few nuances in the lateral decubitus position. More emphasis is put on lateral hip rotation and extension to include the iliofemoral ligament in the effect.

In lateral decubitus (Fig. 5.10)

The patient lies on the side opposite the hip concerned. You place your fingers on the cranial facet of the greater trochanter and ask the patient to extend and laterally rotate his leg. Accompanying lateral rotation targets gluteal muscle fibers that blend with the iliofemoral ligament.

5.4 TENSOR FASCIAE LATAE (FIG 5.11)

This muscle interests us because of its tendinous extension, the iliotibial tract. Tensor fasciae latae is a biarticular muscle.

5.4.1 Review

Origin

- Coxal bone on the anterior superior iliac spine
- Iliac crest in contact with gluteus medius
- Femoral aponeurosis

Direction

- Caudal and slightly lateral

Termination

- Fascia lata, which inserts into iliotibial tract beneath greater trochanter
- Iliotibial tract, a tendinous aponeurosis of the fascia lata
- Infracondylar tubercle (Gerdy's tubercle)
- Various expansions
  - Femoral fascia;
  - Lateral border of the patella;
  - Fibers that join sartorius.

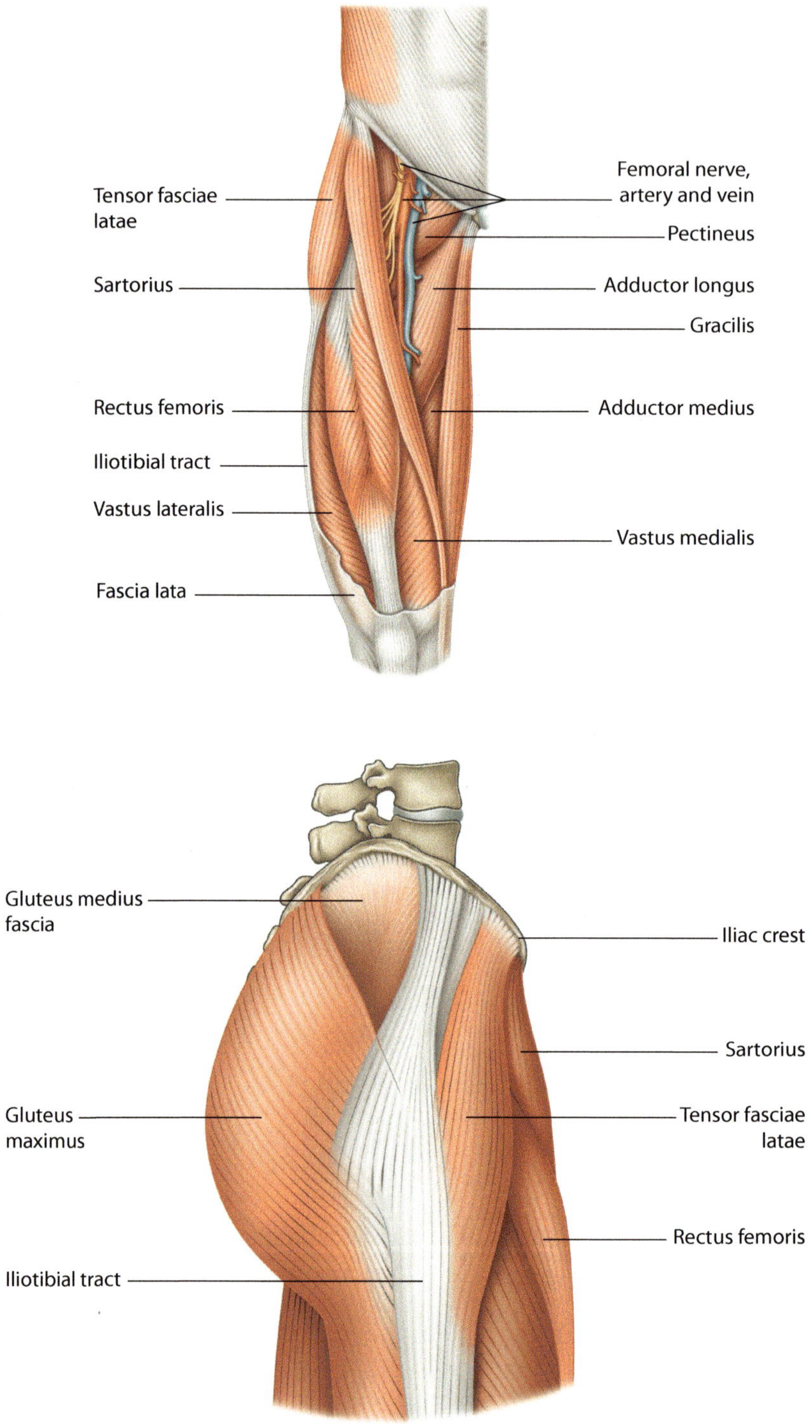

Fig. 5.11 Tensor fasciae latae.

Innervation

- Superior gluteal nerve (L4–L5)

Vascularization

- Superficial circumflex iliac artery

Actions

- Statically:
  - It steadies the pelvis upon the head of the femur.
  - It supports the anteriors of gluteus medius and minimus.
  - It stabilizes the lateral knee.
- Dynamically:
  - The hip is:
    - o flexor;
    - o abductor;
    - o medial rotator.
  - It braces the knee:
    - o in lateral rotation;
    - o in extension.

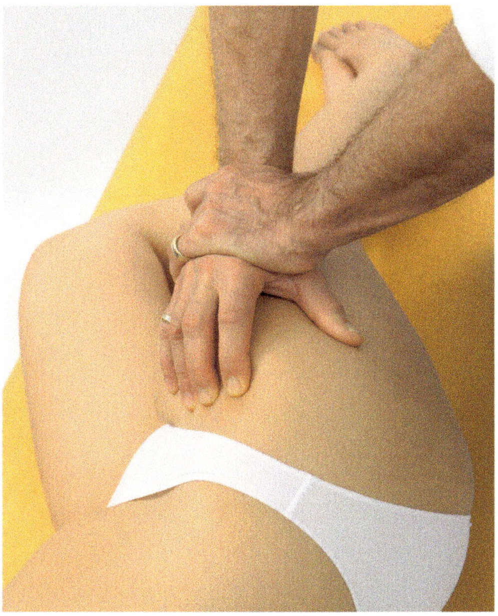

Fig. 5.12 Tensor fasciae latae in lateral decubitus (first method).

Important relationships

- At the hip
  - Fascia lata
  - Biceps femoris
  - Rectus femoris
  - Sartorius
- At the knee
  - Biceps femoris
  - Fibers that radiate into lateral patellar retinaculum
  - Anterior patella

5.4.2 Techniques

Some techniques treat the tensor fasciae latae itself, while others are designed to affect the iliotibial tract.

Tensor fasciae latae in lateral decubitus—first method (Fig. 5.12)

The patient lies on the side opposite the hip concerned, knee slightly flexed. You stand behind the patient and place one thumb or two fingers slightly below the anterior superior iliac spine to feel clearly the fleshy fibers of the tensor fasciae latae. Be careful not to confuse them with rectus femoris and sartorius fibers that lie just medially. Search the muscle for sensitive fibers or areas of microfibrosis.

While the patient extends the hip slightly, stretch the tensor fasciae latae by drawing it first distally and then lateromedially. Keep in mind that when this muscle becomes tight or shortened, cartilage is adversely affected by this abnormal tension.

Tensor fasciae latae in lateral decubitus—second method (Fig. 5.13)

Through the iliotibial band, the tensor fasciae latae has fiber connections to the patella, anterior crural fascia, posterior crural fascia, and infracondylar tubercle.

The patient assumes the same side-lying position as in the preceding method. You place one thumb on the tensor fasciae latae at the hip, while the fingers of your other hand surround the crural fascia on the leg.

Ask the patient to extend his hip and knee, stretching the leg distally. Your proximal thumb serves as a fixed point. Your distal hand stretches the crural fascia distally with some lateral rotation. Complete the maneuver with induction, as usually recommended.

Iliotibial tract (Fig. 5.14)

The iliotibial band is lateral thickening of the fascia lata in the thigh. It plays an important role in stabilizing the lower extremity and also supports periarticular muscles at the knee.

Origin

- Fibrous continuation of the fascia lata

Direction

- Distal from outside of hip to top of knee

Important relationships

The iliotibial band exchanges fibers with the tensor fasciae latae and the gluteus maximus.

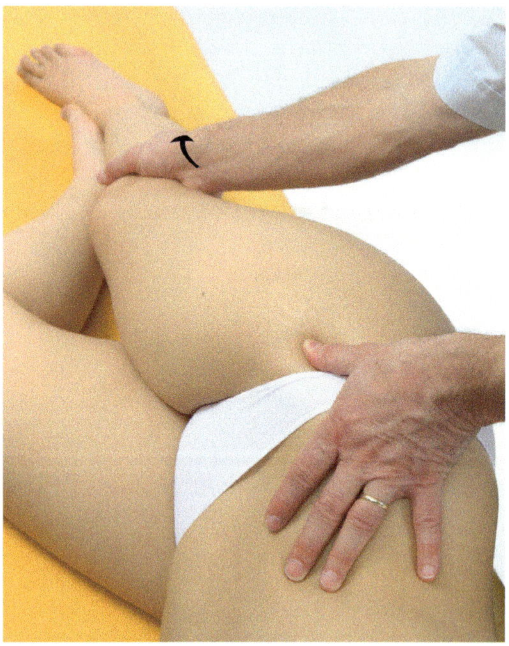

Fig. 5.13 Tensor fasciae latae in lateral decubitus (second method).

Iliotibial-gluteus maximus junction in lateral decubitus (Fig. 5.15)

The patient lies on the side opposite the leg treated, knee slightly flexed. You stand behind the patient and place a flat thumb on the lateral and slightly caudal part of the gluteus maximus. Position your other thumb where muscle joins the iliotibial tract. Bring your thorax to bear directly over your hands; this brings precision to the maneuver without harming your hands. While the patient extends his knee and leg, separate your thumbs by directing them medially and into slight medial rotation.

Reminder: The gluteus maximus aponeurosis inserts fibers into the iliotibial tract. It is important to release restrictions that commonly occur at this junction.

Special note

Bear in mind the perforating branches of the lateral femoral cutaneous nerve. Neural techniques are described in chapter 18.

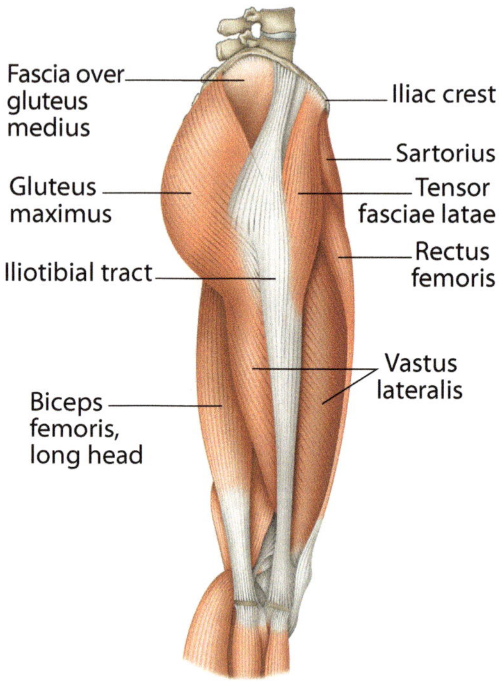

Fig. 5.14 Iliotibial tract.

5.5 SARTORIUS (FIG. 5.16)

The sartorius is a biarticular muscle whose treatment is not particularly effective for the hip. It is a useful muscle, however, to landmark at the hip when locating rectus femoris, iliacus, and pectineus, and at the knee where it forms part of the pes anserinus that we manipulate.

5.5.1 Review

Origin

- Coxal bone, cranial part of the anterior superior iliac spine

Direction

- Oblique caudally and medially: palpable as it courses down the interior medial length of the thigh

Termination

- Curves anterior to insert on the proximal medial part of tibia, just in front of gracilis and semitendinous, with whose tendons it forms the superficial pes anserinus
- Sends expansions to the crural fascia for which it acts as a tensor, like the iliotibial band

Innervation

- Femoral nerve

Vascularization

- Superficial circumflex iliac artery, a branch of the femoral artery
- Perforating branches of the deep femoral artery

Actions

- Hip
  - Flexion
  - Abduction
  - Lateral rotation

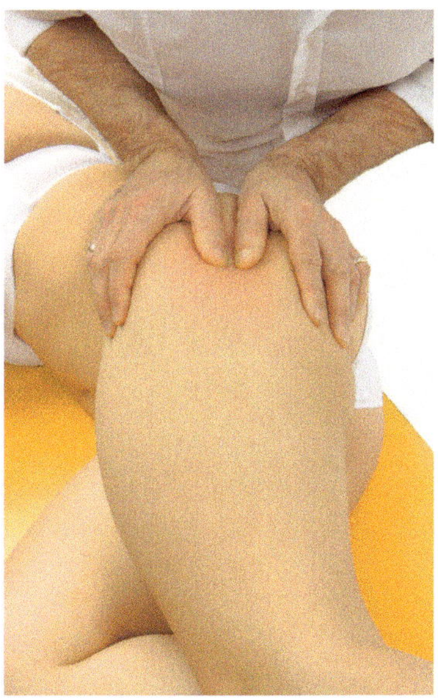

Fig. 5.15 Iliotibial–gluteus maximus junction.

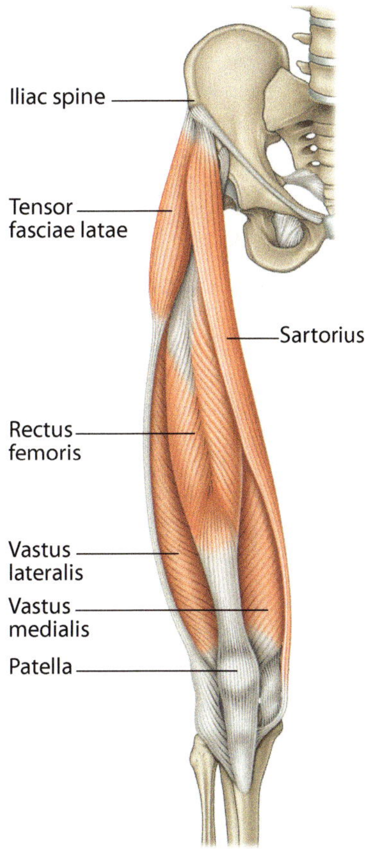

Fig. 5.16 Sartorius.

- Knee
  - Flexion
  - Medial rotation (resists lateral rotation)
- Both joints
  - Dynamic coordination between knee and hip

5.5.2 Techniques

Femoral triangle (Fig. 5.17)

To landmark the sartorius, it is useful to familiarize yourself with the femoral triangle (also known as Scarpa's triangle).

It is bound:

- cranially by the inguinal ligament;
- laterally by the sartorius;
- medially by the gracilis.

The triangle floor is made up laterally to medially by the psoas, pectineus, adductor longus, and adductor magnus.

This triangle contains the neurovascular bundle that runs from the lesser pelvis to the anterior surface of the thigh, beneath the inguinal ligament, and passes through the muscular and vascular lacuna, separated by the iliopectineal arch.

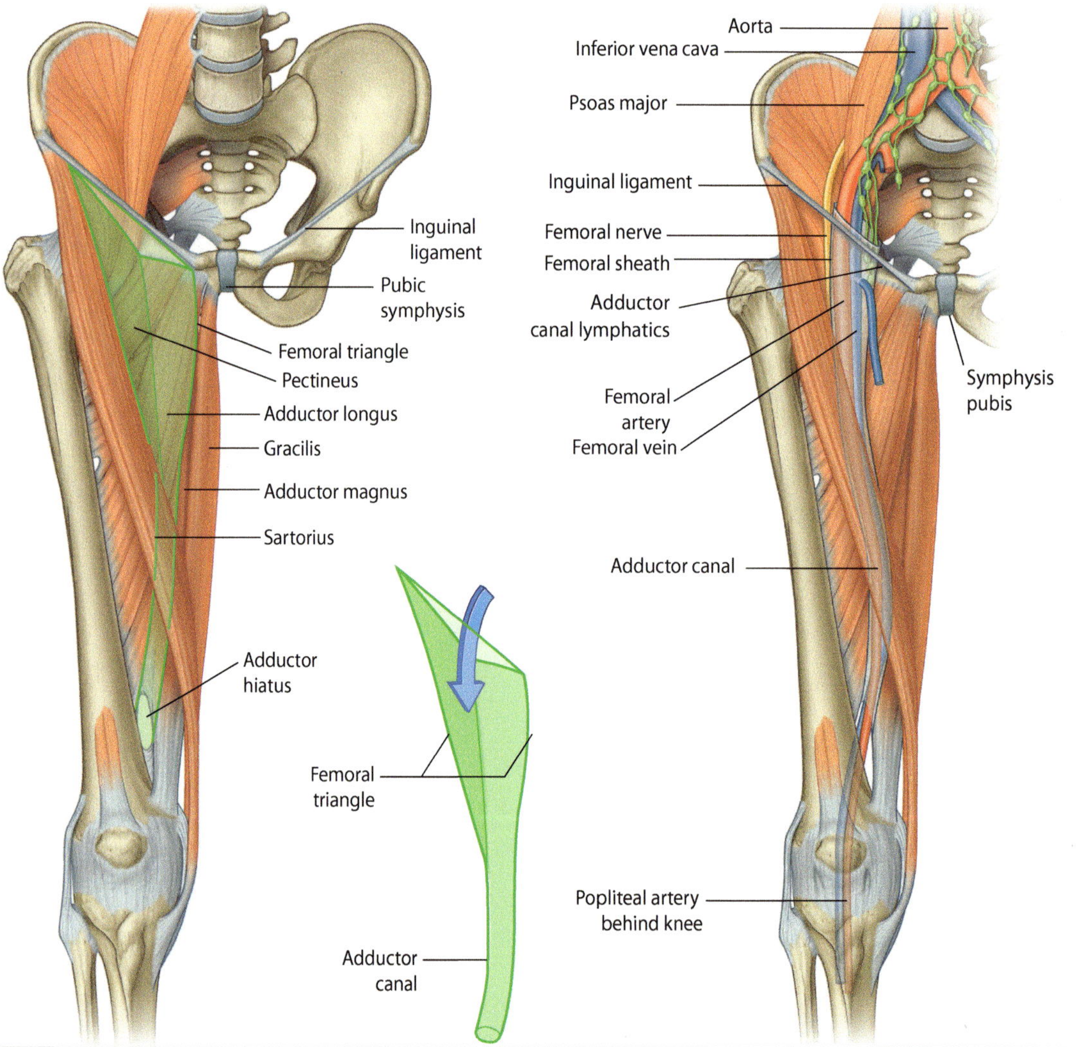

Fig. 5.17 Femoral triangle schema.

Spreading technique below the anterior superior iliac spine, in lateral decubitus (Fig. 5.18)

The patient lies on the side opposite the muscle to be treated. You position yourself behind the patient. Begin medially at the anterior superior iliac spine and progress toward the tensor fasciae latae and rectus femoris, located more distally. Feel for the lateral aspect of the musculotendinous sartorius junction.

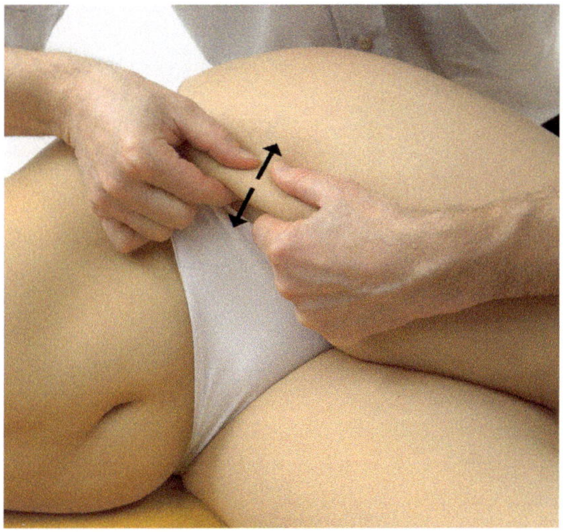

Fig. 5.18 Sartorius in lateral decubitus.

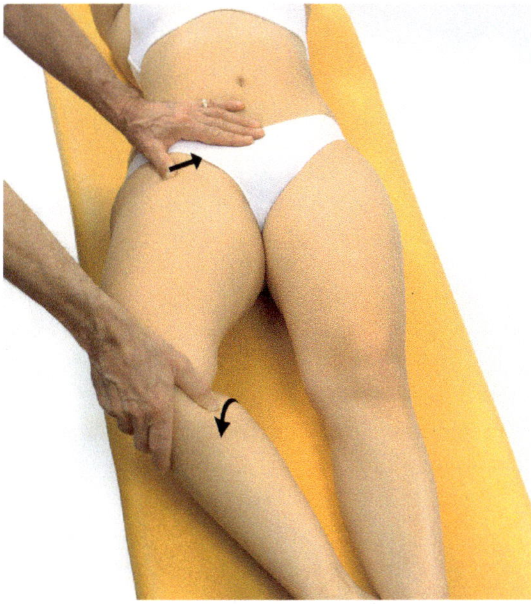

Fig. 5.19 Sartorius in decubitus.

Glide the junction medially and laterally. Concentrate on places that do not glide easily and treat them with stretch-induction. We treat the distal insertion of the sartorius at the pes anserinus ("goose's foot") described in the knee joint chapter.

Spreading technique beneath the anterior superior iliac spine, in decubitus (Fig. 5.19)

The patient lies on the table, leg slightly flexed. You place one thumb on the anterior superior iliac spine, below the inguinal ligament, inside the tensor fasciae latae. Place the other thumb on the anterior part of the goose's foot at the tibia.

Ask the patient to extend his leg, adding a lateral rotation component. The proximal thumb moves the sartorius insertion on the anterior superior iliac spine. The distal thumb increases lateral rotation of the tibia.

5.6 RECTUS FEMORIS (FIG. 5.20)

Rectus femoris is one of the four quadriceps muscles. It is biarticular.

5.6.1 Review

Origin

The muscle arises by three tendons (Fig. 5.21):

- The powerful and round straight tendon arises from the anterior inferior iliac spine.
- The reflected tendon is a thin but strong fibrous expansion arising from a groove above the rim of the acetabulum. The reflected tendon adheres to the cranial part of the capsule.
- The recurrent tendon attaches to the anteromedial aspect of the greater trochanter.

Direction

- Distal and slightly medial

Termination

- Base of the patella

- Spindle-shaped muscle prolonged downward anteriorly to the vastus intermedius, between vastus medialis and vastus lateralis

Important relationships

At its origin, the muscle is covered by the sartorius before departing from it caudally. To access the rectus femoris, we first move the sartorius out of the way, either medially or laterally.

Actions

The rectus femoris keeps the head of the femur in the acetabulum, especially when the hip is extended and the knee flexed. It plays an accessory role in hip flexion.

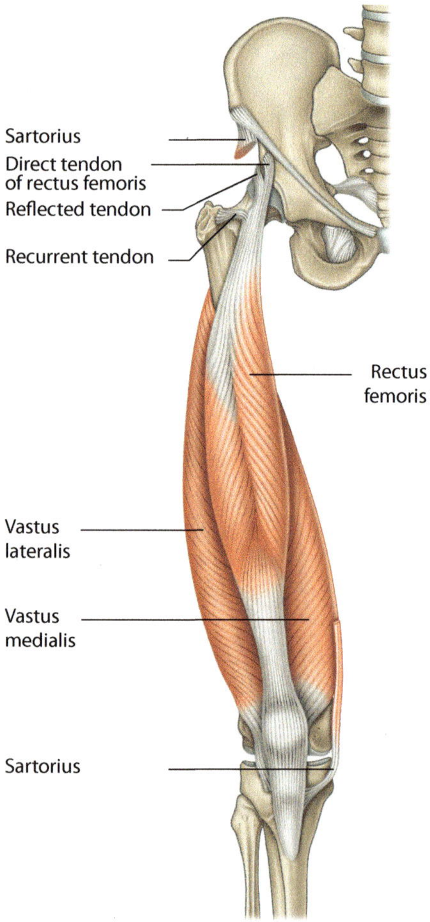

Fig. 5.20 Rectus femoris.

Innervation

- Femoral nerve

Vascularization

- Superior and inferior gluteal arteries

Important relationships

Rectus femoris is of interest because it has a profound action on the coxofemoral joint capsule. It is a capsule strengthener. Manipulating this muscle allows us to have a significant effect on capsular fibers.

5.6.2 Techniques

In lateral decubitus (Fig. 5.22)

The patient lies on the side opposite the joint concerned, top foot positioned behind the other. You place your thumb on the lateral part of the sartorius and mobilize it inside or sometimes outside of the rectus femoris, depending on the shape of the patient, in order to access the anterior inferior iliac spine. Access to the tendon varies according to the angle of the tendinous insertion.

Straight tendon

Place your flat thumb on the tendon as it inserts at the anterior inferior iliac spine. Ask the patient to extend his hip by sliding his top foot behind his other leg until the hip is fully extended. At the point of maximum stretch, ask the patient to push his foot even further, as if wanting to lengthen the leg as far as or beyond the end of the table.

Simultaneously stretch the direct tendon distally with your thumb to affect the joint capsule. You can ask younger, more flexible patients to bend their knee with the hip in extension to increase traction on the rectus femoris muscle by means of the quadriceps tendon. Be careful to avoid cramps that can occur if this manipulation is not performed in a sufficiently progressive manner.

Reflected tendon

This tendon arises from the exterior surface

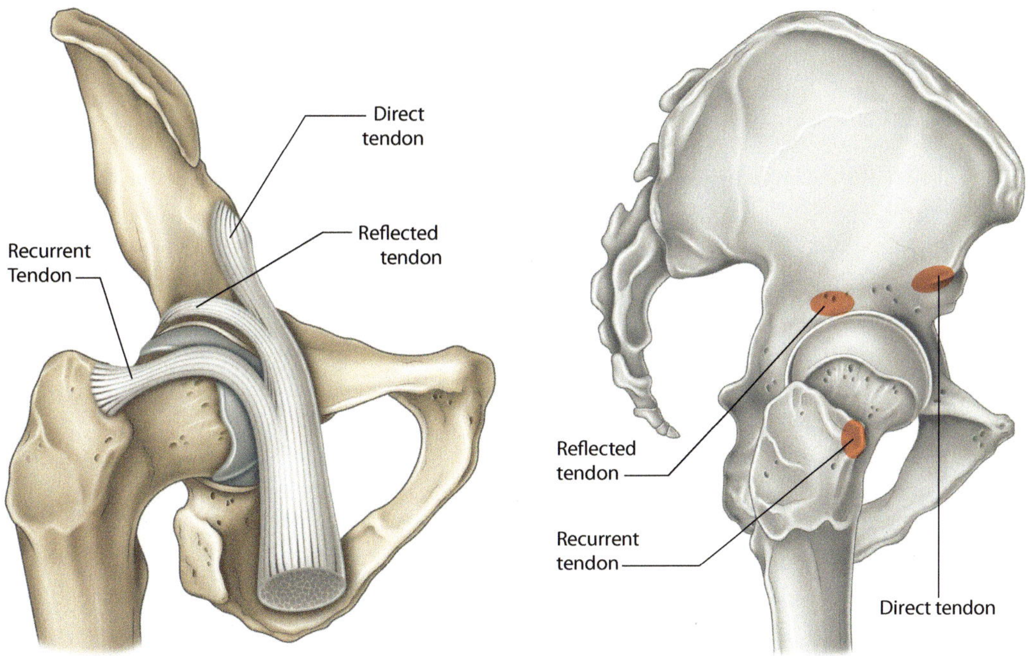

Fig. 5.21 Origins of the rectus femoris muscle.

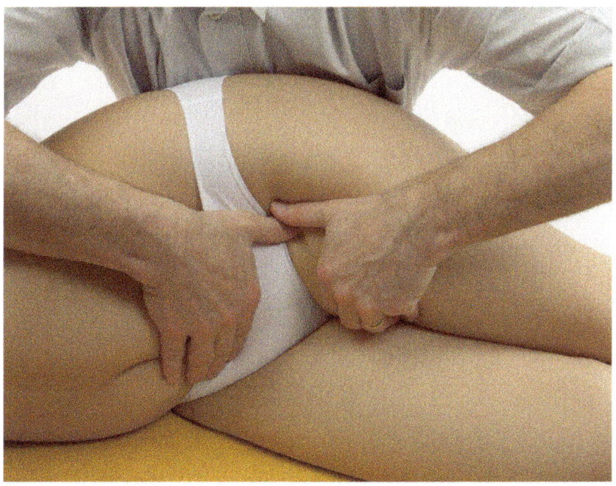

Fig. 5.22 Rectus femoris in lateral decubitus.

of the boney ridge that forms the superior acetabular groove. The patient assumes the same position as above and moves the hip in the same way. You place one thumb against the anterior inferior iliac spine and the other thumb more medially in the direction of the superior acetabular ridge. Depending on the shape of the patient, the tendon can be located nearer to the inferior gluteal line than to the acetabulum. One thumb accompanies the distal push of the leg while the other is directed more medially. Do this 12 times and finish with induction using both thumbs.

Recurrent tendon

In the same position, place one thumb against the anterior inferior iliac spine and the other as cranially as possible on the cranial and medial aspect of the greater trochanter. While the patient moves his hip into extension, pushing the lower extremity inferiorly, stretch the recurrent tendon distally with your anterior inferior iliac spine thumb contact. Your other thumb stretches the femur laterally, accomplishing lateral rotation. While it is not easy to clearly feel the femoral insertion of the recurrent tendon, we can nonetheless stretch along its fiber direction.

5.7 ILIACUS MINOR (ILIOCAPSULARIS) (FIG. 5.23)

Some people are astonished at the very existence of this muscle, let alone the interest generated by it. Iliacus minor is composed of

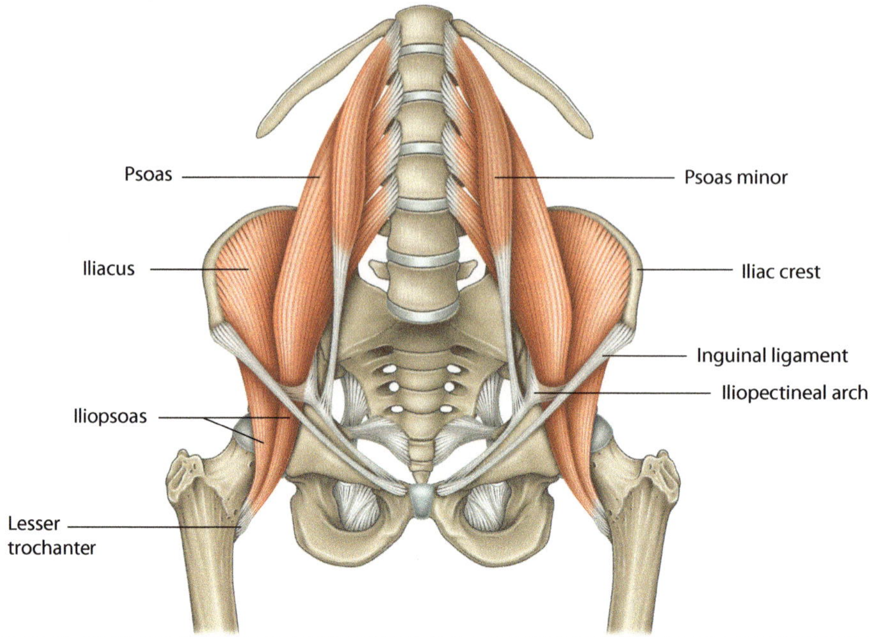

Fig. 5.23 Iliopsoas.

fibers that separate from the iliacus and, as a special feature, join the coxofemoral capsule it overlays.

Iliacus minor is also known as iliocapsularis; this is the capsular relationship that interests us. A great deal has been written about psoas muscle stretches, and for this reason none are included here. Our next book, dedicated to the vertebral column, describes precise psoas muscle stretches in connection with spinal disc techniques.

Iliacus minor is made up of extra pelvic iliopsoas fibers. The nineteenth–century French anatomist Jean Cruveilhier termed this small muscle the ilio-capsulo-trochanteric. In contrast to the inconsistent psoas minor, the iliacus minor is little known but constant.

5.7.1 Review

Origin

- Iliacus minor attaches to:
  - the cranial two-thirds of the internal iliac fossa;
  - the inner lip of the iliac crest;
  - the iliolumbar ligament;
  - the quadratus lumborum (a few fibers);
  - the base of the sacrum;
  - both anterior iliac spines and the notch between them;
  - the anterior medial surface of the hip capsule, which it partially overlays.

Course

Iliacus minor reaches a groove on the anterior rim of the acetabulum between the anterior inferior iliac spine and the iliopectineal eminence.

Termination

A strong tendon attaches iliacus minor to the posterior surface of the lesser trochanter. Lateral and caudal iliacus fibers join the psoas tendon to insert directly onto the femur. Iliacus minor fibers follow along the caudal border of the tendon to insert onto the femur as far as the lesser trochanter, a little distal to the psoas tendon.

Serous bursa of iliopsoas

Iliopsoas is cushioned from the front of the hip joint capsule by a serous bursa that sometimes communicates with the synovial membrane. This explains the sharp hip joint pains that can accompany iliopsoas tendinitis.

As a rule, the sturdy coxofemoral capsule cannot be perforated by the synovium. Remember: Except at its cranial part, the capsule is 8–12 ml thick, which is considerable for a joint capsule. Caudally, however, it measures no more than 2–3 ml. Its anterior portion, between the pubofemoral ligament and the caudal fascicle of the iliofemoral ligament, is invariably thin. This is the site of the iliopsoas serous bursa, where a genuine opening can occur between the bursa and the synovial membrane.

5.7.2 Technique

Palpation in lateral decubitus (Fig. 5.24)

The patient lies on the side opposite the hip to be treated, his top foot on the table, hip abducted. You position yourself behind the patient in line with his hips. Glide the fingers of one hand along the adductor muscles as far as the pectineus, in the space bound by the ischial tuberosity, the superior pubic ramus, and the lesser trochanter. Maneuver progressively until you reach the posterior caudal surface of the lesser trochanter.

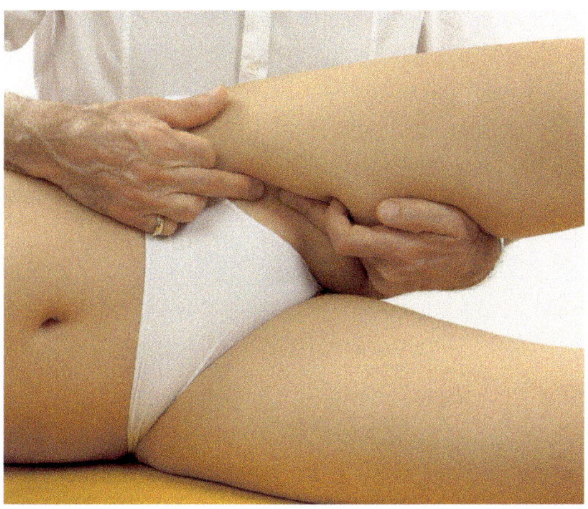

Fig. 5.24 Iliacus minor in decubitus.

Place your free hand between the patient's sacrum and your thorax to counterbalance your hand against the lesser trochanter. Search the iliacus minor where it crosses the lesser trochanter for small irregularities and painful microzones. This technique is performed with induction, incorporating sacral and pelvic movements that allow you deeper access to musculoligamentous fibers.

5.8 OBTURATOR EXTERNUS (FIG. 5.25)

This deep muscle often exchanges fibers with the coxofemoral joint capsule.

5.8.1 Review

Origin

The obturator externus arises at the acetabulum on the:

- lateral perimeter of the obturator foramen;
- obturator membrane;
- inferior pubic ramus.

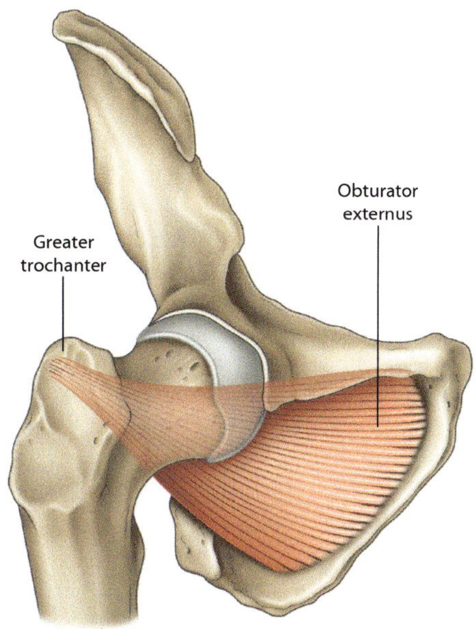

Fig. 5.25 Obturator externus.

Course

- Transversal and slightly cranial

Termination

- On the femur, at the medial aspect of the trochanteric fossa, the fibers have an occasional expansion that reaches the capsule where it winds around the femoral neck.

Innervation

- Obturator nerve (L1–L4)

Vascularization

- Inferior gluteal artery

Important relationships

The obturator internus is a deep muscle visible only when all the neighboring muscles have been separated away. Its proximal insertion is covered by the adductor muscles, while its trajectory is masked by quadratus femoris.

Actions

The obturator externus is static:

- It helps stabilize the hip.
- It supports the pelvis where it crosses the infra-acetabular groove to form an important element of Dolto's hammock together with gemelli.
- It decompresses the coxofemoral joint and preserves the cartilage through the coordinated action of both obturator externus muscles.

The obturator externus is dynamic:

- It acts as a lateral hip rotator and a weak adductor, and it contributes to pelvic anteversion.

5.8.2 Technique

In decubitus (Fig. 5.26)

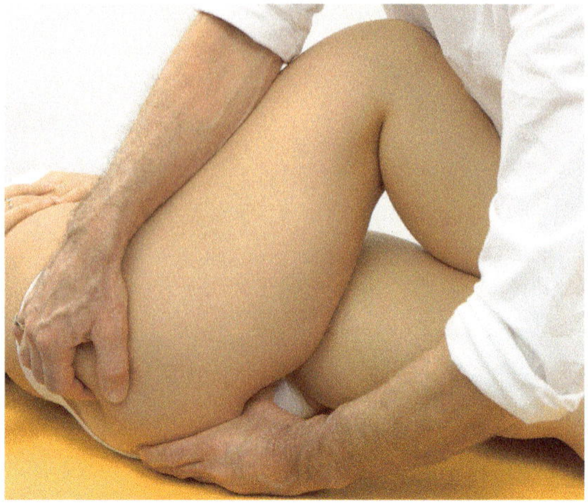

Fig. 5.26 Obturator externus in decubitus.

The patient lies on the table, lower extremity flexed. You situate yourself on the side opposite the hip to be treated. Place the fingers of one hand on the cranial aspect of the trochanteric fossa. Place your other hand on the lateral part of the obturator foramen, just in front of the ischial tuberosity. Ask flexible patients to place their foot across the straight leg in line with the knee.

Progressively draw the thigh medially in adduction using your torso. Amplify the movement by drawing the greater trochanter and the femur toward you. The idea is to relax the soft tissue of the obturator foramen in order to increase the patient's extensibility. When femoral adduction is relaxed, the tissues decompress. When you increase adduction, the tissues tighten.

This is a global technique that involves the other hip rotators. To target obturator externus, focus on the obturator foramen.

5.9 OBTURATOR INTERNUS-GEMELLI COMPLEX (FIG. 5.27)

Judging from their common function and muscle provenance, obturator internus and gemelli can, and have been considered, as a single functional unit called the hip triceps or pelvic triceps. The superior gemellus is distinguished by its attachment on the ischial spine, a key point in our urogenital manipulations.

By way of the obturator internus muscle

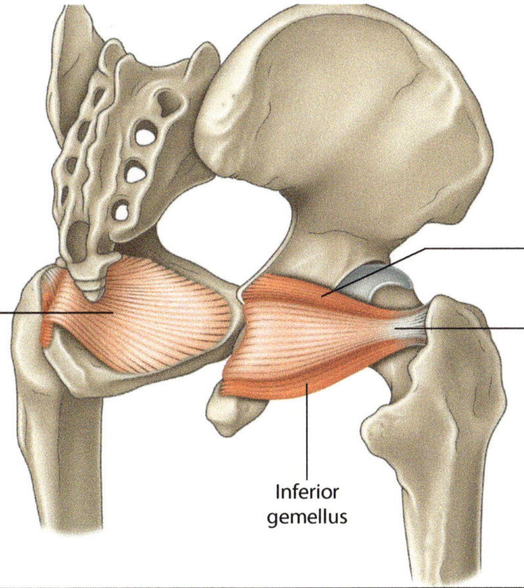

Fig. 5.27 Obturator internus and gemelli.

we can have an effect on the obturator membrane and, through it, the obturator foramen. This muscle is of particular interest in the treatment of the pudendal nerve. Alcock's canal is formed by the obturator internus aponeurosis, which can entrap the pudendal artery and nerve if it becomes thickened.

5.9.1 Review—obturator internus

Origin

- The coxal bone, which arises medially from the perimeter of the obturator foramen and the obturator membrane

Direction

- Essentially transversal

Course

- Exits the pelvic cavity through the lesser sciatic foramen, where it curves around the posterior ischium and courses laterally to reach the greater trochanter

Termination

- The medial surface of the greater trochanter

Remarks

A serous bursa is located over the lesser sciatic foramen to allow muscle glide. Here the musculotendinous junction presents a number of intermediary tendons that lend a grooved appearance to the muscle. This serous bursa facilitates glide where the muscle curves and rides over the medial ischial body.

Innervation

- Inferior gluteal nerve

Vascular supply

- Inferior gluteal artery

Important relationships

- Transverse acetabular ligament
- Coxofemoral capsule
- Sacrotuberous ligament
- Pudendal nerve and artery

5.9.2 Review—gemelli

The gemelli form the hip tricep together with the obturator internus.

Origin

- Superior gemellus: ischial spine
- Inferior gemellus: ischial tuberosity

The ischial spine is an indispensable landmark for many urogenital manipulations. It is located about three fingers above and slightly medial to the ischial tuberosity.

There are other main attachments of this thorny projection:

- on the pointed extremity—the sacrospinous ligament;
- on its internal surface—from posterior to anterior ischiococcygeus and levator ani.

The pudendal nerve curves around the ischial spine.

Termination

- Attaches to the trochanteric fossa merged with the tendinous insertion of obturator internus

Actions

- Acts as powerful lateral hip rotators
- Steadies the femoral heads in the acetabulum

5.9.3 Techniques

In decubitus (Fig. 5.28)

The patient lies on the table, lower limb flexed. The technique resembles piriformis muscle stretches because of their similar trochanteric insertions.

To contact the obturator foramen, place your fingers inside the inferior pubic ramus.

Starting from the medial surface of the ischial tuberosity, direct your fingers forward and medially to serve as a fixed point. Position the fingers of your other hand on the medial surface of the greater trochanter in the trochanteric fossa. Ask the patient to extend his leg, gliding his foot along the outstretched leg. The trochanteric hand amplifies the movement to create a more intense stretch.

For the inferior gemellus, change your pelvic contact by fixing the ischial tuberosity; proceed with the femur in the same manner. For the superior gemellus, place your fingers on either side of the ischial spine and accomplish the same movement. Be sure to place your fingers on either side of the ischial spine so that you do not cause pain. The pudendal nerve curves around the ischial spine and must not be compressed.

5.10 QUADRATUS FEMORIS (FIG. 5.29)

This muscle is worth manipulating for two main reasons:

- It exerts considerable influence over coxofemoral intra-articular pressures, especially at the inferior pole of the femoral head.

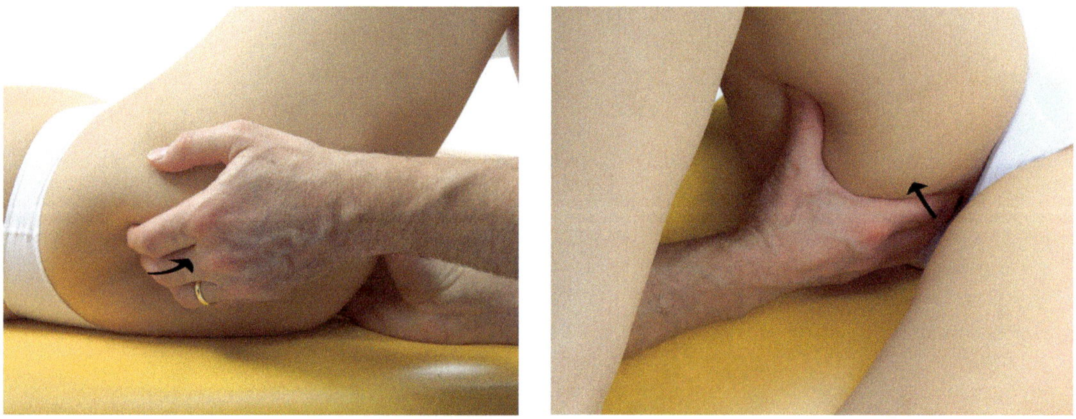

Fig. 5.28 Obturator internus and gemelli in decubitus.

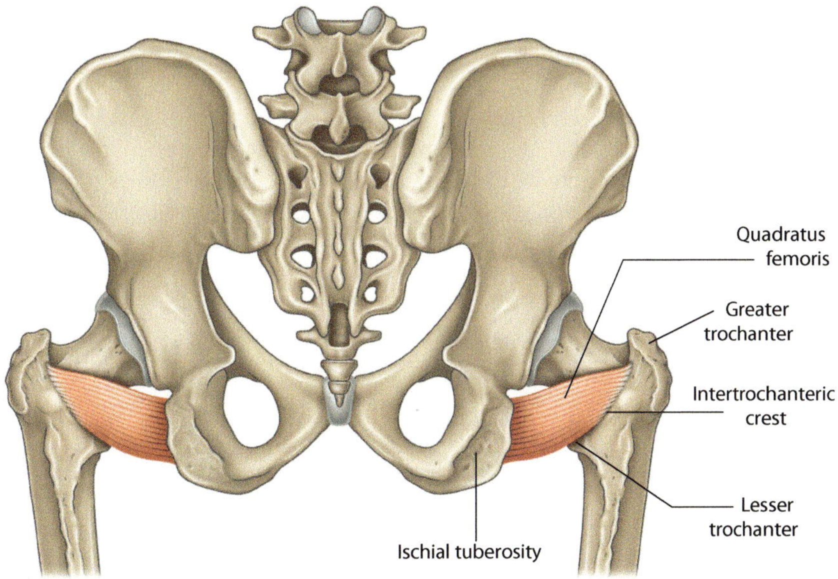

Fig. 5.29 Quadratus femoris.

- It serves as a floor for the sciatic nerve at the bottom of the ischiotrochanteric groove.

5.10.1 Review

Origin

- The ischium, which arises on the lower lateral surface, along the ischial tuberosity, and attaches laterally in relationship to semitendinosus and semimembranosus

Direction

- Runs horizontally and inserts along a vertical line at the base of the neck of the femur

Termination

- Posterior surface of the greater trochanter, on the intertrochanteric crest

Innervation

- Inferior gluteal nerve, arising from the sacral plexus (L5–S2)

Vascular supply

- Inferior gluteal artery and first perforating artery of the thigh

Actions

- Adductor and lateral rotator of the thigh
- A strong lateral rotator together with gluteus maximus and the obturator internus-gemelli complex

Characteristics

- It runs on the same horizontal plane as the adductor magnus, whose principal insertion is more medial. It can either mask or be confused with this muscle.
- Quadratus femoris is the pillow of the sciatic nerve that borders it. It protects the nerve from injury during prolonged sitting.
- It is very often tight. Most of us can benefit from having it stretched.

5.10.2 Techniques

In decubitus (Fig. 5.30)

The patient lies supine with his leg flexed.

You place one hand on the posterior part of the greater trochanter and the other hand on the lateral aspect of the ischial tuberosity. Gently spread the bones apart while the patient glides his foot distally. Separate your hands to keep maximum tension on the quadratus femoris throughout the entire maneuver. The technique is more effective performed in supine than in side lying.

The technique can cause muscle sensitivity or even pain during the stretch. Progress slowly using induction to avoid causing harm.

In lateral decubitus (Fig. 5.31)

The patient lies on the side opposite the treatment, with the knee against your abdomen. You place your thumb on the lateral part of the ischium; place the fingers of your other hand against the posterior surface of the greater trochanter.

Ask the patient to push his leg against your abdomen. Amplify the movement by fixing the ischium and drawing the greater trochanter toward you in flexion. Repeat 12 or so times.

5.11 PIRIFORMIS (FIG. 5.32)

This muscle assumes great importance for the hip, not just because of its mechanical role but also due to its intimate relations with the lumbosacral plexus and the urogenital system.

Piriformis manipulation is essential in treating a number of conditions:

- lumbosacral pain;
- sciatica and pudendal neuralgia;
- coxofemoral joint problems;
- static and dynamic pelvic organ dysfunctions;
- intrapelvic circulatory disorders.

5.11.1 Review

Pelvic origin

- Ventral sacrum between S2–S3–S4
- Lateral of the anterior sacral foramen
- Superior margin of the greater sciatic notch of the ilium

Direction

- Lateral and somewhat caudal as it passes through the greater sciatic notch

Termination

- Medial surface of the superior facet of the trochanter

Innervation

- Sacral plexus (L5–S2)

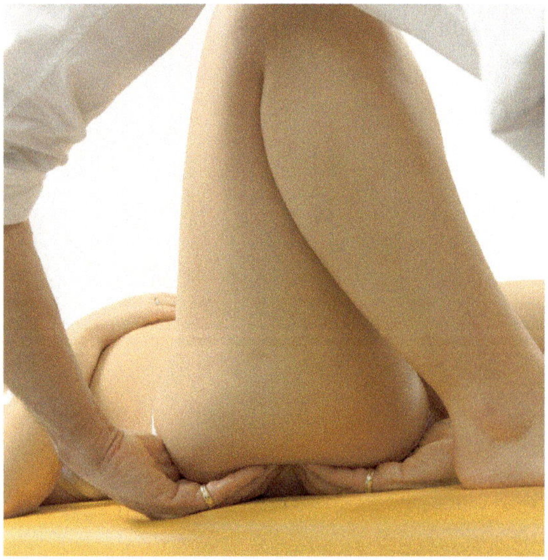

Fig. 5.30 Quadratus femoris in decubitus.

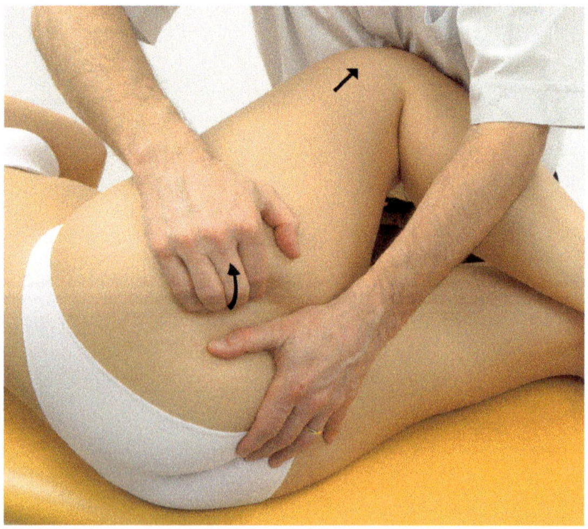

Fig. 5.31 Quadratus femoris in lateral decubitus.

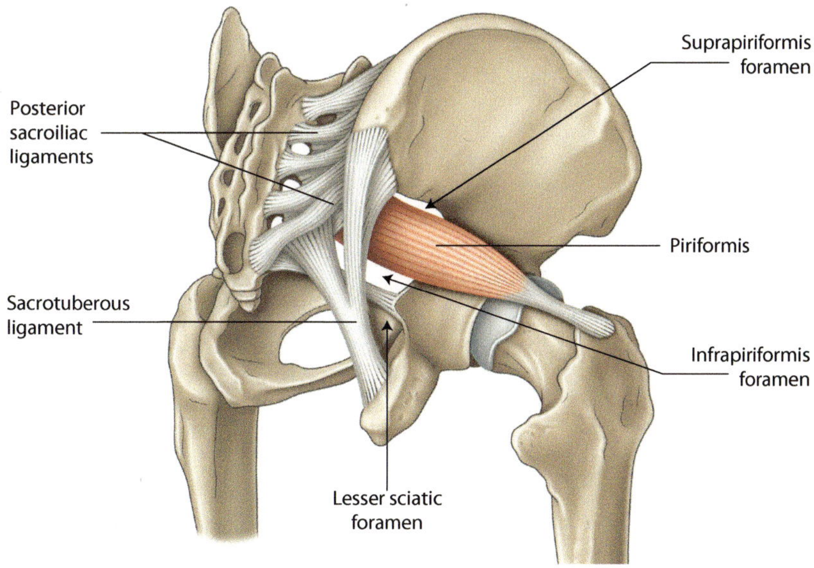

Fig. 5.32 Piriformis.

Vascular supply

- Superior and inferior gluteal arteries

Actions

- Lateral hip rotation
- Hip abduction
- Sacrum retroversion
- Foot orientation to optimize footing
- Femoropelvic joint stabilization

Useful relationships

- Piriformis covered by gluteus maximus
- Muscle runs above ischial spine
- Muscle fills the greater sciatic notch or greater sciatic foramen

Special note

- It is important to recognize the protective role piriformis plays for the sciatic nerve.
- The sciatic nerve appears at its caudal border. One could say that piriformis is the "roof" of the sciatic nerve, while quadratus femoris is its "pillow."
- A tight or fibrosed piriformis can create mechanical irritation for the sciatic, inferior gluteal, posterior femoral cutaneous, and pudendal nerves.

5.11.2 Techniques

In decubitus—first method (Fig. 5.33)

The lower limb is flexed in abduction in order to stabilize the sacrum. Place two fingers in the cranial part of the trochanteric fossa. Ask the patient to glide his foot down the opposite leg. Direct the path of the lower limb by placing your hand on the knee.

At the start of the glide, the leg naturally moves into abduction-lateral rotation. Encourage this movement with your trochanteric finger contact. As the foot slides further down the leg, the coxofemoral joint naturally moves into extension, adduction, and medial rotation. The hand on the knee does nothing more than guide the movement to ensure that the foot glides along the opposite leg while staying in contact with the table. For heavyset patients, support your fingers in the trochanteric fossa with the fingers of your other hand.

Before beginning, warn the patient that the maneuver can be uncomfortable. Proceed progressively to avoid pain.

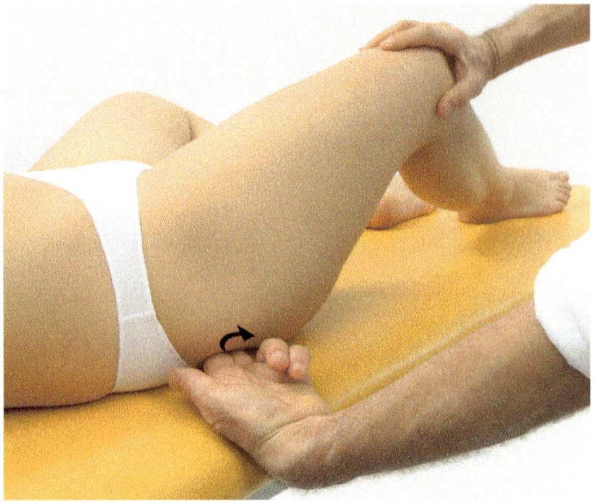

Fig. 5.33 Piriformis in decubitus (first method).

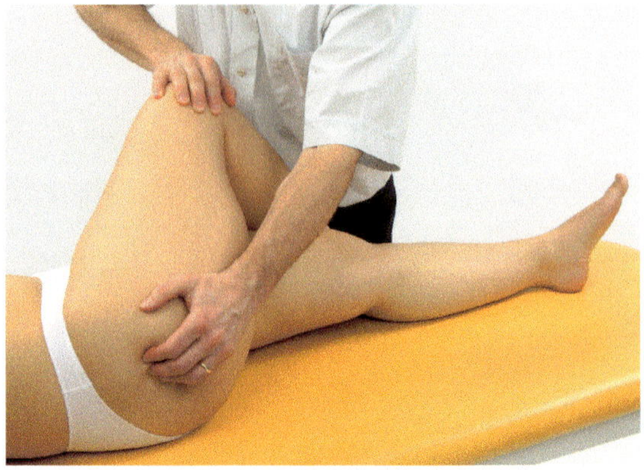

Fig. 5.34 Piriformis in decubitus (second method).

In decubitus—second method (Fig. 5.34)

You can ask very flexible patients to begin with their flexed leg positioned over the straight leg. Standing across from the hip in question, firmly grasp the trochanteric fossa and draw the piriformis laterally. Augment this adduction of the hip by placing your hand on the patient's knee to pull the caudal part of the femur toward you, alternating between tension and relaxation. This very effective maneuver is best performed after the first method.

In lateral decubitus (Fig. 5.35)

The patient lies on the side opposite the hip being treated, the knee resting against your belly. The underlying leg is slightly flexed. Standing in front of the patient, place two or three fingers as cranially as possible in the trochanteric fossa. Ask the patient to push his knee against your belly. Accompany and amplify the movement with your fingers, drawing the trochanter toward you.

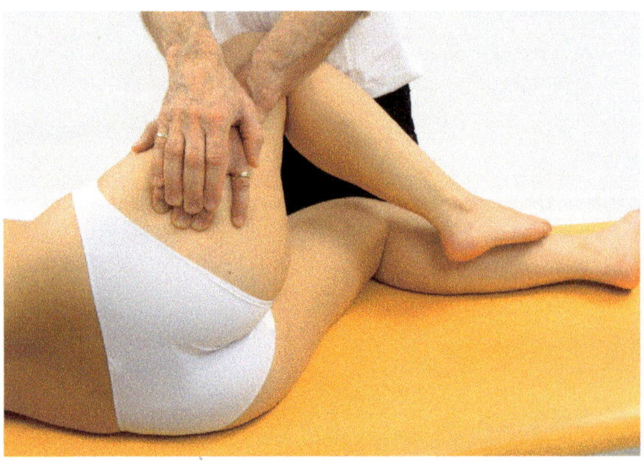

Fig. 5.35 Piriformis in lateral decubitus.

When the greater trochanter is pulled as far as possible toward you, complete the stretch by adding some hip flexion. Let off the stretch, maintaining the coxofemoral joint in adduction, to affect the sacrum and the sacroiliac junction. Finally, keeping adduction, push the knee back toward the hip as you return to the initial position.

Precaution: Position the patient so that the opposite hip rests firmly on the table to stabilize the sacrum. Even when it causes slight discomfort, this technique is well received by patients as they feel the piriformis gradually stretch. It also gives them awareness of just how stiff the piriformis had become.

Stretching specific sacral attachments (Fig. 5.36)

A variation on the above technique involves altering the degree of flexion according to sacral insertions. More hip flexion focuses on the lower sacrum and stretches the caudal fibers of the piriformis. Less flexion puts the cranial fibers under more stretch.

As we have highlighted, releasing the piriformis muscle is a priority in cases of intrapelvic organ dysfunction, especially:

- urinary stress incontinence;
- premenstrual syndrome;

- pudendal neuralgia;
- intrapelvic circulatory problems.

Piriformis stretches are also indicated for sciatica, pubic pain, and mechanical problems of the lower extremity.

5.12 PECTINEUS (FIG. 5.37)

While the pectineus is not the most worthwhile of muscles to manipulate, sensory nerves located on its anterior surface have a remarkable reflexogenic effect on the genital region. Pectineus is the most cranially situated of the adductor muscles.

5.12.1 Review

Origin

- The coxal bone at the superior pubic ramus and the pectin pubis (pectineal line) between the Iliopectineal eminence and the pubic tubercle

Direction

- Caudal and lateral

Termination

- Posterior surface of the femur behind the lesser trochanter along the cranial pectineal line of the linea aspera

Innervation

- Femoral nerve (L2–L3)
- Obturator nerve, anterior branch (L2–L4)

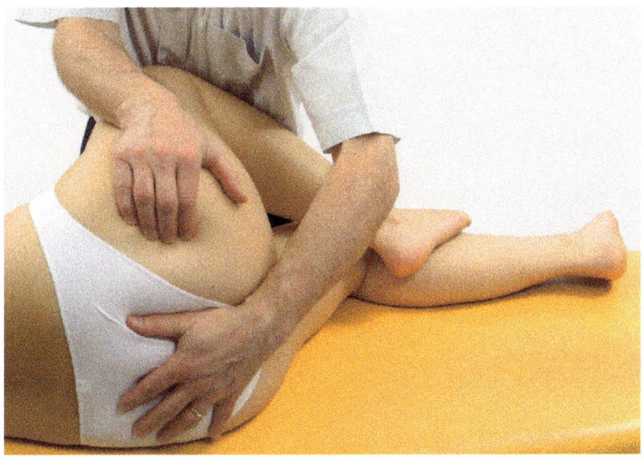

Fig. 5.36 Piriformis: stretching the sacral attachments.

Vascular supply

- Femoral artery

Important relationships

- Medially, adductor longus and gracilis
- Laterally, psoas

Special note

The skin over the pectineus is innervated by the ilioinguinal and iliohypogastric nerves. Manipulation of the muscle has an effect on the femoral nerve as well as an effect through the skin on the two aforementioned nerves. The pectineus is found medially of the sartorius and laterally of the adductor brevis.

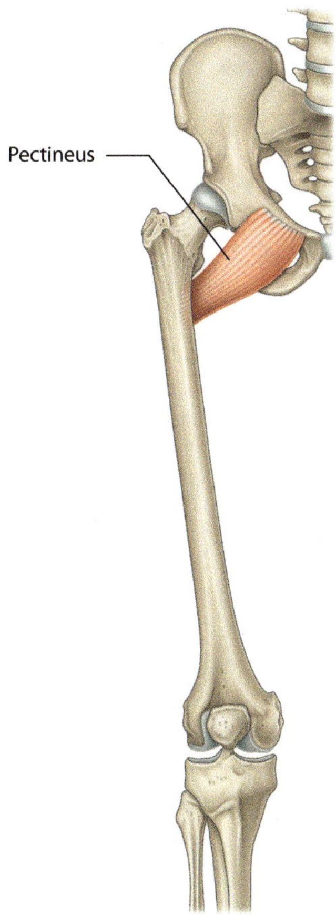

Fig. 5.37 Pectineus.

Actions

- Statically:
  - It is a medial hip stabilizer.
- Dynamically:
  - It is primarily a hip flexor.
  - It adducts, helps medially rotate the thigh.

5.12.2 Techniques

In decubitus (Fig. 5.38)

The patient lies on the table, leg slightly flexed. You place one thumb on the superior pubic ramus, lateral of the pubic tubercle. The palm of your other hand lies flat on the adductor muscle mass, with the thumb pointing toward the lesser trochanter.

Ask the patient to flex and adduct the leg while you spread the fibers of the pectineus between your two hands. Search for microadhesions or fibrosed areas on the pubic attachments.

Complete the treatment by lightening your touch to focus superficially on the skin overlaying the muscle. The ilioinguinal and iliohypogastric nerves are released by rolling the overlaying skin.

While this maneuver is often very sensitive at the outset, pain tends to fade and disappear after just a few manipulations. It is worthwhile to check this zone in an athlete suffering from athletic chronic groin pain (pubalgia). It is also an effective treatment for pudendal neuralgia, even though we are not acting directly on the sensitive pudendal nerve fibers.

Variation (Fig. 5.39)

The pectineus can also be manipulated at its distal insertion. Maintain the same anterior palm contact on the proximal insertion at the pubis. Place the thumb of your other hand behind the thigh on the cephalad part of the linea aspera, near the base of the lesser trochanter. Stretch the pectineus with induction to release the fibers near their distal insertion.

5.13 ADDUCTORS LONGUS AND BREVIS

We prefer to group these muscles together, as they operate in close coordination and their manipulation differs little. They often exchange muscle fibers and can even be considered to constitute one muscle.

5.13.1 Review—adductor longus (Fig. 5.40)

Origin

- Coxal bone at the body of pubis, just lateral of symphysis, inferior and medial to pubic tubercle

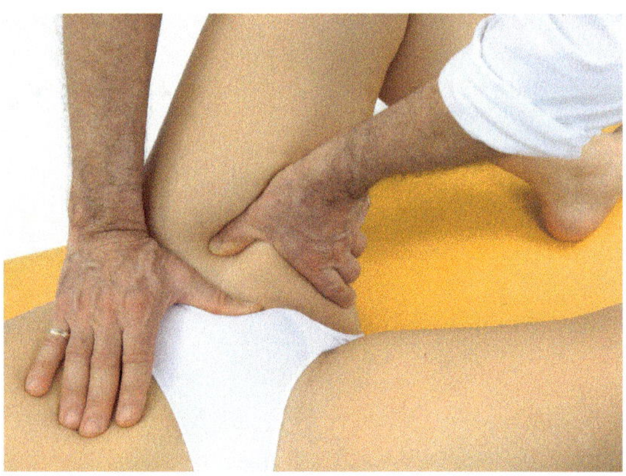

Fig. 5.38 Pectineus in decubitus.

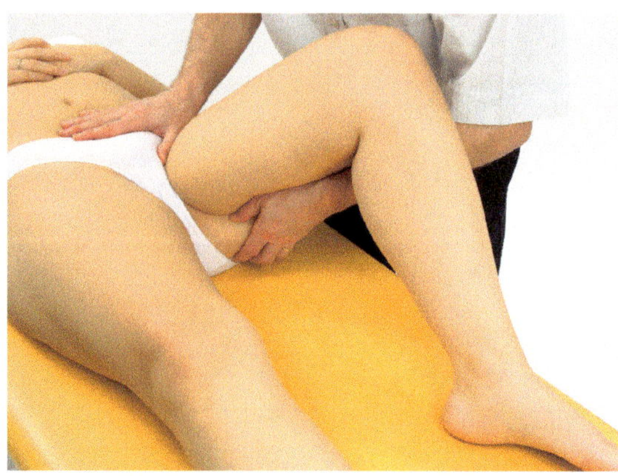

Fig. 5.39 Pectineus by the linea aspera.

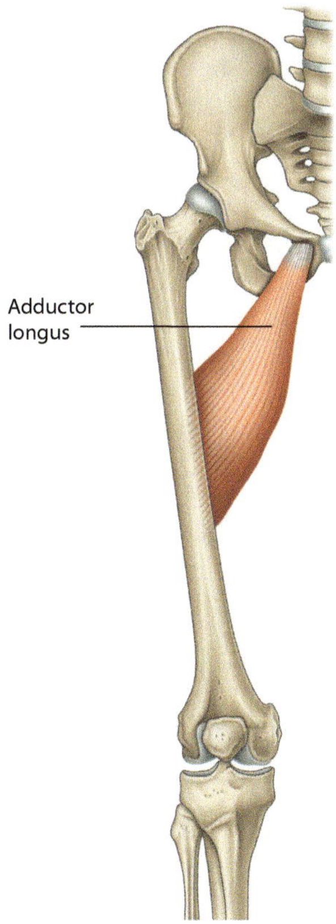

Fig. 5.40 Adductor longus.

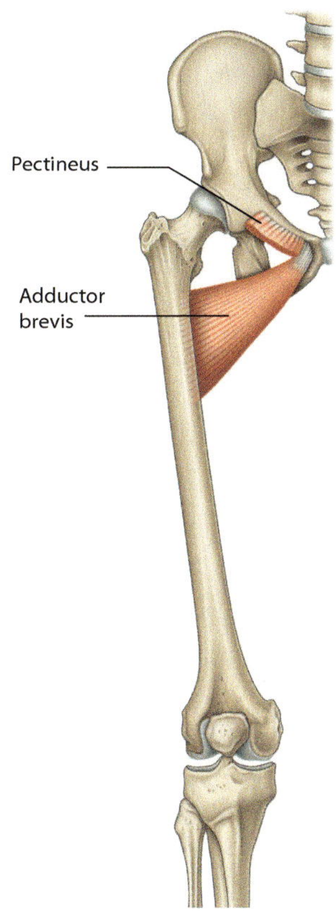

Fig. 5.41 Adductor brevis.

Direction

- Caudal and slightly lateral

Termination

- Middle third of the linea aspera of the femur along the medial lip

Innervation

- Obturator nerve

Vascular supply

- Deep femoral artery, muscle branch

Actions

- Statically:
  - It stabilizes the symphysis pubis.
- Dynamically:
  - It adducts the leg, providing some medial rotation.

Special note

- The adductor longus is the most superficial of the adductor muscle group.
- It runs ventrally to the adductor magnus.
- Some fibers reach the adductor canal to reinforce the adductor magnus. The saphenous nerve passes through this canal.
- It forms the femoral triangle together with the sartorius and the inguinal ligament.

5.13.2 Review—adductor brevis (Fig. 5.41)

Origin

- Coxal bone at the inferior pubic ramus and lateral surface of pubic body

Direction

- Caudal and slightly lateral

Termination

- On the femur at the upper third of the linea aspera at the medial lip

Characteristics

- Situated dorsally to adductor longus, to which it is closely related

Innervation

- Obturator nerve, anterior branch (L2–L4)

Vascular supply

- Deep femoral artery, muscular branch

Actions

- Adduction with some lateral rotation and slight hip flexion

5.13.3 Technique

In decubitus (Fig. 5.42)

The technique is common to adductors brevis and longus. The patient lies with his leg outstretched in slight medial rotation. You place your thumb where the body of the pubis meets its inferior ramus. Position the fingers of your other hand on the femur, near the linea aspera.

Draw the leg into lateral rotation to stretch the adductor while fixing the pubis. Search the muscle between your thumbs for micro-adhesions near the femoral insertion, and release them in induction. Ask the patient to lengthen his leg while you increase the distance between the pubis and the femur. This technique is very similar to treatment of the adductor magnus.

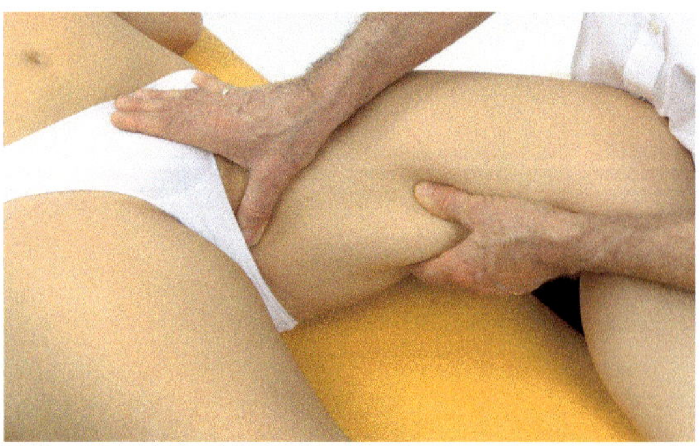

Fig. 5.42 Adductors longus and brevis in decubitus.

5.14 GRACILIS (FIG. 5.43)

This is the only biarticular muscle of the adductor group. It is a main contributor in the formation of the superficial "goose's foot" (pes anserinus) on the tibia, which makes it of interest to us. It is also the most medial of the adductor muscles.

5.14.1 Review

Origin

- Coxal bone on the inferior pubic ramus and lower half of the body of the pubis, very near the symphyses

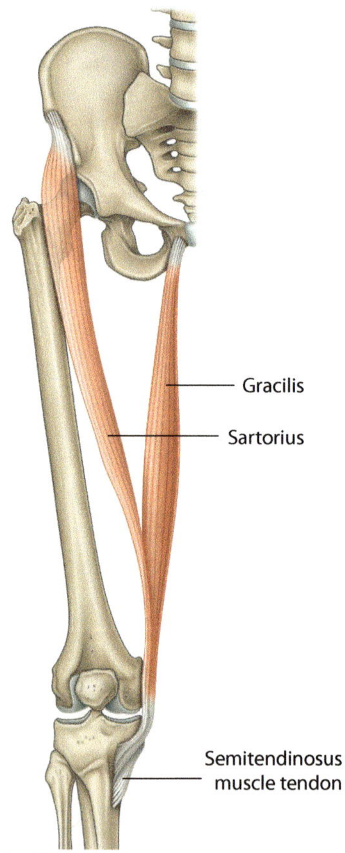

Fig. 5.43 Gracilis.

Direction

- Caudal vertically, a little more medially as it curves around the tibia

Termination

- Medial surface of the tibia, behind the sartorius and cranial to the semitendinosus with which it forms the superficial pes anserinus.

Actions

- Statically:
  - It stabilizes the knee medially (counters valgus deformity).
- Dynamically:
  - It provides hip adduction and flexion when the knee extended.
  - It provides medial rotation and flexion of the knee.

Innervation

- Obturator nerve (L2–L4)

Vascular supply

- Medial circumflex femoral artery and muscular branches of the deep femoral artery

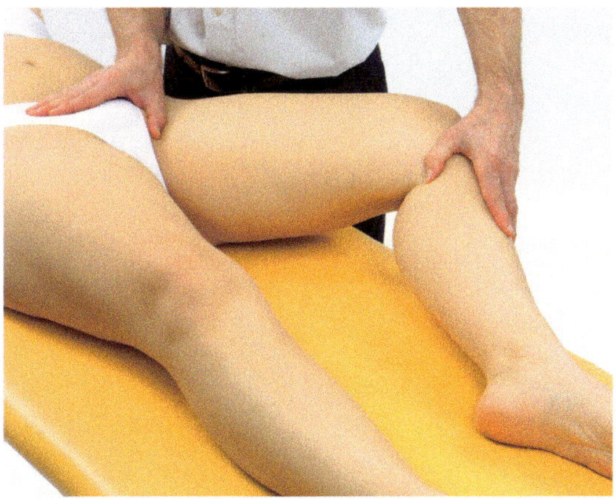

Fig. 5.44 Gracilis in decubitus.

Special note

A serous bursa, called the bursa anserinum, is interposed between the superficial pes anserinus and the muscle tendons that form it. Certain patients, especially athletes, suffer from bursitis of the pes anserinus. This type of tendinopathy is difficult to alleviate and involves a fair length of treatment time. The pelvis, pelvic organs, and the mechanical balance of the entire lower extremity must all be addressed.

5.14.2 Techniques

In decubitus (Fig. 5.44)

The patient lies on the table with his lower limb slightly flexed in abduction and lateral rotation. You place one thumb close to the symphysis pubis on the inferior pubic ramus. Position your other thumb on the cranial part of the pes anserinus, located on the medial tibial epicondyle.

Ask the patient to gradually extend his leg. Your proximal thumb fixes the gracilis, while your distal thumb concentrates on stretching the leg, following the direction shown by induction.

Superficial pes anserinus

The muscles of the pes anserinus are treated by placing one or two fingers beneath the gracilis tendon, just before its boney insertion at the anterior medial proximal tibia. Maintain the tendon in stretch induction to obtain an effect on the sub muscular serous bursa. We return to the superficial pes anserinus in the knee section of this book.

In lateral decubitus (Fig. 5.45)

The patient lies on the side of the limb in question, knee slightly flexed. Glide your thumb along the medial tibia to reach the three tendons as they insert. To release adhesions between tendons, ask the patient to make small flexion-extension movements while you alternately lift and release the tendons.

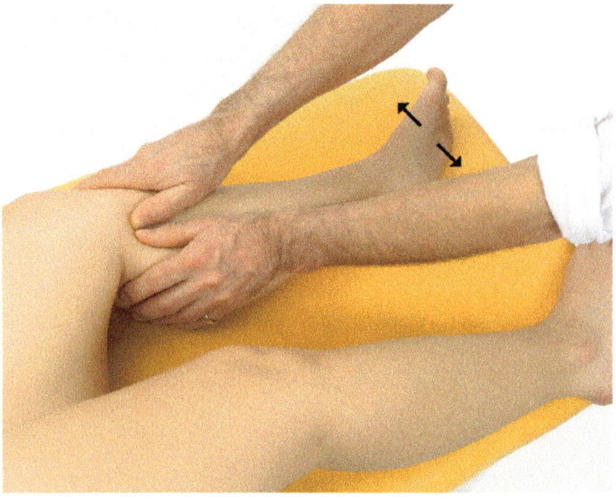

Fig. 5.45 Gracilis in lateral decubitus.

5.15 BICEPS FEMORIS (FIG. 5.46)

The biceps femoris muscle has a biarticular long head and a monoarticular short head. The biarticular part provides a junction between the hip and the knee. Its relationships with the sacrotuberous and collateral fibular ligaments make it of special interest in treating the hip joint.

Hamstrings

There are three hamstring muscles on the posterior thigh: biceps femoris, semitendinosus, and semimembranosus. Their mechanical role is to control the hip when we bend forward. Their main action flexes the knee and inwardly rotates the leg when the knee is bent.

The hamstrings are familiar to people because they tend to stiffen up due to their high concentration of collagen fibers in proportion to their elastin component. This natural deficit of elasticity is what allows us to lean forward without any great stabilizing effort. Modern daily life exempts us from extreme positions such as forward bending, which would call for hamstring retraction.

5.15.1 Review

Origin

- Long head: ischial tuberosity (by a tendon in common with semitendinosus)
- Short head
  - Lateral lip of the linea aspera on the mid-femur
  - Lateral intermuscular septum

Direction

- Caudal and lateral

Termination

- Posterior lateral side of the head of the fibula, lateral to the fibular collateral ligament
- Tibiofibular capsule
- Lateral condyle of the tibia
- Crural fascia

Innervation

- Tibial nerve for the long head (L5–S2)
- Common fibular nerve for the short head (S1–S2)

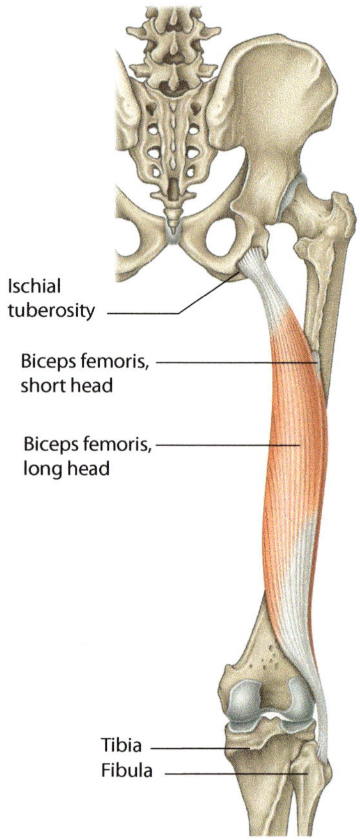

Fig. 5.46 Biceps femoris.

Vascular supply

- Inferior gluteal artery
- Deep femoral artery, first perforating branches

Noteworthy relationships

- The sacrotuberous ligament, which exchanges fibers with the long head at the ischial tuberosity
- The iliotibial tract, with which it stabilizes the lateral leg
- The sciatic nerve, which crosses the biceps femoris laterally as it descends
- The biceps, which form the lateral cranial part of the popliteal fossa
- The biceps femoris, which wraps around the fibular collateral ligament at the fibular insertion that is separated by a serous bursa

Actions

- Statically:
  - It stabilizes the hip in trunk flexion.
  - It provides posterior lateral stability to the tibia.
  - It strengthens the tibiofibular capsule.
  - It tenses the crural fascia.
- Dynamically:
  - It extends the thigh.
  - It flexes the knee and laterally rotates the leg.

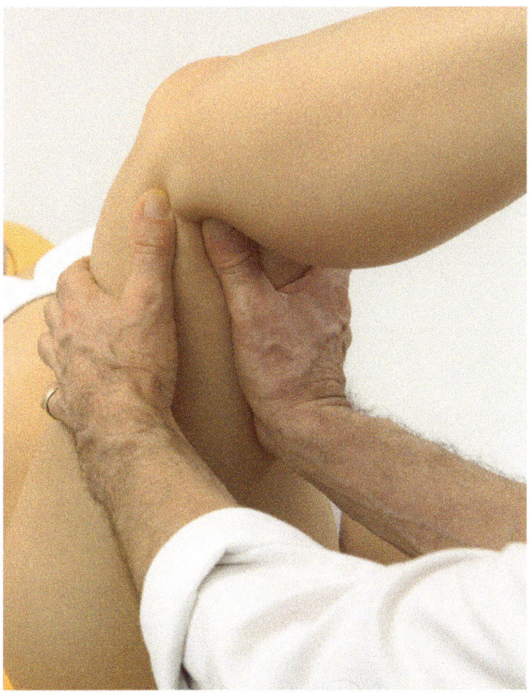

Fig. 5.47 Biceps femoris in decubitus.

Special note

From both a mechanical and visceral perspective, the biceps femoris connects the pelvis and the leg. All abdominal pelvic tension can eventually have repercussions for the head of the fibula through the sacrotuberous ligament as intermediary. A good number of femoral head fixations are a long way from being simply mechanical. Their high level of recurrence, with no obvious link to mechanical stress, advocates in favor of a visceral connection. Very often this visceral connection is the intestines.

5.15.2 Techniques

The following maneuvers focus on the fibular attachment.

In decubitus (Fig. 5.47)

The patient lies on the table with his foot resting on your shoulder. Place your thumbs on either side of the biceps tendon, slightly above the fibular attachment. Mobilize the tendon medially and laterally. While you lengthen the leg in extension, continue to gently mobilize the tendon medially and laterally.

Reposition your fingers after several rounds. First, mobilize the junction between the long and short heads of the biceps. Next, move more cranially to mobilize the connection between the semitendinosus and the long head of biceps.

In lateral decubitus (Fig. 5.48)

The patient lies on the side opposite the knee concerned, leg slightly flexed. You place one thumb proximally at the junction of the biceps and semitendinosus muscle bodies; place the other thumb on the head of the fibula. Gently spread the fibular tendinous insertion laterally, working your two thumbs in induction. Finally, ask the patient to make very small flexion-extension movements at the knee to better feel and free up areas of fixation.

Special note

Manipulation of the insertions on the ischial ramus yields unconvincing results.

5.16 SEMITENDINOSUS (FIG. 5.49)

Semitendinosus is an important muscle for medial knee stability in contrast to biceps femoris, which provides lateral stability.

5.16.1 Review

Origin

- Ischial tuberosity by common tendon with biceps femoris

Direction

- Caudal, medially curving distally

Termination

- Medial condyle of the tibia
- Lies behind sartorius and below gracilis; unites with the sartorius and gracilis to form the pes anserinus
- Crural fascia tensor

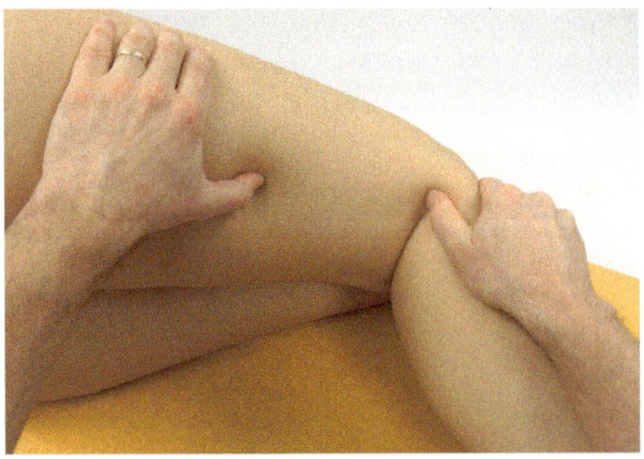

Fig. 5.48 Biceps femoris in lateral decubitus.

Innervation

- Tibial nerve (L5–S2)

Vascular supply

- Deep femoral artery, first perforating branch
- Superior gluteal artery, supplies cranial part of muscle

Actions

- Statically:
  - It counters forward bending at the hips.
  - It stabilizes posterior medial knee together with semimembranosus.
  - It tenses crural fascia.
- Dynamically:
  - It flexes and medially rotates the knee.
  - It weakly, mediallly rotates the hip.

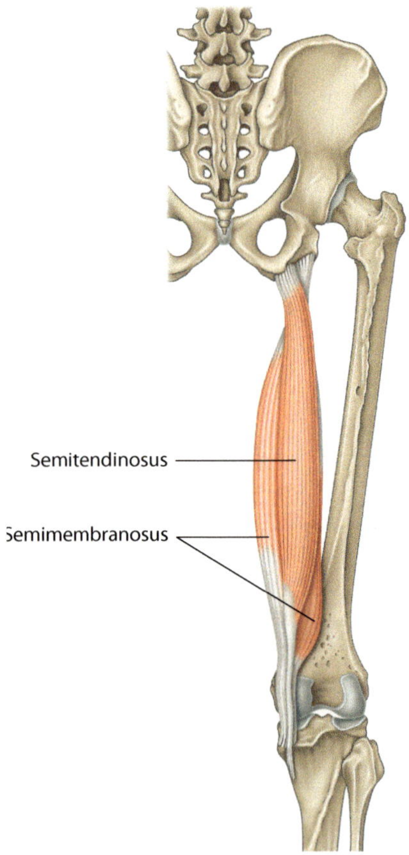

Fig. 5.49 Semitendinosus.

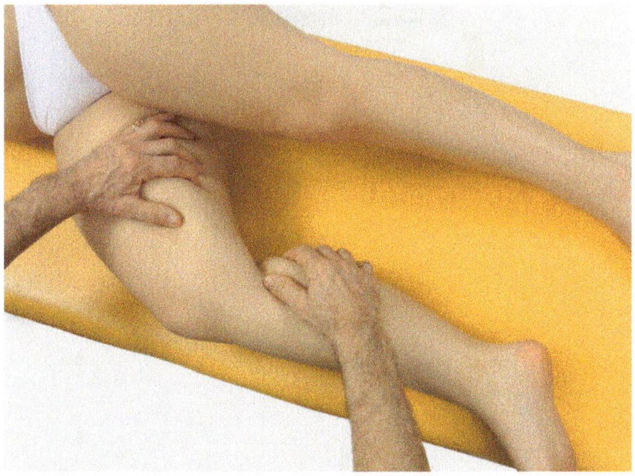

Fig. 5.50 Semitendinosus in lateral decubitus.

Special note

As described earlier, the large bursa between the tendons of the pes anserinus (bursa anserina) and the medial tibial condyle can become irritated. Incapacitating bursitis can combine with tendinitis of the pes anserinus and be difficult to resolve. When this occurs in athletes, it is often secondary to a foot or lumbosacral problem.

5.16.2 Techniques

In lateral decubitus (Fig. 5.50)

The patient lies on the side of the leg to be treated, knee slightly flexed. You place one thumb on the posterior part of the superficial pes anserinus. Position two or three fingers of your other hand on the lateral aspect of the musculotendinous junction formed at mid-thigh by the semitendinosus, gracilis, and sartorius.

The thumb works the tibial insertion while your finger simultaneously lifts and stretches the musculotendinous junctions as it follows the listening. The goal is to reduce fibrosis at the tenoperiosteal junction and at the bursa anserinus.

In decubitus (Fig. 5.51)

The patient lies on his back, hip and knee flexed, his foot resting on your shoulder. This technique can be applied equally to semimembranosus. Mobility test the ischial and musculotendinous attachments of the semitendinosus.

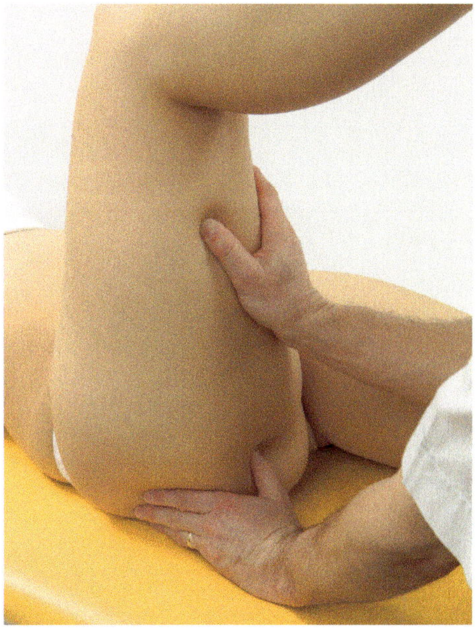

Fig. 5.51 Semitendinosus in decubitus.

Next, look to mobilize the semitendinosus medially and laterally in relation to the semimembranosus. Over time and with accumulated strains due to trauma, these muscles have a tendency to shorten to a point of creating adhesions between themselves.

5.17 SEMIMEMBRANOSUS (FIG. 5.52)

This muscle is primarily treated at the knee, where it is a capsuloligamentous strengthener. We will study this muscle in greater detail in the knee section. For the moment, we include it from a global perspective as the most medial of the three hamstrings muscles.

5.17.1 Review

Origin

- Ischial tuberosity, medial to semitendinosus

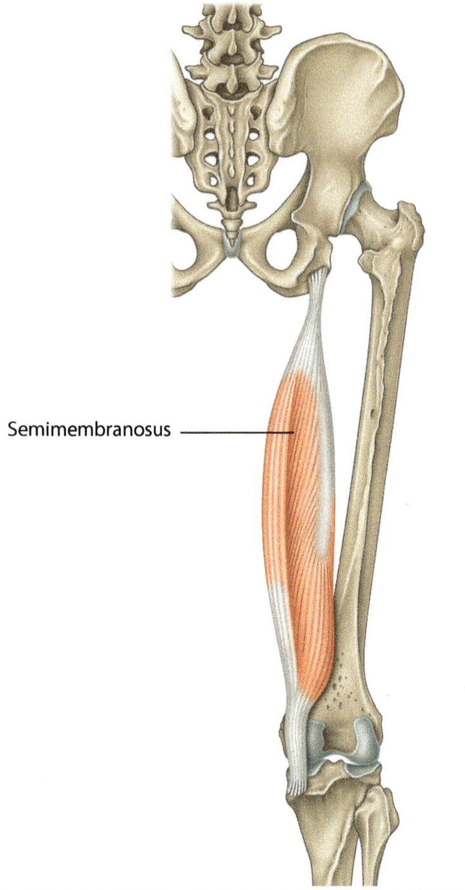

Fig. 5.52 Semimembranosus.

Direction

- Distal, toward the medial surface of the tibial tuberosity

Termination

- Under the tibial collateral ligament
- Distal tendon, comprised of three tendon trains that prolong onto the
  - Medial tibial condyle
  - Fascia of the popliteus muscle posterior lateral part of the capsule, where it forms the oblique popliteal ligament

This tendon arrangement is known as the pes anserinus profundus, whereas the conjoined tendons of semitendinosus, gracilis, and sartorius are termed the pes anserinus superficialis.

Innervation

- Tibial nerve (L5–S2)

Vascular supply

- Branches of the deep femoral artery

Actions

- Statically:
  - It maintains the hip in trunk flexion and provides pelvic retroversion.
  - It stabilizes the posterior medial compartment of the knee.
- Dynamically:
  - It flexes and medially rotates the knee.
  - It helps extend the hip.

Special note

Like the other hamstrings, this muscle has a tendency to become chronically tight and fibrosed. The semimembranosus stabilizes the lumbopelvic hip complex in flexion. It definitely should be included in the treatment of many knee pathologies.

5.17.2 Techniques

In lateral decubitus (Fig. 5.53)

The patient lies on the side to be treated, leg slightly flexed. You stand facing him. With your thumb on the ischial attachment, explore the tendon for painful or fibrosed zones. With your other hand, squeeze the semimembranosus between your thumb and index finger. Follow up the length of the

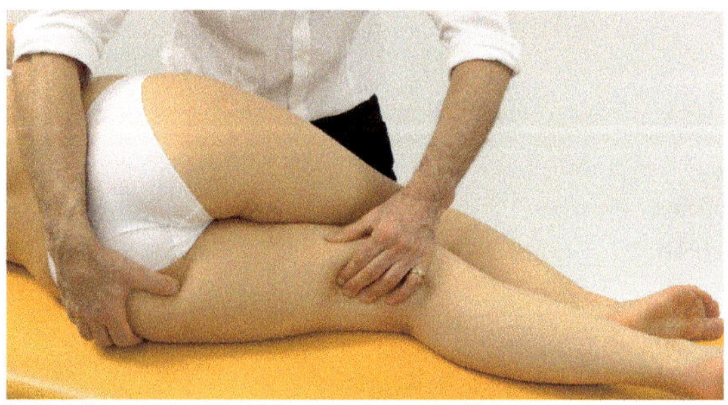

Fig. 5.53 Semimembranosus in lateral decubitus.

semimembranosus, mobilizing the muscle and tendon medially and laterally, searching out areas of retraction or adhesion.

The knee section contains techniques for the distal tendon attachments that should be included in comprehensive treatment.

In decubitus (Fig. 5.54)

The patient lies on his back, hip and knee flexed, foot resting on your shoulder. You use both your thumbs to mobilize the ischial tendon insertion, the muscle body, and the distal musculotendinous junction mediolaterally. The concept is to mobilize the semimembranosus on the semitendinosus, and vice versa.

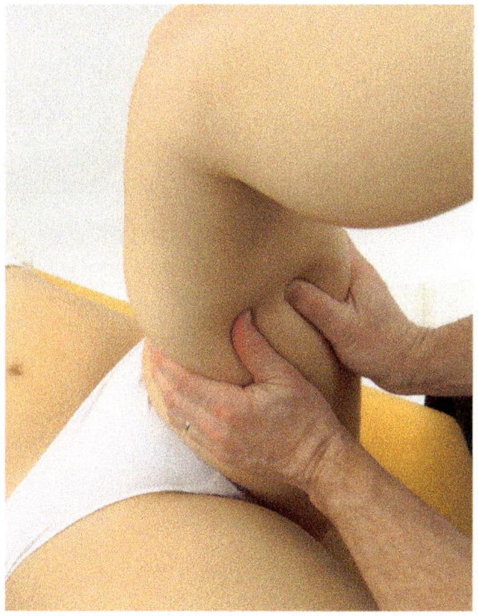

Fig. 5.54 Semimembranosus in decubitus.

Treatment of the passive stabilizers

6

6.1 CAPSULOLIGAMENTOUS TECHNIQUES

The capsule is treated by way of the coxofemoral ligaments as intermediary. These bands surround the hip and form the capsule from which they cannot be dissociated.

All joints benefit from focusing on their ligaments. In practice, effective treatment usually involves several ligaments. We have separated them here in the interest of clarity.

6.1.1 Review—coxofemoral joint capsule

The joint capsule is strong, tough, and strengthened by powerful ligaments. Being that the hip joint is open to the front, the most powerful ligaments are located anteriorly and reinforced by the rectus femoris muscle (Fig. 6.1.)

Origin

- Coxal bone
  - Boney acetabular rim and the supra-acetabular ligament
  - Outer margins of the fibrocartilage labrum
  - Transverse acetabular ligament

Direction

- Caudal and lateral, with variations as a function of capsular insertions

Termination

- Femur encloses the femoral head and most of its neck, attaching anteriorly at the intertrochanteric line, in front of the obturator externus groove. Posteriorly, the lateral half of the femoral neck is extracapsular.
- Psoas minor and iliacus minor contribute fibers to the capsule. Psoas minor is often absent, while iliacus minor is constant for the most part.

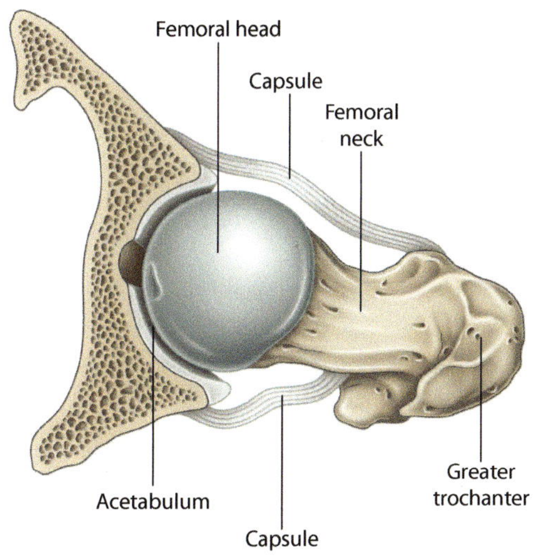

Fig. 6.1 Relationships between the femoral neck and capsular fibers.

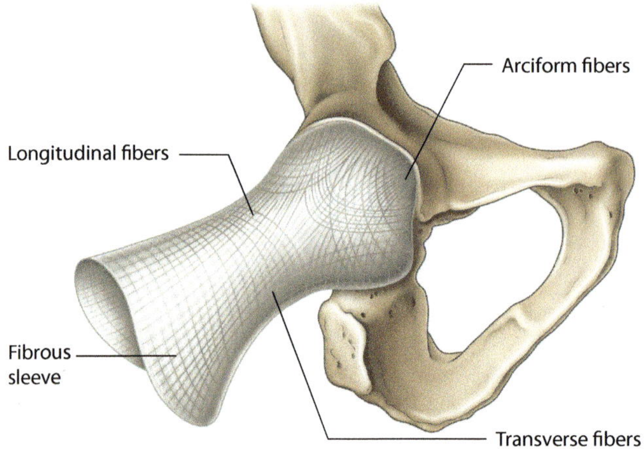

Fig. 6.2 Coxofemoral joint capsule (fibers).

Structure

Capsular fibers (Fig. 6.2) have various orientations. There are four distinct fiber types:

- Longitudinal fibers run from the coxal bone to the femur.
- Circular fibers or orbicular fibers form a collar around the subcapital part of the capsule, securing the head of the femur, much like the knot of a tie.
- Arciform fibers leave the coxal bone, only to turn back to hold the head of the femur firmly in the acetabular socket.
- Inferior folds are called capsular brakes.

Labrum

The labrum or fibrous collar is intimately linked to the capsule. It floats freely in the joint cavity. It is covered in cartilage that is generally thicker at the periphery.

This rubbery cartilage:

- deepens the socket, increasing acetabular surface by as much as 30%, thereby enhancing boney fit;
- acts as a shock absorber interposed between the hardness of the bone and flexibility of the capsule.

Synovial membrane

The synovial membrane lines the inner surface of the capsule. At the center of the acetabulum it forms a cylindrical reflection to unsheathe the ligament of the femoral head.

Innervation

The capsule is supplied by:

- the femoral nerve in front;
- the obturator nerve caudally and medially;
- the sciatic nerve behind and laterally.

Vascularization of the capsule

- Branches of the deep femoral artery, namely:
  - the lateral and medial circumflex arteries;
  - the transverse branch of lateral circumflex femoral artery.

6.2 ILIOFEMORAL LIGAMENT (FIG. 6.3)

6.2.1 Review

- The iliofemoral band is the strongest ligament in the human body, with a tensile strength exceeding 350 kilos.
- Once upon a time, dislocated hips were reset with the help of a horse pulling on the lower limb!
- This ligament is about 10 mm thick.

Origin

- Coxal bone
  - Lower part of the anterior inferior iliac spine (AIIS)

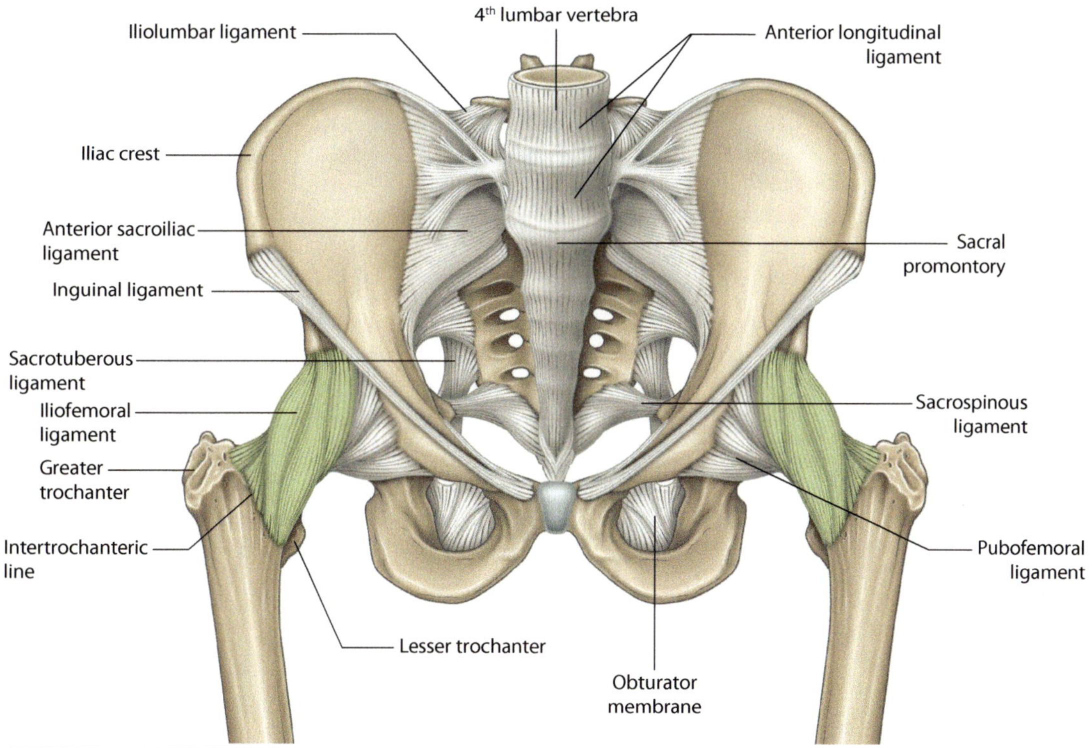

Fig. 6.3 Anterior ligaments: iliofemoral. (After Testut.)

- Beneath the reflected tendon of the rectus femoris muscle
- Rim of the acetabulum

Direction

- Caudal and lateral

Trajectory

This ligament divides into two bands:

- The transverse part above is strong and runs parallel to the axis of the femoral neck.
- The more caudal descending part is weaker and runs parallel to the axis of the femoral shaft.

Termination

- Femur
  - The strongest fibers cover the anterior surface of the cranial end of the femur.
  - More proximal fibers run downward and laterally and attach to the superior tubercle of the intertrochanteric line.
  - The most distal fibers pass downward to fix on the inferior tubercle.

Special note

The iliofemoral ligament receives reinforcements from the gluteus minimus and the reflected tendon of the rectus femoris. Manipulation of these muscles complements treatment of the iliofemoral ligament. Treating these structures together obtains good results for all the anterior ligaments of the hip.

Actions

- This ligament allows us to maintain upright posture without the need for muscle activity. It prevents the trunk from falling backward over the lower extremities.
- It keeps the femoral head pressed into the acetabulum.
- It provides joint vigilance during weight transfer.
- In flexion, the ligament slackens to permit a greater range of motion.

- In extension, the band tenses to resist hyperextension.
- The cranial or transverse part is strong; it controls lateral rotation and femoral abduction.
- Its caudal part or descending part is weaker and limits medial rotation.

6.2.2 Techniques

In lateral decubitus (Fig. 6.4)

This technique blends together with manipulation of the rectus femoris muscle. The patient lies on the side opposite the hip in question. The inferior limb rests on the table, knee slightly flexed and positioned behind the limb lying directly on the table.

Standing behind the patient, you stabilize the sacrum and pelvis between your thorax and hand. Place your free hand on the greater trochanter or the most cranial aspect of the femur, depending on the shape and size of your patient. Ask the patient to gradually extend his hip by gliding his foot posteriorly. The foot must remain on the table.

Accompany the movement using your hand to move the greater trochanter posteriorly, caudally, and somewhat laterally. These combined movements eventually bring the femoral head forward in relation to the iliofemoral part of the capsule. Repeat the movement a dozen times, finishing with induction.

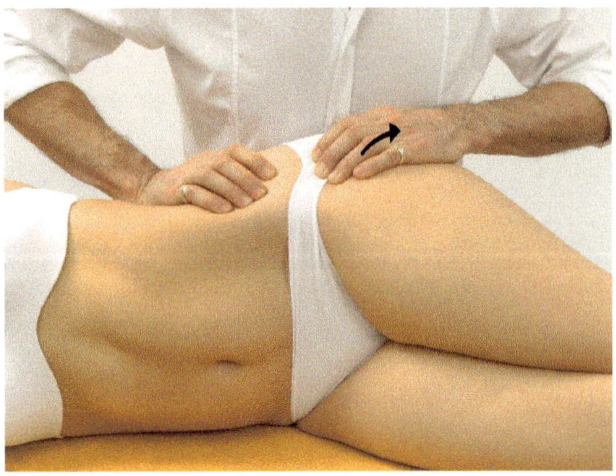

Fig. 6.4 Manipulation of the iliofemoral ligament in lateral decubitus.

In decubitus (Fig. 6.5)

The patient lies on the table, lower extremity slightly flexed in lateral rotation. Have the patient place one hand beneath the greater trochanter to anteriorize the upper femur and the coxofemoral joint.

With one hand you fix the AIIS, either directly or through the rectus femoris. With the other hand you contact the anterior part of the greater trochanter and draw it into lateral rotation while the patient outwardly rotates the thigh. At the end of the movement, ask the patient to stretch out his leg as if wanting it to grow longer.

This technique can also be done by placing your proximal hand underneath the dorsal greater trochanter. Proceed as if wanting to anteriorize the greater trochanter.

6.3 PUBOFEMORAL LIGAMENT AND OBTURATOR FORAMEN

6.3.1 Review—pubofemoral ligament (Fig. 6.6)

This is the weakest of the hip ligaments. It is little more than a simple capsular reinforcement.

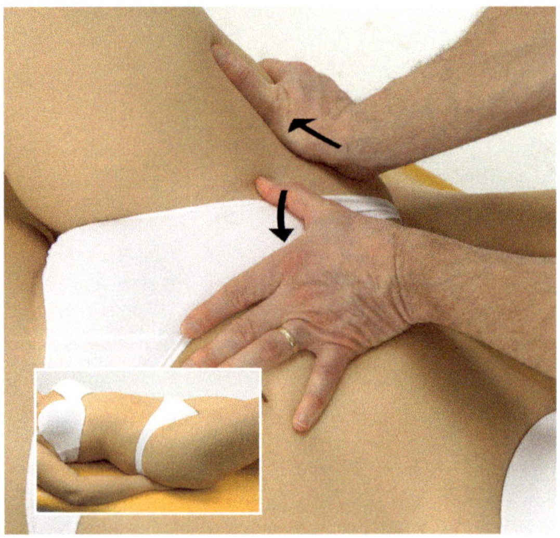

Fig. 6.5 Manipulation of the iliofemoral ligament in decubitus.

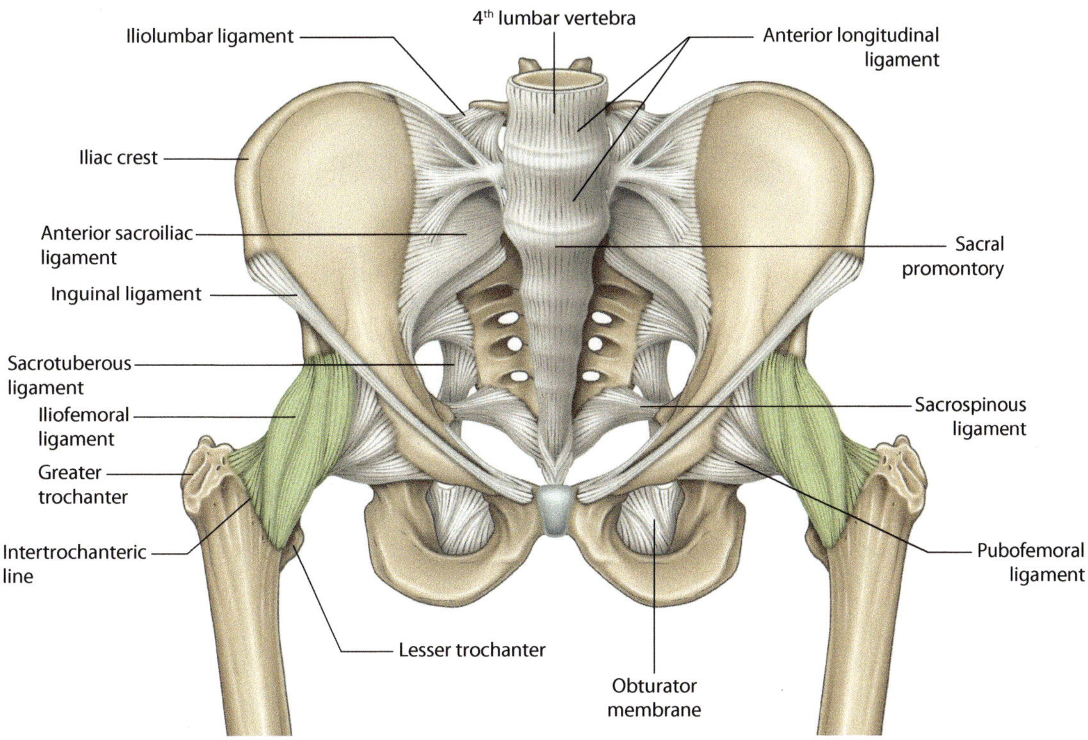

Fig. 6.6 Anterior ligaments of the hip (pubofemoral ligament).

Origin

- Coxal bone
  - Extends from the superior pubic ramus and the obturator crest to the acetabulum
  - The pectineal crest
  - The obturator membrane

Direction

- Caudal and lateral (narrows caudally)

Termination

- Femur
  - Anterior surface of its cranial extremity
  - Behind the inferior tubercle of the intertrochanteric line, near the iliopsoas muscle

Actions

- Limits abduction and resists overabduction

Remarks

The iliopubic ligament is much less powerful than the iliofemoral ligament. It is of interest to us because it exchanges fibers with the zona obicularis surrounding the capsule.

6.3.2 Review—obturator foramen (Fig. 6.7)

This boney foramen gives insertion to the internal and external obturator membranes and muscles.

Form

The periphery is shaped like a key ring. It is more triangular in men, broader in women. On the superior ramus there is a deep groove, the obturator groove, which runs from the pelvis obliquely, medially, and caudally.

Obturator canal

The obturator groove is converted into a

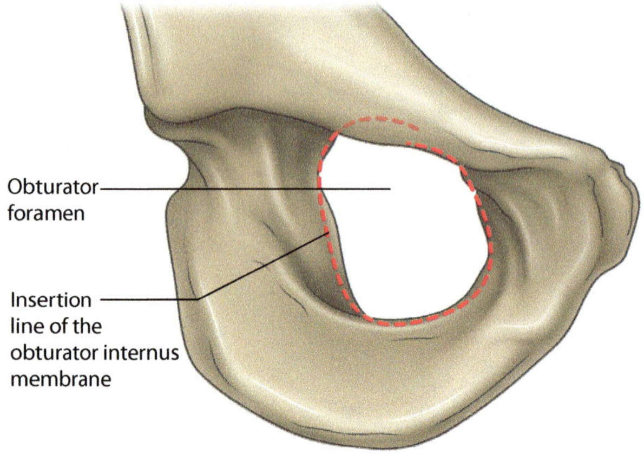

Fig. 6.7 Obturator foramen.

canal by the internal obturator membrane. This passageway transmits the obturator artery, vein, and nerve (Fig. 6.8).

6.3.3 Techniques

Pubofemoral ligament in decubitus

This technique mainly affects the obturator membrane and the joint capsule. The patient assumes the same position as for the iliofemoral ligament outlined above.

Change the proximal contact by stabilizing the superior pubic ramus with one or both of your hands. Broaden your contact by including the pectineal crest that borders the obturator membrane.

Ask the patient to rotate his hip laterally a little; exaggerate this motion with your distal hand on the greater trochanter. The patient glides his foot on the table. At the end of the movement he tightens his leg as if wanting it to grow longer.

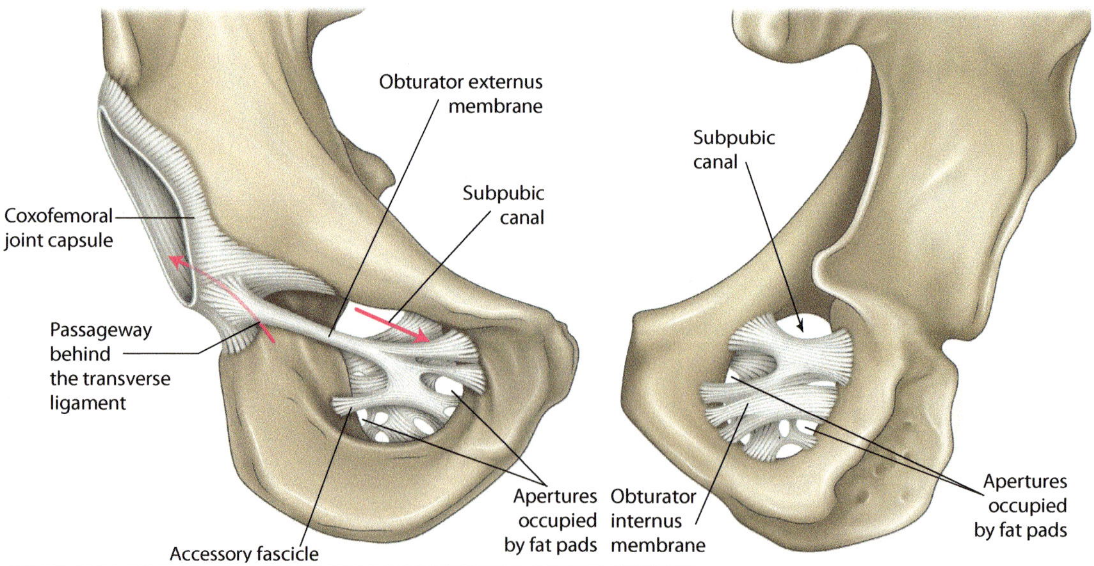

Fig. 6.8 Obturator membranes and obturator canal. (After Testut.)

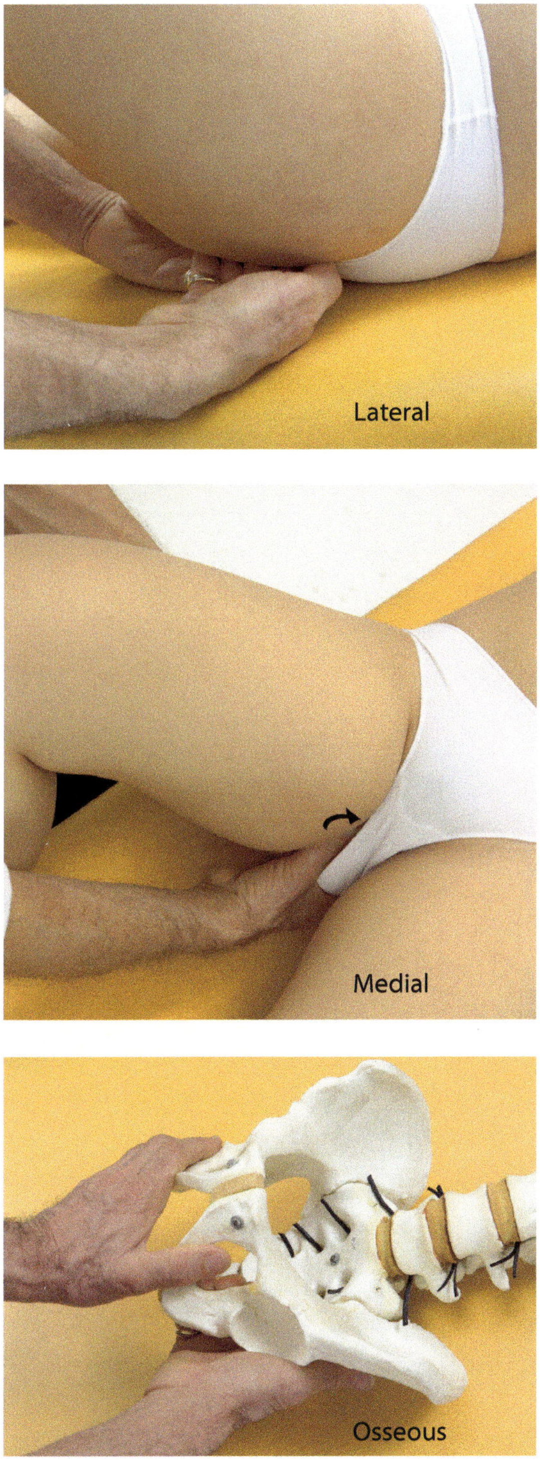

Fig. 6.9 Obturator membrane in decubitus.

Exploration of the obturator foramen

It is important to explore the entire obturator foramen region, searching for sensitive, adhered, or fibrosed fibers. The obturator foramen consists of the united inferior rami of the pubis and ischium.

- The external (exopelvic) surface of the ramus serves as muscle attachment for:
  - the quadratus femoris;
  - the gracilis;
  - the adductor brevis;
  - the adductor longus.
- On the cranial part: the obturator internus membrane

Obturator membrane technique in decubitus (Fig. 6.9)

The patient lies on the table on the side of the pubofemoral ligament to be treated; his lower limb is flexed. Place the fingers of one of your hands on the medial part of the ischial tuberosity and gradually trace along the inferior ramus of the pubis. Direct your fingers on the endopelvic surface of the obturator foramen to contact the obturator membrane. Here we meet the attachments of the obturator internus, some fibers of the levator ani, and the sacrotuberous ligament.

Place the thumb of your other hand on the lateral surface of the obturator foramen between the pectineus and adductor longus. Here you are very close to the obturator nerve as it emerges from the canal. The membrane will be between your two hands. Work the membrane like the skin of a drum that you would like to soften. Search carefully for irregularities and hardened zones within the obturator membrane, and then manipulate them in induction. Areas of reduced elasticity are commonly found in athletic individuals and in women who have had children.

To complete the maneuver, ask the patient to extend his leg while you compress the obturator membrane. This boosts the stretch effect.

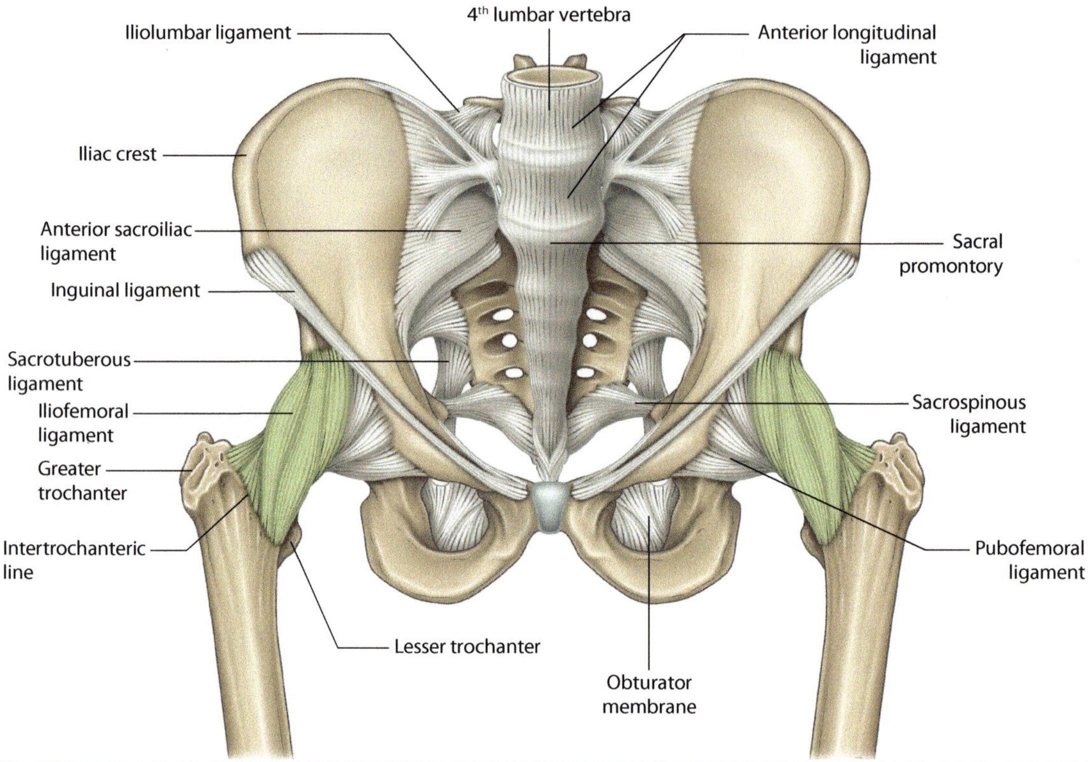

Fig. 6.10 Ischiofemoral ligament.

> **Comment**
>
> **Dividends of obturator membrane manipulation**
> The obturator plays a key role in distributing intrapelvic pressures. It is important to release it, as even a little fibrosis has repercussions for the pelvic organs (the bladder, in particular) and the coxofemoral joint. It also needs to be manipulated because of its relationship to the pubofemoral ligament. The membrane is closely connected to the transverse acetabular ligament and thus indirectly to Alcock's canal.
>
> We have remarked that when great pressure variations occur in the visceral cavities, such as during a cough or sneeze, the obturator foramen and the thoracic inlet are conjointly solicited to absorb and distribute excessive force. This means that a stiffening of the soft tissues in the thoracic inlet can, in the long run, have consequences for the obturator foramen and vice versa.

6.4 ISCHIOFEMORAL LIGAMENT (FIG. 6.10)

6.4.1 Review

Origin

- Coxal bone on the ischium at a point below and behind the acetabulum

Direction

- Lateral and slightly caudal

Termination

It varies according to fibers.

- The cranial fascicle terminates on the medial surface of the greater trochanter to merge with the iliofemoral ligament.
- The middle fascicle attaches to the posterior part of the capsule.
- The caudal fascicle joins the caudal part of the capsule.

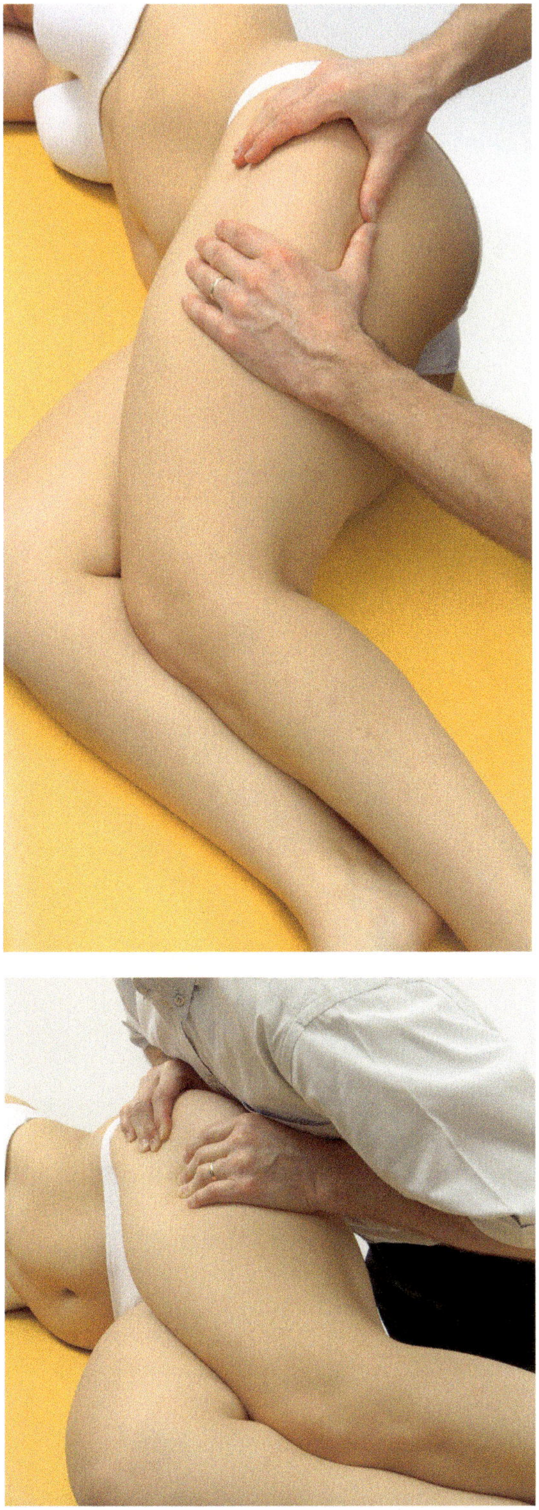

Fig. 6.11 Ischiofemoral ligament in lateral decubitus.

The circular ligament of the zona orbicularis

The zona orbicularis is made up of circular fibers that wrap around the neck of the femur like a tie. Orbicular derives from the Latin meaning "circular in form." The ischiofemoral ligament strongly reinforces this part of the capsule together with other stabilizing ligaments. In the zona orbicularis, the head of the femur is secured to the hip socket like a button in its buttonhole. In a non-weight-bearing situation, this reinforcement occurs thanks to the labrum, negative intra-articular pressure, and the work of certain hip muscles that keep the femoral head in contact with the acetabulum.

Actions

- Limits hip abduction and medial rotation

6.4.2 Technique

The ischiofemoral ligament is mainly manipulated because of its connection to the zona orbicularis, whose circular fibers are such a key element in hip stability.

In lateral decubitus (Fig. 6.11)

The patient lies on the side opposite the treatment, top foot resting behind the other leg on the table. Stand behind the patient and press your body on your hands. Place one thumb at the ischium, as close as possible to the coxofemoral joint. Your other hand draws the greater trochanter into medial rotation and flexion. The patient simultaneously extends his leg in medial rotation by gliding his foot along the table. On the return, you bring the trochanter into lateral rotation extension. Think of it as moving the femoral head clockwise and counterclockwise, as if screwing on and unscrewing the hip, to act on the ligament and the capsule.

Note

Use the weight of your body to bring the necessary power to the manipulation. This allows you to be powerful, soft, and gradual without great effort on your part.

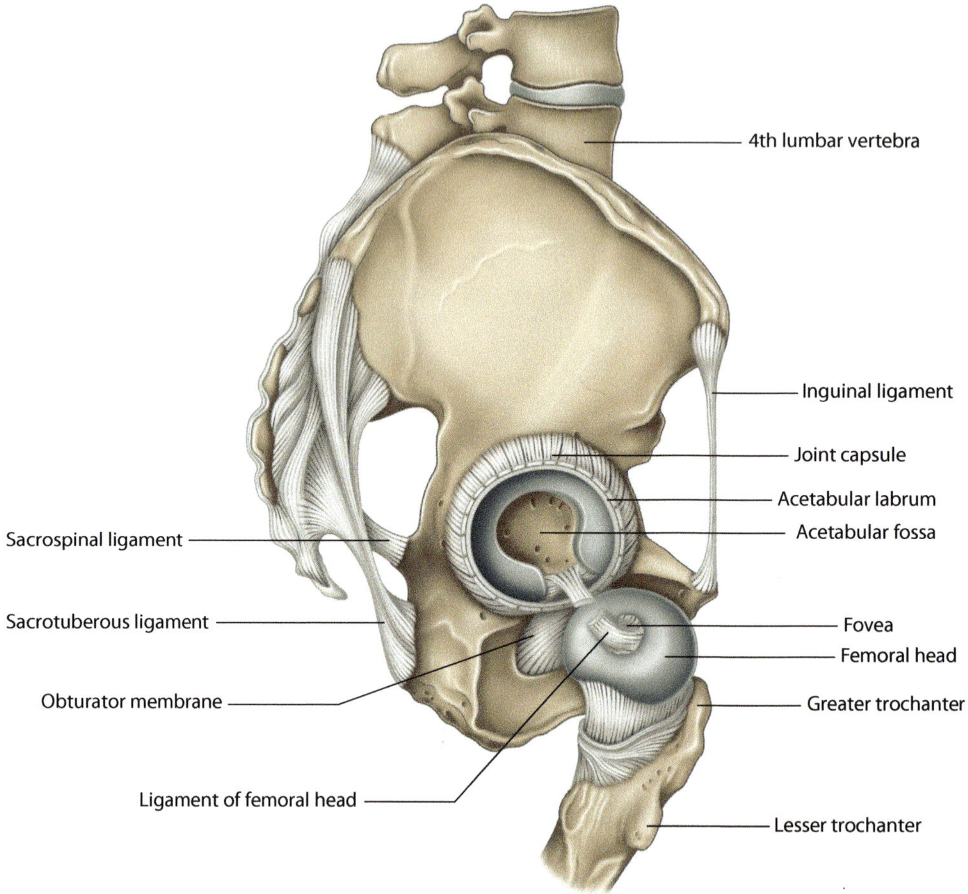

Fig. 6.12 Ischiofemoral ligament.

6.5 LIGAMENT OF THE FEMORAL HEAD (FIG. 6.12).

6.5.1 Review

Generalities

- The ligament of the femoral head (round ligament) is the hip's only intracapsular ligament, although in some sense it can also be considered extra-articular. The "tent of the round ligament" is a synovial fold that ensheathes the ligament, excluding it from the joint cavity.
- This ligament contains an artery, which we will address further in the book.
- The round ligament is 3–5 cm long and just under 1 cm wide.

Origin

- On the coxal bone, more precisely the acetabular notch, by three insertions:
  - one anterior, behind the anterior horn;
  - one middle, at the cranial border of the transverse acetabular ligament;
  - one posterior, behind the posterior horn.

Termination

- Fovea capitis of the femoral head

Actions

- The round ligament is a powerful intra-articular ligament with tripodal roots. While classically deemed to have a modest mechanical role, this ligament is fairly strong.

- It is made tense when the thigh is semiflexed and outwardly rotated. Check extreme rotation.
- It can be considered an accessory brake on abduction.

The artery of the ligament of the femoral head

The great feature of this ligament is that it contains an important slender artery that vascularizes the subchondral bone of the superior pole of the femur. We have seen patients develop osteonecrosis of the femoral head at the very site of this artery. Such an interruption of blood supply tends to arise in the aftermath of a direct fall on the heel, where the collisional forces land on the head of the femur. More rarely, femoral bone necrosis follows an incident of extreme rotation and adduction.

The artery of the femoral head arises from the obturator artery, a branch of the internal iliac artery. This underscores the importance of this iliac artery, not just in terms of pelvic organs but also for the hip joint and the aftermath of hip trauma.

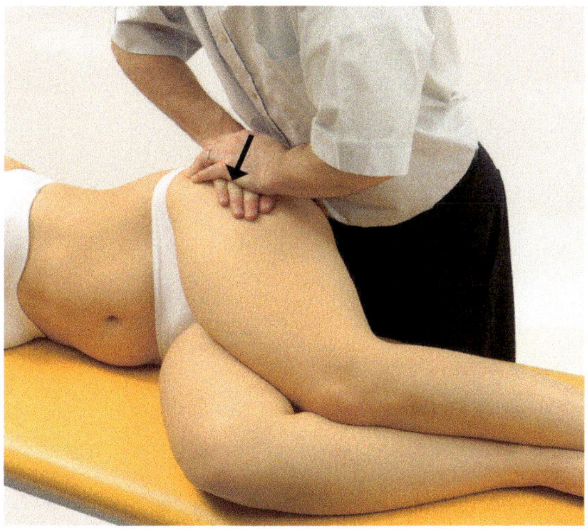

Fig. 6.13 Ligament of the head of the femur in lateral decubitus.

Innervation of the ligament of the femoral head

The round ligament is innervated by a branch of the obturator nerve. It plays a reflexogenic role that is rarely talked about. To be convinced of this, according to Ficat et al. (1967), one only needs to observe thigh muscle contractions during electrocautery coagulation of the femoral fosset into which the ligament is implanted. This is observable during hip replacement surgery.

6.5.2 Techniques

Advantages of the maneuver

This maneuver attempts to achieve both a vascular effect on the artery of the ligament and a proprioceptive gain for the intra-articular ligamentous structure itself. Compression traumas involving forced abduction of the coxofemoral joint can have a nociceptive effect on the artery. This translates into ischemia with disastrous effects for the femoral head.

As we said at the start, little function has classically been imputed to this vessel. Personal observations, however, have shown us that such an arterial lesion can have delayed effects. In our experience, one or two years often go by after a trauma before osteochondrosis appears at the femoral head.

In lateral decubitus (Fig. 6.13)

The patient lies on the side opposite the hip treated, with the lower limb semiflexed. Standing behind the patient, you place your palms one on top of the other over the greater trochanter. Bring in your thorax to increase compression forces along the axis of the femoral neck. Compress the greater trochanter medially and slightly cranially.

Do this as if you want to push the head of the femur into the acetabulum, and then let off and allow the femur to come back into its viscoelasticity. The difference between this technique and the one for the ischiofemoral ligament is that no medial rotation component is involved with this technique, and the pressure direction stays in line with the neck of the femur.

At the end of the compression phase, follow the tissular listening that often indicates slight rotation. The round ligament blends with the transverse acetabular ligament at three places. This might explain why the listening can direct the movement more caudally or more cranially.

Repeat the technique five or six times, proceeding slowly and precisely. Remember to perform induction at the end of the movement.

Treatment of the gliding apparatus

7

7.1 LABRUM (FIG. 7.1)

7.1.1 Review

Anatomy

The acetabular labrum is a triangular fibrocartilaginous ring that attaches to the boney rim of the hip socket. It spans the acetabular notch by its fibrous continuation, the transverse acetabular ligament. The labrum is anchored to the hip at two levels: the deep and the peripheral acetabular surfaces. Its height ranges from 6–10 mm depending on anatomists' descriptions.

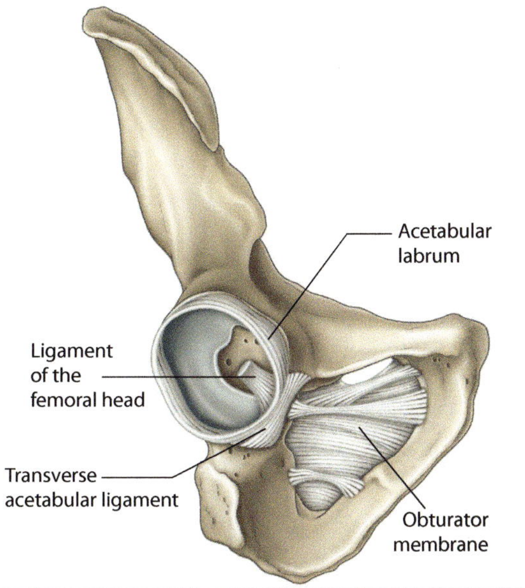

Fig. 7.1 Acetabular labrum.

The labrum has three surfaces:

- The medial surface inserts on the deep articular surface of the acetabulum. The attachments extend through a transition zone of cartilage, except where an attachment is indirect.
- The lateral surface contacts the cartilage on the head of the femur.
- The convex peripheral surface attaches directly to the acetabulum; it interconnects with the joint capsule, and has a good blood supply.

Vascular supply (Fig. 7.2)

Generally, the peripheral labrum is richly vascularized.

- The anterior inferior labrum is supplied by the posterior or external branches of the obturator artery. This posterior branch gives an ascending or acetabular branch that further subdivides.
- The ischial artery furnishes several branches to the posterior surface of the joint, particularly the acetabular rim.
- The superior gluteal artery supplies the upper region of the acetabulum, extending from the posterior border of the gluteus minimus to terminate at the intertubercular groove. Along its course, this artery distributes ascending branches to the gluteal muscles, while descending vessels pierce the gluteus minimus, destined for the joint—specifically the superior acetabulum and labrum.

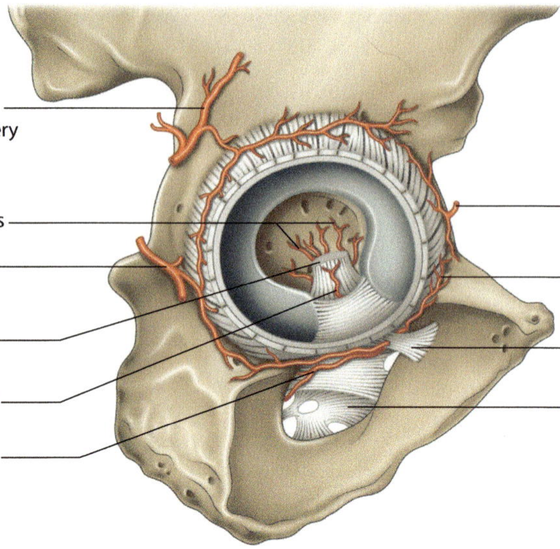

Fig. 7.2 Vascular supply of labrum.

Innervation

Labrum innervation is rich and complex. The obturator nerve, the principal nerve of the hip joint, furnishes a constant branch called the joint nerve of the hip, and an inconstant subpubic articular branch. The joint nerve of the hip is the more important and the largest nerve of the hip. It issues two smaller nerves, whose labral branch reaches the joint by passing under the transverse acetabular ligament in company with the acetabular artery.

- The accessory obturator nerve (Schmidt) is a small inconsistent nerve that distributes filaments to the anterior surface of the joint and the labrum.
- The nerve to the quadratus femoris and to the inferior gemellus branches into one or more articular filaments. It supplies the posterior surface of the joint together with the posterior segment of the labrum.
- The inconsistent articular nerve arises from the sciatic nerve. It stands in for the nerve supplying the quadratus femoris and the inferior gemellus when it is absent.

Functions

Congruence

The labrum increases the surface area of the acetabular socket by more than 25%. Like other fibrocartilages, it improves joint coupling; in this case, fitting together of the femoral head and the acetabulum.

Shock absorption

The labrum cushions contact stress between the hard surfaces of the femur, the pelvis, and the capsule. It increases the depth of the acetabulum and provides the acetabular rim a degree of softness it would otherwise lack. It is generally the medial part that poses problems, and it is where we target our techniques.

Sealing

The labrum functions as a sort of circular joint seal, which, in maintaining negative fluid pressure, creates a "vacuum" effect favorable to coxofemoral joint physiology.

Joint centering

Philippe Chiron (2001) considered the labrum to have a joint-centering role. The circumference of its free border is slightly smaller than the boney acetabulum, burying the femur slightly deeper in the socket.

Lateral and vertical movements within the acetabulum are reduced. This dynamic stabilization happens during weight bearing. When the hip is in the extension phase, the capsule twists on itself and tightens around the labrum, stabilizing and re-centering the femoral head.

Lubricating and cushioning intra-articular pressures

Studies show a pressure difference between the peripheral and the deep hip. The labrum is thereby able to diminish joint strain by momentarily doubling up joint fluid when the hip is under load. This system has two major advantages:

- It allows the synovial membrane to spread during hip movement.
- Fluid exchanges between the deep and the peripheral hip function as shock absorbers.

Simulated labral ablation experiments demonstrate that a reduced labrum increases strain at the femoral head.

Canine experiments have shown that progressive wearing away of the developing labrum causes acetabular dysplasia and early arthritis.

Proprioception and nociception

The labrum is sensitive to pain, touch, and temperature (Kim 1995). Here one finds Vater-Pacini and Golgi-Mazzoni corpuscles that sense vibration and pressure, together with Ruffini corpuscles that transmit information about deep pressure and temperature.

7.1.2 Techniques

Test in decubitus

The patient lies on the table, the coxofemoral joint forming a 90-degree angle. You stand on the same side, first testing the hip in flexion-adduction and then in flexion-abduction. At the end of each adduction/abduction range, compress the femur in the proximal direction without changing your adduction or abduction angle. You will often feel the femoral head drop distally or posteriorly. When a labrum or cartilage problem exists, compression can be sensitive.

Note: The above test works for cartilage, too.

Maneuver in procubitus (Fig. 7.3)

The patient allows his thigh to drop off the side of the table, knee flexed and foot touching the floor. You stand to the side of the patient and stabilize the pelvis by placing your hand on the sacrum. With your other hand on the greater trochanter, mobilize the hip in two directions: forward distally and medially, and backward distally and laterally.

Do this a dozen times, performing the last few rounds in induction. Work carefully, as this rather powerful, very impressive technique must be done gradually. To increase the effect, maintain the trochanter for a few seconds when the joint is at the end of its course.

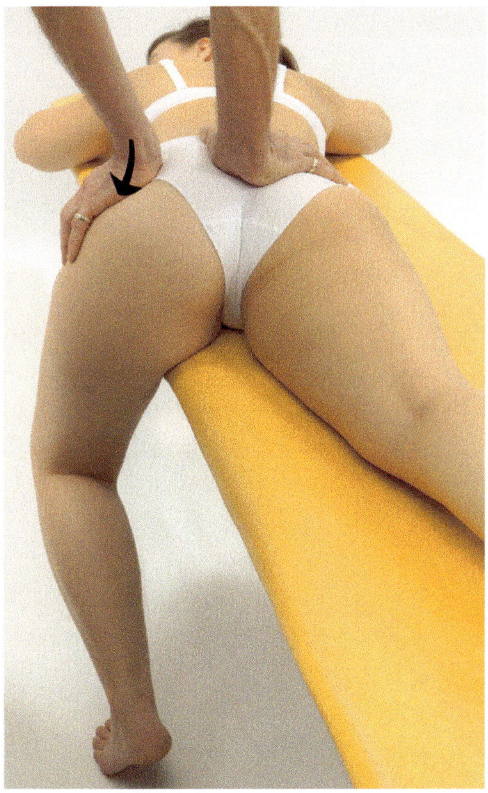

Fig. 7.3 Acetabular labrum in procubitus.

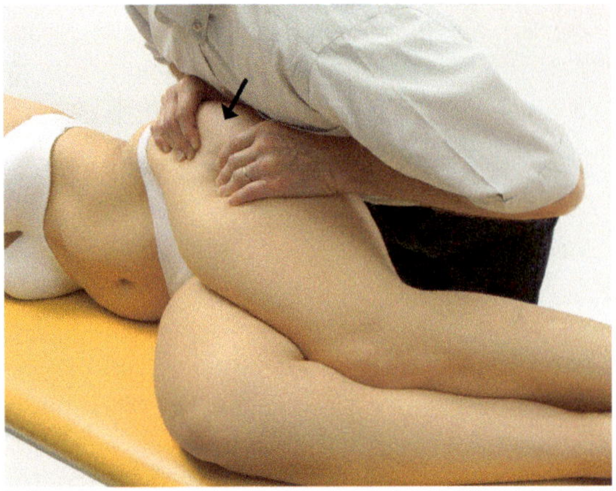

Fig. 7.4 Cartilage polishing in lateral decubitus.

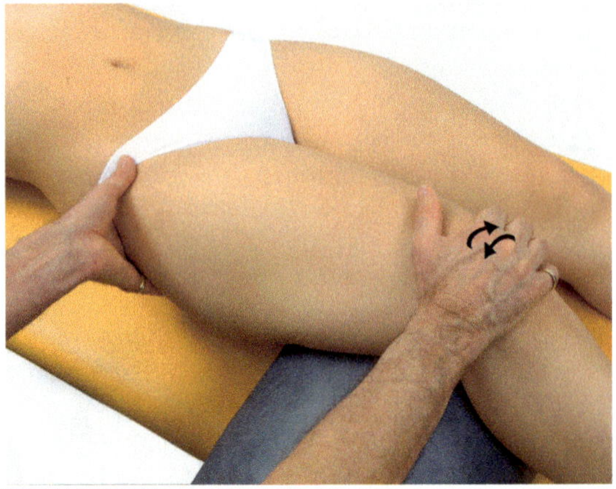

Fig. 7.5 Cartilage polishing in decubitus.

7.2 CARTILAGE

7.2.1 Techniques

Cartilage polishing in lateral decubitus (Fig. 7.4)

This technique affects both joint cartilage and labrum. The labrum cartilage is thicker peripherally.

The patient lies on the side opposite the hip concerned. You place your hands over the greater trochanter. Bear down on your hands with your thorax. Compress the femoral head into the acetabulum, transmitting pressure through the greater trochanter and the femoral neck. Vary your angle to find roughened zones on which to focus the technique. Maintain the compression and ask the patient to flex and extend his leg by gliding his foot along the table.

While the head of the femur compresses as the leg moves, the acetabular cartilage will be experiencing "polishing." Perform this maneuver gradually and at the end of a session. It must not cause pain.

Cartilage polishing in decubitus (Fig. 7.5)

The patient lies supine, lower limb slightly flexed, with a cushion under the knee. Grasp the greater trochanter with one hand and draw it into medial rotation. At the same time, place the other hand on the knee to accentuate the rotation. Keep a good grasp on the knee joint to avoid any motion between the tibia and the femur.

Alternate rotational movements as if "screwing on" and "unscrewing" the hip joint. By emphasizing medial and lateral rotation of the greater trochanter, you are compressing and decompressing the femoral head in the acetabulum.

Treatment of osseous elements

8

The main goal of these osseous techniques is to restore a degree of the coxal bone's innate elasticity and malleability. Astonishing as it may seem, the acetabulum is a deformable structure. Understanding this makes it easy to see that osseous techniques are designed to improve shock absorption qualities that are vital to the health of femoral and acetabular cartilage.

Note specifically that these osseous techniques call for forces that engender micromovements aimed at restoring tissular elasticity and deformability, not large-scale movements.

8.1 BIOMECHANICAL REVIEW

8.1.1 Acetabular formation

Three bones of the coxal bone unite in the formation of the acetabulum, which means "little vinegar cup" in Latin. The ilium, pubis, and ischium all contribute to the construction of the acetabular cavity or hip socket. The Y-shaped growth plate that separates them persists through childhood and fuses definitively between the ages of 14 and 15 (Schuenke et al. 2010).

8.1.2 Dynamic memory

The distinctive embryological constitution and singular form of the acetabulum provide very specific dynamics throughout life. Studies have been done on fresh cadavers whose capsular ligamentous systems remain intact. Experiments looked at areas of contact stress between cartilaginous surfaces of the acetabulum and the femoral head during hip joint loading and unloading (Greenwald 1974). Strain gauge measurement analysis showed that surface contact between the hip socket and femur varied and developed with load demands.

The roof of the acetabulum is, in fact, flexible.

- With a weak load, contact is limited to interacetabular horn spread.
- When pressure is increased, the acetabular roof comes into play, and the horns close up.
- Once the pressure is let off, the femoral heads "spring back."

8.1.3 Variable acetabular geometry

In the course of walking, the acetabulum comes into contact with the femoral head during the weight-bearing phase. In the swing phase, only the anterior and posterior parts of the acetabulum remain in contact with the head of the femur. The movement remains consistently modest, in the range of 10 to 90 μm, depending on bone quality and joint configuration. Nevertheless, some authors go as far as describing a "geometric variable" to characterize this phenomenon and demonstrate osseous plasticity.

8.1.4 Weight-bearing and non-weight-bearing zones

A. Seth Greenwald (1974) describes types of joint zones:

- Zones in constant contact irrespective of load are located at the anterior and posterior parts of the acetabulum and at the femoral head.
- Zones of intermittent contact depend on the degree of load. This is the case at the top of the acetabulum.
- No acetabular joint contact exists at the lower part of the femoral head, as well as none at the area around the fovea capitis.

Very few areas of intermittent contact remain evident in the elderly. This signifies greater joint congruence and a loss of inter-osseous elasticity.

The acetabulum is in constant contact with the femoral head, onto which a tremendous amount of force can land. Pressures can amount to 15 times body weight within the acetabulum (Freeman et al. 1979). Cadaver observations confirm significant wear at the acetabular roof in the aged population.

It is easy to appreciate the usefulness of treating the boney elements of the coxal bone. By restoring flexibility to osseous tissue, we can help the acetabulum better adapt to the constraints that inevitably land on it.

Summary

- The acetabulum deforms as a function of load bearing.
- Acetabular horns function like an opening clamp whose movement is limited by the acetabular labrum and the transverse acetabular ligament.

8.1.5 Hardening of the subchondral bone

Our colleague and friend Olivier Bazin (1998) has done some excellent research on arthritis of the hip. He emphasizes that a dense bone puts greater strain on cartilage than does a more flexible bone. Failure of the subchondral bone can thus be the start of arthritic changes.

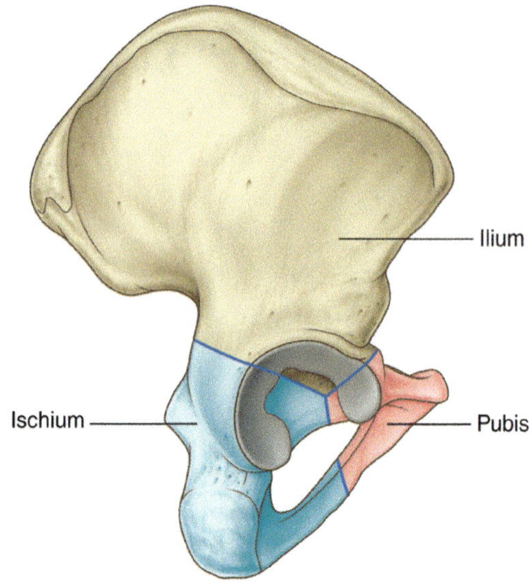

Fig. 8.1 Test of hip bone elasticity.

Experimental evidence shows that relative hardening of subchondral bone is harmful to the vitality of adjacent cartilage. In addition, fibrillar cartilage wears down only if the subchondral bone hardens. In other words, even if cartilage is not in great shape, arthritis depends on bone hardness. This finding adds another dimension to the value of intraosseous techniques geared to restoring bone malleability.

8.1.6 Techniques

Osseous technique for the coxal bone in lateral decubitus

The patient lies on the side opposite the hip concerned, and you locate yourself behind the patient. Your cephalad hand grasps the iliac crest between the heel of your hand and your fingers. Your fingers glide on the endopelvic slope of the iliac crest. Firmly grasp the ischiopubic ramus with the heel of your other hand, which is placed on the lateral buttock with the finger pads in the ischiorectal fossa.

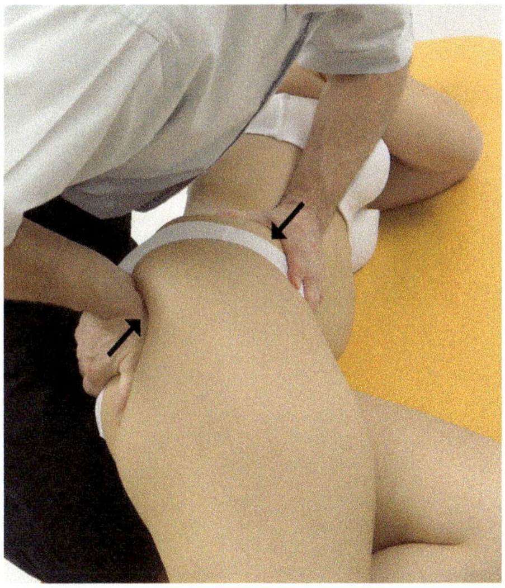

Fig. 8.2 Osseous technique for the coxal bone.

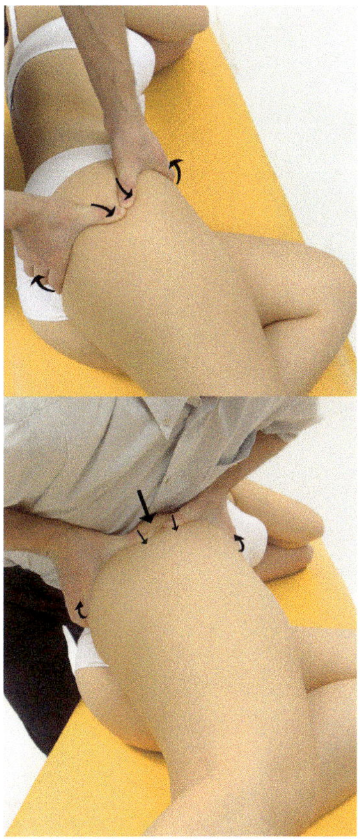

Fig. 8.3 Combined technique for the femoral neck and the coxal bone.

Place the knee of your distal leg on the table; this serves to reinforce your pressure without strain. Using both hands, compress and decompress the bone longitudinally in the direction of the acetabular socket, as if wanting to reduce the coxal bone slightly in height. Repeat two or three times. Work with your knee against your hand to increase and decrease this longitudinal compression.

The test (Fig. 8.1)

Allow your hands to follow the listening as a guide to the interosseous restrictions. With practice you will feel them quickly. Trained hands can feel where there is a loss of boney elasticity and how they are arranged. Until this sense becomes automatic, however, we begin by deconstructing and visualizing the task:

- Pretend you want to "fold" the coxal bone from front to back and from back to front.
- With each fold, analyze which phase of the deformation is limited or absent—the bend or the return?

The technique itself (Fig. 8.2)

If you find a restriction, bend the bone in the direction of ease until you perceive a certain "softening" of the dense osseous structure. Until you become aware of this, accompany the coxal bone without force in the chosen direction, following the tissular listening as closely as you can. At the end of the bending action, allow the bone to slowly return to the starting point. Follow with a new listening. With practice you will easily feel areas of lost elasticity around which you can begin to feel and encourage tissue restructuring.

Combined technique for the coxal bone and the femoral head in lateral decubitus (Fig. 8.3)

The patient assumes the same position as above, with you situated behind him. Delicately hook the iliac crest with the finger pads of one hand. Clasp the ischial tuberosity with the fingers of your other hand. Join your thumbs on the lateral surface of the greater trochanter and reinforce them with your thorax.

Lift the iliac crest and the ischial tuberosity together; simultaneously bring your thumb pressure to bear on the greater trochanter. The pressure should fall directly along the axis of the femoral neck. You can gauge the elasticity of the coxal bone using this combination of forces, which essentially simulate (if minimally) the flexibility demands made on the acetabulum during weight bearing in real life. Try to visualize the coxal bone "unfolding" and then "folding" again when you let up your pressure. Work with these parameters in induction to restore the elastic quality of the bone.

Neural manipulations

9

9.1 REVIEW

While subject to individual variation, all nerves of the hip derive from two sources: lumbar and sacral plexuses.

9.1.1 Lumbar plexus

The lumbar plexus supplies the anterior hip.

Femoral nerve

The articular branches derive from the nerves to the pectineus and quadriceps.

Obturator nerve

The anterior articular nerve supplies the subpubic hip. The obturator nerve sometimes gives off an articular branch through the obturator canal, as well.

Accessory obturator nerve (Schmidt)

This small, inconstant nerve distributes to the anterior hip.

9.1.2 Sacral plexus

The sacral plexus supplies the posterior hip.

Nerve of quadratus femoris and inferior gemellus

The nerve to these muscles gives a branch to the hip joint called the posterior articular nerve. This nerve is sometimes split.

Sciatic nerve

The sciatic nerve distributes to the posterior joint.

9.2 CLINICAL PICTURE

Occasionally, nerves that pass near the hip create pain that can be mistaken for other problems.

- The femoral nerve produces pain in the groin and often in the upper thigh. This is classic cruralgia (pain in the thigh). The femoral nerve trunk is located immediately beneath the inguinal ligament, just outside the femoral artery.
- The lateral femoral cutaneous nerve is a sensory nerve that can cause tingling, numbness, and pain on the outer thigh (meralgia paresthetica). Terrible burning pain can arise as the nerve passes through the outer part of the inguinal ligament, just inside the ASIS.
- The obturator nerve can create pain that mimics pubalgia (athletic groin injury), radiating to the adductors and deep part of the inner thigh. This nerve can sometimes produce medial knee pain.
- The sciatic nerve produces the well-known pain that radiates down the back of the leg, sometimes as far as the foot. Curiously, it sometimes produces pain confined to the buttock region, limited to the ischiofemoral groove at the posterior surface of the joint capsule. It is here that

the sciatic nerve delivers capsular branches to the coxofemoral joint.
- The superior gluteal nerve can cause pain deep in the buttocks, often mistaken for tendonitis of the gluteus medius. The superior gluteal nerve relates to piriformis. Because piriformis reacts to pelvic congestion, pain in the superior gluteal nerve often coincides with the menstrual cycle.

9.2.1 Techniques

Neural techniques for the lower extremity are described in our books devoted to the peripheral nerves (Barral et al. 2004). We highly recommend this text to our readers as a valuable reference for treating patients.

Vascular manipulations

10

10.1 ARTERIES OF THE HIP

10.1.1 Review—hip circulation

Vascular supply to the femoral head and neck

Various arteries irrigate the femoral head and neck:

- medial circumflex femoral artery, behind;
- lateral femoral circumflex artery, in front;
- superior and inferior gluteal arteries;
- artery of the femoral head, which derives from the obturator artery that branches off the internal iliac artery (artery sometimes arises from the medial circumflex femoral artery).

Vascularization of the acetabulum

The blood is supplied to the acetabulum by:

- the obturator artery that gives off ascending and descending acetabular branches, which further subdivide;
- the acetabular artery that furnishes several branches to the posterior surface of the joint, particularly the acetabular rim;
- the superior gluteal artery that supplies a branch to the roof of the acetabulum. This vessel passes out of the pelvis posterior to the gluteus minimus and terminates at the intertubercular sulcus. It continues with descending osteoarticular branches that distribute to the superior acetabulum.

The origin of all these arteries divides into two vascular distributions from the common iliac artery: the external iliac artery and the internal iliac artery.

10.1.2 Review—external iliac artery (Fig. 10.1)

The external iliac artery becomes the femoral artery and the deep femoral artery.

The deep femoral artery

This artery furnishes:

- the medial circumflex artery of the thigh as it supplies blood to the adductors and the femoral head;
- the lateral circumflex artery as it supplies the greater trochanter, and the neck and head of the femur.

The artery continues as three perforating branches; the third is the terminal.

Terminal perforating artery

This artery pierces the adductor magnus in the adductor hiatus formed by the adductor longus, adductor magnus, and vastus medialis.

The adductor canal joins the adductor hiatus, which essentially is formed by fibers of the adductor magnus. The adductor magnus inserts onto the femur by two fascicles:

- The proximal fibers insert on the linea aspera.
- The distal portion of the muscle inserts on the adductor tubercle of the medial femoral condyle.

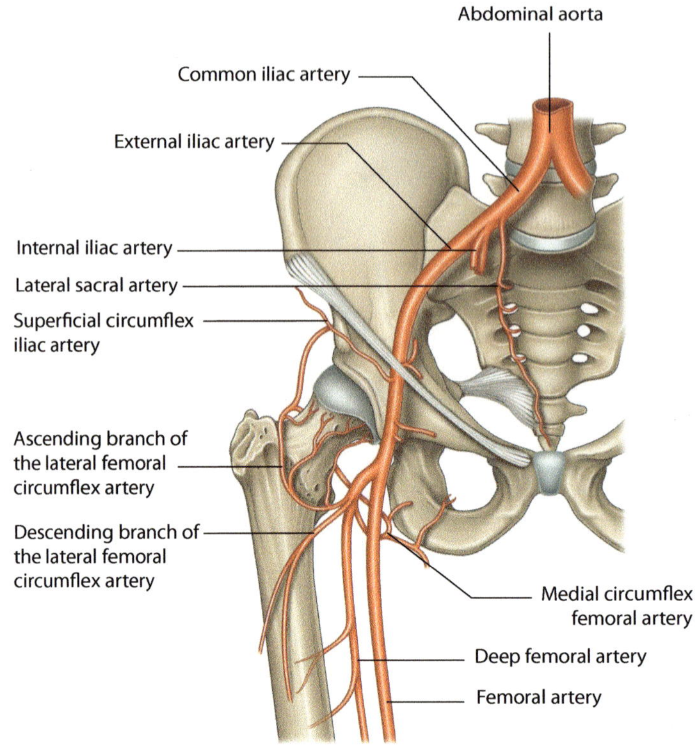

Fig. 10.1 External iliac artery.

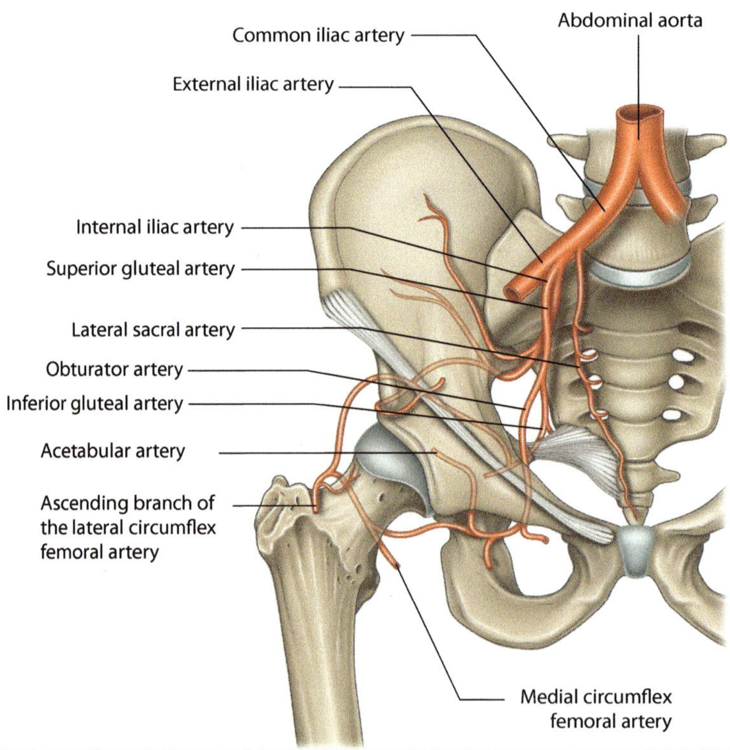

Fig. 10.2 Internal iliac artery.

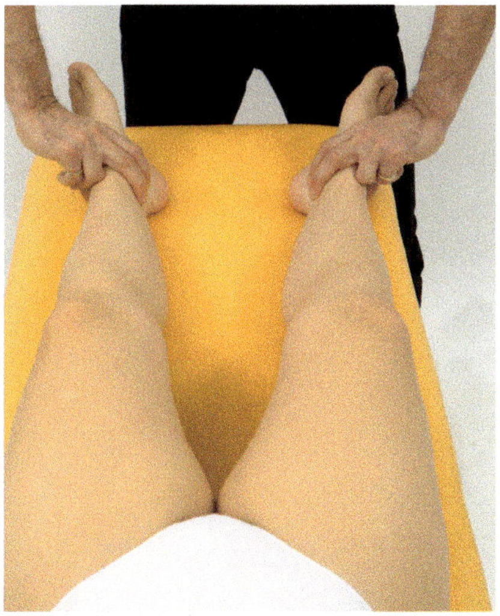

Fig. 10.3 Witness pulse of the posterior tibial arteries.

The adductor hiatus is found in the gap between these two femoral insertions and the femur.

10.1.3 Review—internal iliac artery (Fig. 10.2)

This artery divides into the following arteries:

- obturator;
- sciatic;
- gluteal;
- pudendal.

The obturator artery supplies the artery contained within the round ligament of the femoral head.

10.1.4 Techniques

We have obtained our best results from stretching the main arterial trunks, such as the internal and external iliac vessels, as well as the femoral artery. Other arteries are difficult to feel and not easy to mobilize. In cases of major coxofemoral joint dysfunction it is beneficial to treat the medial circumflex artery. In any event, we always compare the posterior tibial pulses.

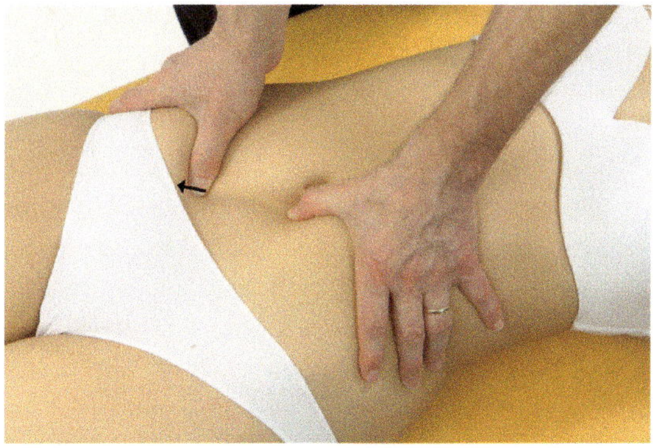

Fig. 10.4 Manipulation of the external iliac artery.

The posterior tibial arteries as witness pulses

The patient is supine, legs extended. Place two of your finger pads of each hand behind the tibial malleoli. Slide your fingers slightly posteriorly. You will easily feel the posterior tibial pulses (Fig. 10.3).

A weak pulse can signify different things:

- a problem with the main abdominal trunks (aorta, common iliac artery, or external vessels);
- a femoral artery restriction or even compression of the posterior tibial artery in the leg.

To discover the arterial segment involved, slightly compress the suspected artery. The compression that noticeably diminishes the tibial pulse is the site of the problem. When in doubt—particularly in the presence of risk factors—ask your patient to consult his physician or a blood vessel specialist.

External iliac artery (Fig. 10.4)

The patient is supine, legs extended. Depending on patient morphology, you might want to glide a pillow under the lumbar spine to tilt the pelvis and render the artery more superficial and accessible.

Landmark the abdominal aorta at the umbilicus. Following an oblique 45° axis in a lateral and caudal direction, feel for the nearby pulse of the common iliac artery.

Place one thumb on the common iliac artery near the umbilicus; place the other thumb on its extension, the external iliac artery. Fix the upper end of the artery and stretch the vessel distally with your other contact.

Be attentive: As with nerve treatment, your fingers must exert a minimum of compression. Elongation of the artery wall is what affects the mechanoreceptors. The goal is to regulate local arterial flux and, from this stimulation, obtain a central retroactive effect.

Internal iliac artery (Fig. 10.5)

This artery can be landmarked in two ways:

- Starting from the beat of the abdominal aorta at the umbilical region, search for the internal iliac pulse located slightly laterally of the umbilicopubic line, a little above the bilateral line.
- Starting from the external iliac artery, feel medially for the internal iliac artery pulse, about a hand's width from the umbilicus.

Perform the elongation technique with both thumbs. Place one thumb on the bifurcation with the external iliac artery; place the other thumb next to it to stretch the internal iliac artery in a medial direction.

Femoral artery

The most effective manipulation is performed at the saphenous hiatus.

Saphenous hiatus (Fig. 10.6)

The fascia lata is tough, strong, and not very extensible, except where it opens to form the saphenous hiatus in the iliopectineal fossa of the upper thigh.

Here, instead of being continuous and tough, the fascia lata forms an orifice inferior to the medial part of the inguinal ligament. A perforated superficial layer called the cribriform fascia spreads over the saphenous opening and encloses it.

At the cribriform fascia level, the saphenous hiatus is bounded by superior and inferior horns, which are fascia reinforcements that maintain a gap in the hiatus.

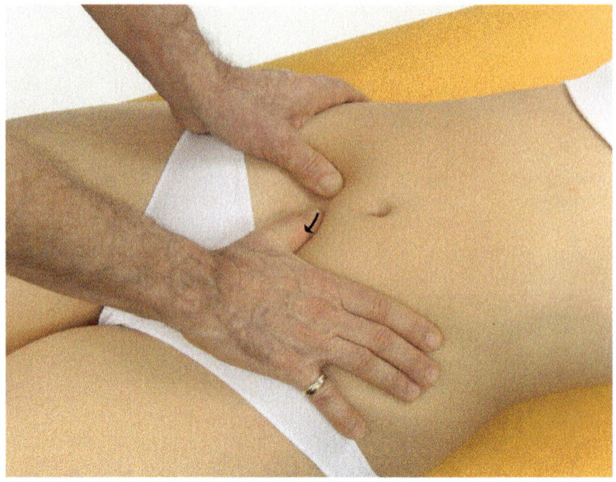

Fig. 10.5 Manipulation of the interna iliac artery.

The main structures passing through the saphenous opening are:

- the great saphenous vein;
- the external pudendal nerves (more medial);
- the superficial epigastric vein (more cranial);
- the lymph nodes;
- the cutaneous branches of the femoral and genitofemoral nerves.

The deep femoral artery is located deeply in the hiatus, situated laterally and posteriorly in relation to the femoral vein.

Technique in lateral decubitus (Fig. 10.7)

The patient lies on the side opposite the hip concerned. Position yourself behind him and place two fingers of each hand very flatly on the saphenous hiatus. First find the femoral pulse, which is easy to feel with the hip in extension. The common mistake is to search for the pulse with the hip in flexion, which automatically renders the artery deeper and less accessible.

Once you find the pulse, create two points of contact with your fingers and stretch the artery distally. We remind you again that your compression must be as light as possible and the stretch done progressively. The elongation can be augmented by having the patient extend his leg distally, his foot pushing behind the immobile leg. Proceed in induction until the end of the leg movement.

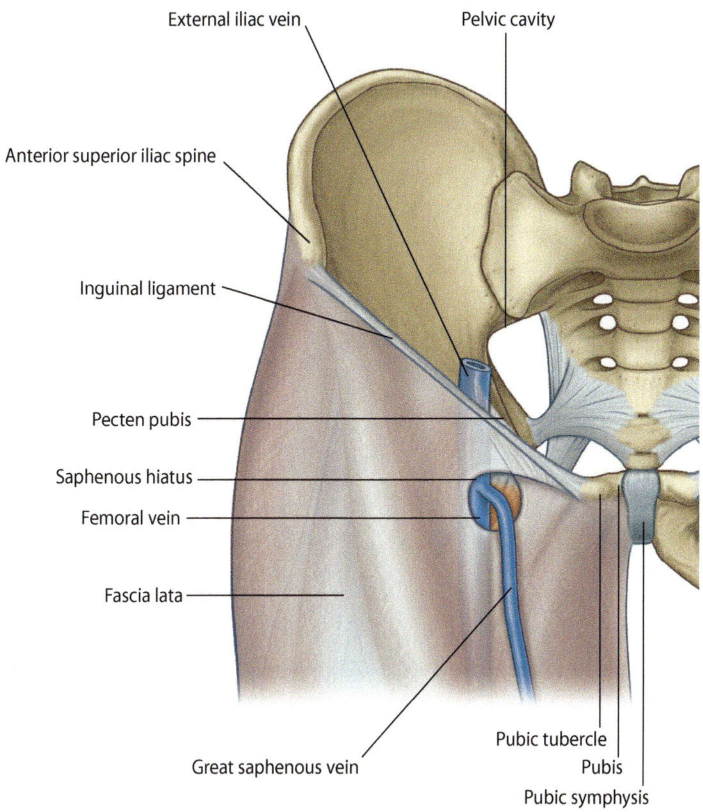

Fig. 10.6 Saphenous hiatus.

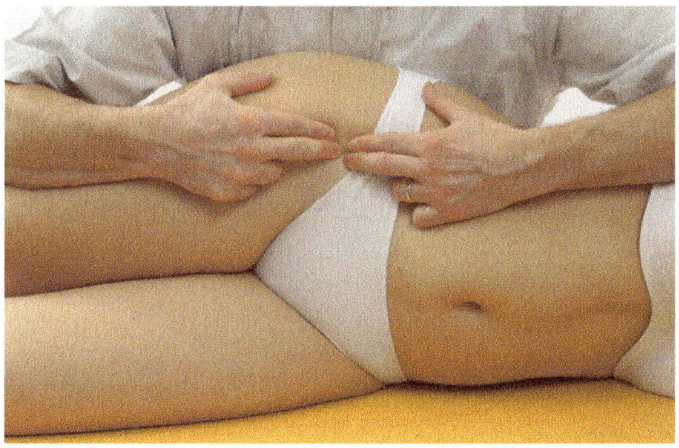

Fig. 10.7 Saphenous hiatus technique.

Medial circumflex artery (Figs. 10.8 and 10.9)

The medial circumflex artery is especially important for the hip joint. It arises from the medial posterior surface of the femoral artery, infiltrating deeply as it passes between the pectineus medially and the psoas laterally.

Sit on the side of the manipulation on a stool a little lower than the table. The patient lies supine, knee sufficiently flexed to bring the hip to about 60° of flexion. Pass one hand under the thigh in order to position your fingertips on the medial surface of the femoral artery, just above the superior border of sartorius. Place the fingertips of your other hand on the lateral side of the artery. Next, search a little more deeply in the psoas tendon with the lateral hand, and search in the pectineus muscle with your medial hand to find the pulse of the medial circumflex artery.

While taking the pulse, perform small spreading induction maneuvers between these muscles, as if wanting to delicately separate them. If you are truly following induction, the pulse should increase under your fingers. Maintain for several seconds the direction that increases the pulse. Release and recommence three or four times. This maneuver has tre-

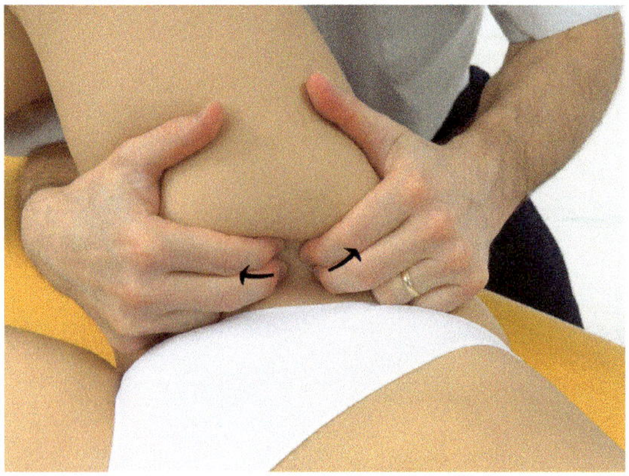

Fig. 10.9 Medial circumflex artery technique.

mendous impact on hip circulation and relieves the deep pain that can come about from joint overuse or overload.

10.2 INGUINAL LIGAMENT AND ILIOPECTINEAL ARCH (FIG. 10.10)

These two structures give passage to the femoral neurovascular bundle. Their retraction and fibrosis harms the coxofemoral joint indirectly through compression of the femoral artery, vein, and nerve.

10.2.1 Review

Inguinal ligament

This band stretches from the medial part of the anterior superior iliac spine to the pubis.

Special note

The ligament surrounds the anterior rectus abdominis muscle and lateral femoral nerve at its iliac spine attachment.

Iliopectineal arch

This arch extends from the inguinal ligament to the iliopubic eminence of the hip bone. It separates the iliopsoas muscle and the femoral nerve from the vascular compartment of the femoral artery and vein.

Femoral triangle and inguinal region

The femoral triangle and the vascular and muscular lacuna are located below the inguinal ligament. The femoral triangle is composed of the inguinal ligament, the sartorius, and the adductor longus.

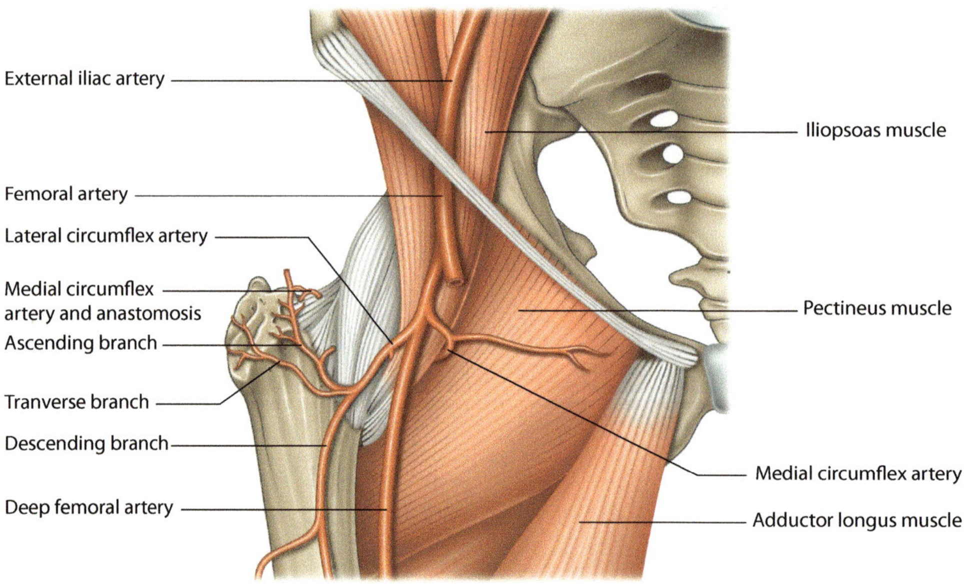

Fig. 10.8 Medial circumflex artery.

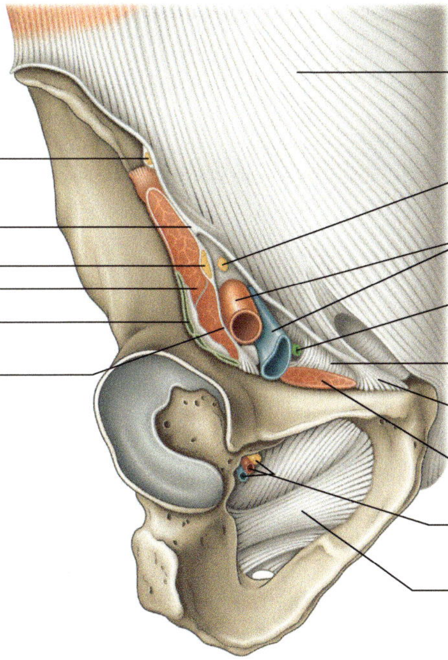

Fig. 10.10 Inguinal ligament and iliopectineal arch.

Vascular lacuna

This compartment is bounded by the inguinal ligament, the lacunar ligament, and the iliopectineal arch. This space comprises (laterally to medially):

- the femoral branch of the genitofemoral nerve;
- the femoral artery;
- the femoral vein;
- the Rosenmüller lymph node, which is important to palpate whenever there is any suspicion that pain might not be of mechanical origin.

Muscular lacuna

This more lateral compartment is located between the pelvic bone and the iliopectineal arch. Through it passes the iliopsoas muscle, femoral nerve, and lateral femoral cutaneous nerve.

Special note

The iliopectineal serous bursa lies beneath the iliopsoas muscle. The largest serous bursa of the hip, it sometimes communicates with the coxofemoral joint. Pay attention to avoid irritating it with any type of compression.

10.2.2 Technique in lateral decubitus (Fig. 10.11)

The patient lies on the side opposite the treatment hip, leg flexed, top knee resting on the table behind the other leg. Position yourself behind the patient and accentuate the pelvic concavity using your thorax to push the pelvis medially.

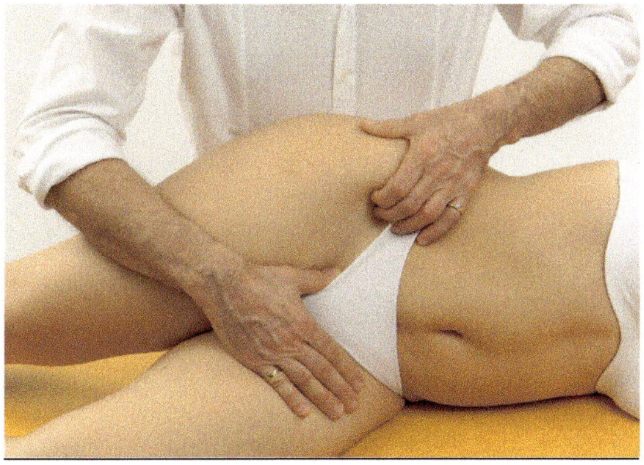

Fig. 10.11 Inguinal ligament and iliopectineal arch in lateral decubitus.

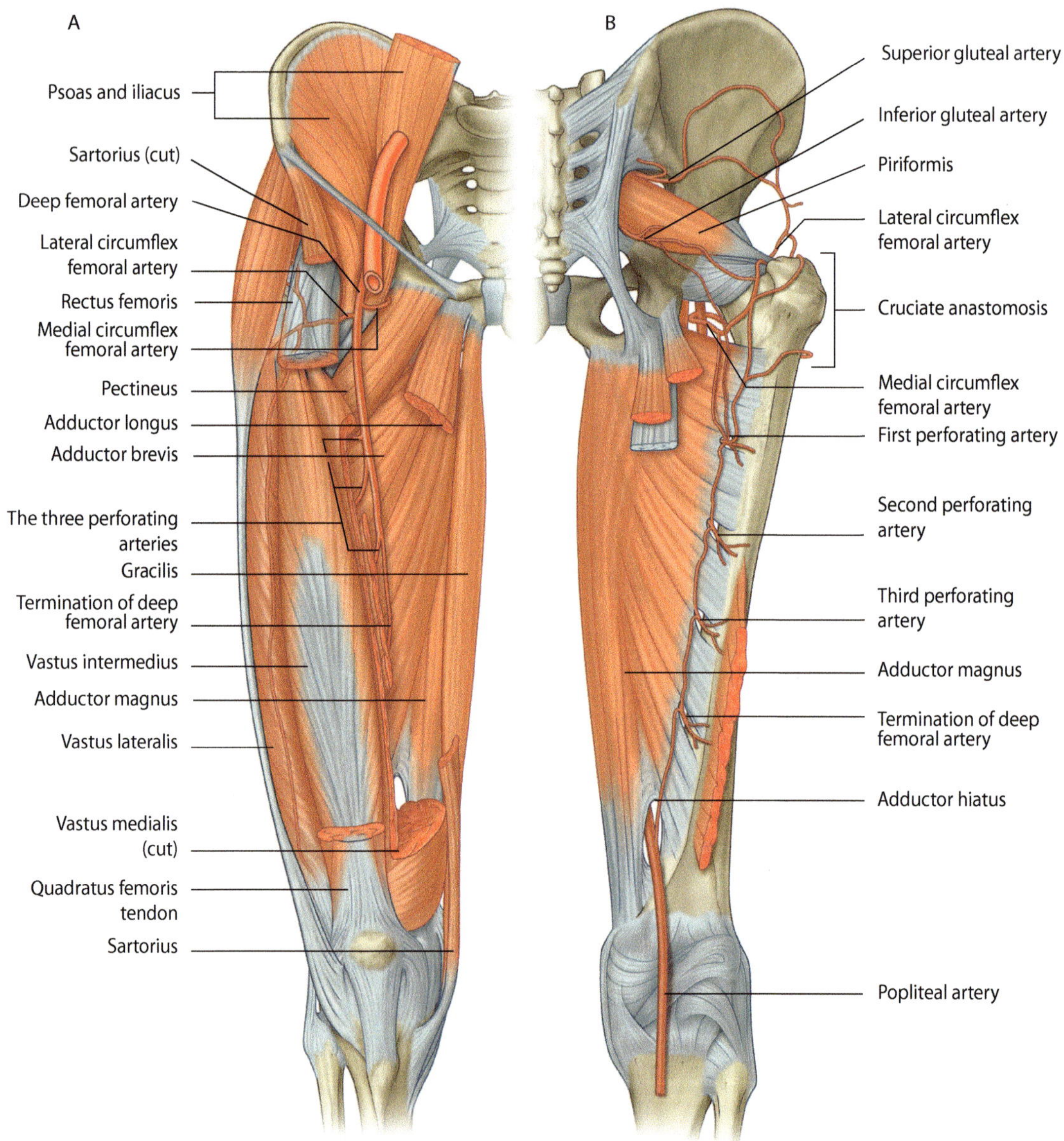

Fig. 10.12 Linea aspera of the femur.

Inguinal ligament

Place your fingers and thumb along the inguinal ligament between the anterior superior iliac spine and the pubic tubercle to tighten or slacken directly in the transverse and longitudinal directions. Finish with a progressive induction maneuver.

Iliopectineal arch

Glide your fingers along the inguinal ligament beginning at the anterior superior iliac spine. You will meet a perpendicular resistance, something firm against your fingers. This is the iliopectineal arch. Gently draw the arch laterally and craniocaudally several times. Allow your fingers to be attracted in the direction of the listening, and work the ligament in induction.

Remark

This manipulation has a neurovascular purpose. It is the first step in releasing the femoral artery and vein from fascial constraint. As with all our arterial and neural techniques, you must scrupulously avoid overcompressing the structures. It is by stretch and elongation that you release them.

10.3 LINEA ASPERA OF THE FEMUR

The linea aspera is a convergence point for the adductor muscles. These muscles of the medial thigh compartment are intimately linked to the circulatory function of the hip, and they continue to the entire lower extremity. The linea aspera is a remarkable site to treat in order to improve blood flow to the hip and leg.

10.3.1 Review—topographical landmarks

To simplify the anatomy, the linea aspera can be divided into medial and lateral parts to which the muscles of the lower extremity and pelvis attach (Fig. 10.12).

- To the lateral surface
  - Vastus medialis
  - Gluteus maximus, medially and cranially
  - Biceps femoris (short head) caudally
- To the medial surface
  - Adductor magnus that separates into medial and lateral attachments
  - Vastus medialis
  - Adductor longus and brevis

10.3.2 Technique

In the knee section you will find another technique aimed at freeing the femoral artery as it passes under the distal femoral insertion of adductor magnus (see "palpation of the hiatus" in chapter 19). We use the same approach to affect branches of the perforating artery as they perforate the tendon

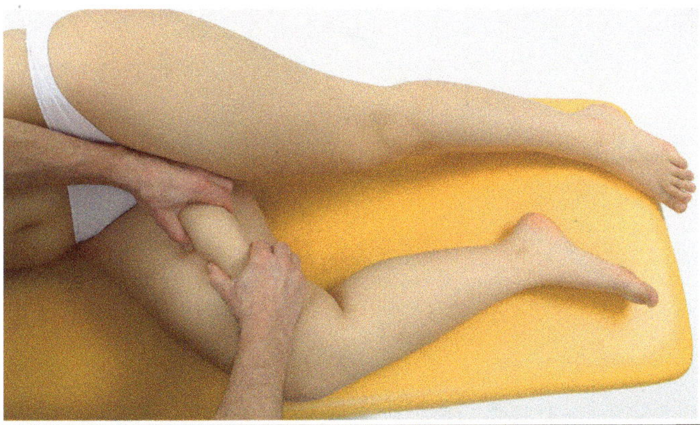

Fig. 10.13 Vascular manipulation on the linea aspera.

of the adductor magnus to reach the back of the thigh. This technique benefits both the hip and the knee.

In lateral decubitus (Fig. 10.13)

The patient lies on the side of the lower extremity to be treated. Position yourself facing the patient. For the medial muscle insertions, place your thumbs on the medial surface of the thigh as close to the bone as possible, while your fingers grasp the most prominent part of the adductors. While your fingers draw the adductor muscle mass medially, your thumbs stretch the femoral muscle insertions laterally. It is as if you want to drag the insertion away from the femur.

To treat the lateral insertions, use your laterally and posteriorly placed fingers to lift off and "detach" the adductor muscular insertions at the femur; direct them medially. Search along the linea aspera for areas that are more stuck down or that feel fibrotic in any way. At the end, perform a lifting induction and maintain the detachment for 12 seconds.

Comment: Adductors

We are all familiar with the primary action of the adductor muscles, which is to squeeze the thighs together. Adductors are hip flexors when the hip is in extension, and they act as extensors when the hip is in flexion. These muscles also balance the pelvis by controlling pelvic rotation on the femoral heads. They provide sexual protection; in fact, they were once whimsically termed custodes virginitatis, "guardians of virginity." The adductors are vital to the vascular system because venous drainage occurs along the linea aspera. Anterior and posterior venous channels meet across the adductors in the thigh. Alternating muscle contraction and relaxation, compress and decompress the veins, somewhat like a sponge that you might squeeze and release. Balanced adductor tensions guarantee good venous circulation in the lower extremities. Ficat et al. (1987) noted that the venous capacity of the hip is six to eight times greater than arterial flow. This is the main reason we encourage you to release the adductor muscles, including where they affix at the linea aspera.

The emotional hip

11

Many people, the majority of them women, suffer from degenerative osteoarthritis of the coxofemoral joint. We have studied the most commonly associated behavioral and psychoemotional features and have highlighted the principle traits.

We have witnessed remarkable postural and emotional changes in patients following hip surgery. While a new hip in no way alters a person's fundamental nature, it can truly transform certain behaviors.

After studying many hundreds of patients, we have compiled a list of psychological components and behaviors that seem to associate specifically with hip degeneration. Feeling the need for, or loss of, stability emerges as a key feature of "hip replacement" people. We offer a case example below.

The hip tends to represent:

- anchorage to the ground or to people;
- need for roots and foundations;
- territorial stability;
- need of attachment;
- defined boundaries;
- belonging to a group;
- familiar landmarks;
- geographical and psychological territory;
- urge for geographical and emotional stability—hip people require their inner circle, their little world, around them;
- familial attachment;
- need to return to their origins;
- dread of change;
- trepidation in altering routine or moving households;
- fear of novelty;
- sense of practicality;
- the concrete;
- constancy;
- determination, even stubbornness;
- need for constant reassurance;
- link to tradition, the past;
- timidity (when out of their environment);
- emotional withdrawal;
- suspicion;
- need for family connection;
- loyalty;
- helping others.

The Swiss have a saying that aptly describes "hip" people: "The church must be at the center of the village." "Hip" people feel at their best and most confident in their own little worlds. They become mistrustful and quite reserved whenever they must be away from their familiar surroundings.

11.1 A POST–SURGICAL TRANSFORMATION

One particular patient had a great need for secure territorial landmarks. Her life was a good illustration of the dictum: "The church must be at the center of the village." She required her family and friends to be around her, and she felt the need to visit them often.

Little by little she developed arthritis in her hip, which impeded her walking any great distance. Geographical confinement closed her off psychologically, as well. She loved to be of service, but she gradually became sour and grumpy to the point of becoming unrecognizable, to the detriment of her relationships.

Once coxarthroses was diagnosed, she underwent successful hip surgery. She reverted to her former self and returned to visiting and being of service to others. She regained her jovial temperament.

While this story is rather extreme, we can nevertheless vouch for similar, more subtle psychological changes that have occurred after applying manual therapy techniques described in this book.

Once the messages of the body become positive, our psychological attitudes and behavior often follow suit. On the other hand, when the brain receives negative messages from the body, it "negates" all information it receives and sends out.

3
The Knee

Functional anatomy

12

The knee is a paradoxical joint. On one hand its bones are massive and solid, giving it a sturdy build. On the other hand it is relatively weak mechanically because of the somewhat incongruent nature of its articular surfaces.

Few high-performance athletes have escaped ligamentous knee injury. While this joint has finally adapted itself to erect posture, it is easily susceptible to trauma that can endure a long time if the joint is ever pushed beyond its natural limits.

The knee relies on a rich and effective proprioceptive system to compensate for any frailty in its makeup. Proprioception is provided by muscles—more exactly, tendons—that surround the knee, allowing it to defend itself through subtle adjustments and enabling it to withstand the multiple aggressions to which it is victim.

12.1 ANATOMICAL REVIEW

12.1.1 Bones and joint surfaces

The knee joint consists of two articulations: one between the femur and the tibia and one between the femur and the patella.

Femorotibial joint

The femorotibial joint joins the distal femur and proximal tibia. This bicondylar junction has a medial and lateral compartment. Two menisci further subdivide the joint spaces at the periphery:

- The meniscofemoral is between the femoral condyle and the proximal surface of the meniscus.
- The meniscotibial is between the distal surface of the meniscus and the proximal surface of the tibial condyle.

Femoropatellar articulation

This joint unites the anterior surface of the caudal end of the femur with the posterior surface of the patella. The patella is a sesamoid bone that plays a role in knee extension. As such it operates under strong constraint and compression. The femur, tibia, and patella are surrounded by a single synovial membrane. While the proximal tibiofibular joint is anatomically part of the knee, this articulation belongs functionally to the ankle (Fig. 12.1). (This will be covered further in the ankle section.)

12.1.2 Articular capsule

Like all joint capsules, this synovial and fibrous structure is important to proprioception. To stay mobile and avoid being folded, the capsule is retracted by the articular muscle of the knee, otherwise known as the subcrural muscle. The capsule is wide, lax, and reinforced by ligaments.

Form (Fig. 12.2)

"The general shape of the knee capsule can be easily understood if you compare it to a cylinder whose posterior surface is misshapen by depression" (Kapandji 1991).

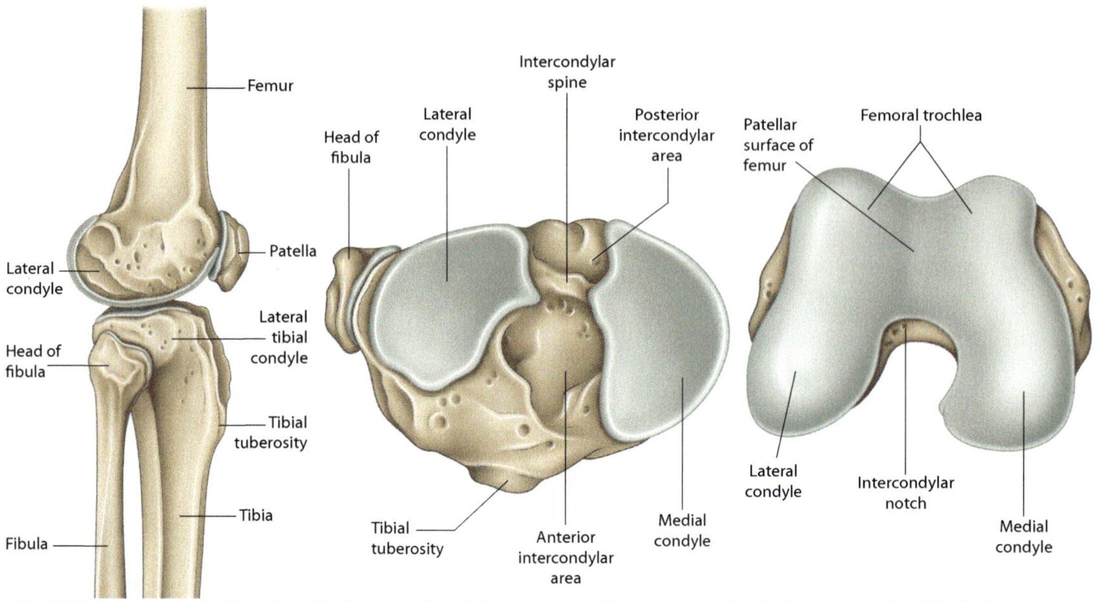

Fig. 12.1 Articular surface of the knee.

Insertions (Fig. 12.3)

On the femur

- The anterior surface
- The posterior surface
- Lateral borders of the condyles

On the patella

- The perimeter of the cartilage, except where it is separated from the synovial membrane, leaves the apex free.
- As a sesamoid bone, the patella is continuous with the fibrous capsule.

On the tibia

- The condylar perimeters

On the menisci

- The capsule adheres to their peripheral surfaces.

On the collateral ligaments

- The medial collateral ligament is intricately linked with the capsule.
- The lateral collateral ligament does not exchange fibers with the lateral surface of the capsule.

Features

The capsule is lax sagittally and more taut laterally. It forms a subquadricipital cul-de-sac, where it is put under tension by the articular muscle of the knee.

Functions

The capsule needs to be under tension to:

- perform its proprioceptive role;
- distribute synovial fluid;
- accommodate the extremes of flexion and extension.

Curiously, several surgeons we interviewed attributed little or no importance to preventing capsular folds. Palpation of the functional knee is, of course, in no way similar to that of a knee receiving surgery, be it open or arthroscopic. The capsule forms a suprameniscal fold laterally called the "capsular ramp." The capsule is reinforced posteriorly by fibers from the gastrocnemius muscle that form posterior thickenings behind the femoral condyles (Fig. 12.4).

Capsular tensors and strengtheners

- In front by the articular muscle of the knee (subcrural muscle)
- Behind by the popliteal, biceps femoris, and gastrocnemius
- Anterior laterally by an expansion from the iliotibial band

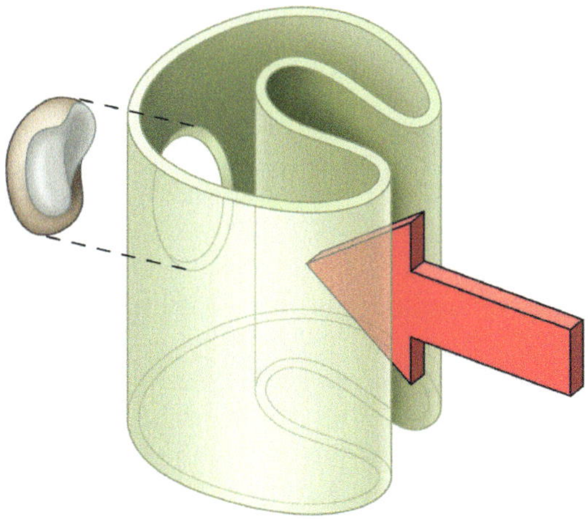

Fig. 12.2 General form of the knee capsule.

- Posterior medially by fibers from semimembranosus that create the oblique popliteal ligament

12.1.3 Ligaments

The articular ligaments are the cruciate, collateral, and capsular bands.

Cruciate ligaments

The cruciate ligaments are identified by the way they cross over each other like an X. The cruciate ligaments control shearing motion and guide flexion and extension.

Anterior cruciate ligament

This ligament arises from the anterior intercondylar area, within the notch of the distal femur, and extends superiorly, posteriorly, and laterally toward the lateral femoral condyle. The insertions and direction of the anterior cruciate ligament help to stabilize the knee in extension, preventing hyperextension of the joint.

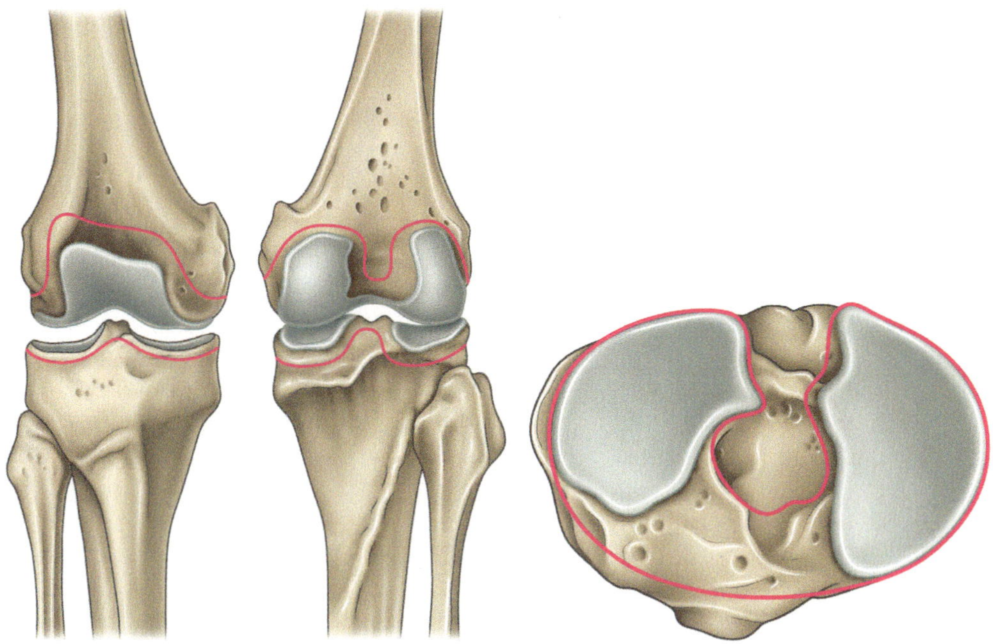

Fig. 12.3 Capsular insertions of the knee.

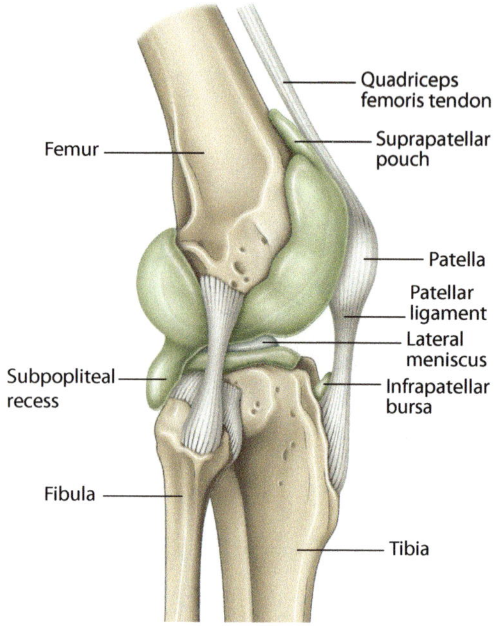

Fig. 12.4 Capsular cul-de-sac and folds.

Posterior cruciate ligament

This ligament arises from the posterior intercondylar area of the tibia and runs superiorly, anteriorly, proximally, and medially to the medial condyle of the femur. The posterior cruciate ligament prevents excessive medial rotation of the tibia on the femur.

Collateral ligaments

Collateral ligaments control sideways motion of the knee.

Medial collateral ligament

This ligament divides into two planes:

- The deep plane has anterior, middle, and posterior fibers that attach to the capsule and the medial meniscus.
- The superficial ligament extends from the medial femoral condyle proximally to the medial border of the tibia distally.

Lateral collateral ligament

This band stretches from the tuberosity of the lateral femoral condyle to the head of the fibula. Its inferior lateral surface is covered by the biceps tendon. It is separated from the lateral surface of the capsule by the popliteal muscle that runs deeply to it.

12.1.4 Special features

Fabella

The fabella is an inconsistent sesamoid bone located behind the knee. When it is absent, one finds capsular thickening in the form of a fibrous nodule in its place. The fabella is located just above the tibiofemoral joint line and articulates with the lateral femoral condyle. The popliteal tendon passes by caudally.

Popliteal tendon

This tendon passes through a hiatus on the posterior lateral capsule of which it is a part.

Condylar shells

Condylar shells are thickenings of the posterior capsule. The two shells separate to allow passage to the posterior cruciate ligament. The medial condylar shell sometimes opens to the extent that it communicates with the synovial membrane.

Synovial membrane

The anterior part of the synovial membrane and the capsule form small folds or "plicatas" that can stick together after trauma or surgery. These capsular cul-de-sacs catch between the femur and the kneecap.

Cruciate ligament sheathes

A synovial membrane fold ensheathes the cruciate ligaments in the intercondylar fossa, separating them from the joint cavity.

12.1.5 Muscles

The knee is a powerful and stable joint, thanks to the strength and action of long muscles that cross the joint. Superior insertions are situated on the pelvis or the femoral shaft. Distal insertions are distal to the knee or on the foot. Muscles pertaining to the knee are classified into four groups: the anterior, posterior, lateral, and medial.

The anterior group includes the extensors represented by the quadriceps or four-headed muscle. These extensors are the vastus medialis, vastus lateralis, and vastus intermedius that arise from the femur. Rectus femoris is a polyarticular muscle that acts on the hip.

The posterior group includes the flexors at the back of the thigh that both flex and rotate the knee. The medial set contains semimembranosus and semitendinosus muscles that inwardly rotate the lower leg on the femur when the knee is flexed.

The lateral group is composed of the powerful biceps femoris. Both heads of the biceps femoris rotate the knee slightly outwardly when the joint is flexed. The medial and lateral gastrocnemius muscles are also in this group. They are considered knee flexors during open kinetic chain exercises; they are extensors when the foot is on the ground and the leg is weight bearing. The lateral group includes the abductors whose main action is to stabilize the lateral knee against bowleg. The iliotibial tract is connected to the hip abductors, specifically the gluteus maximus and the tensor fasciae latae.

The medial group of knee muscles includes the muscles whose tendons elongate on the tibia like the foot of a goose. These muscles are the semitendinosus, gracilis, and sartorius. Their main action is to prevent valgus strain on the knee (knock knee) and protect the medial collateral ligament.

12.2 JOINT PHYSIOLOGY

The knee joint is the largest and most complicated synovial joint in the body. It is constantly dealing with conflicting imperatives: stability and mobility.

12.2.1 Mobility

Knee movement is customarily described as flexion-extension together with a measure of rotation.

Rotation and gliding

In the sagittal section, the anterior-posterior length of the tibial plateau is much smaller than the arc of the femoral condyles. Instead of a purely rolling motion in flexion, the femur slides anteriorly at the same time as it rolls posteriorly, keeping it from rolling off the back of the tibia. Hinging at the knee is not the simple action it appears to be at first glance. Flexion-extension involves small amounts of obligatory rotation as well as slide between femoral and tibial surfaces.

Ligament arrangement

The capsuloligamentous system plays a pivotal role in femoral tibial kinematics. Condylar rotation and glide is a product of the way ligaments are arranged to regulate movement possibilities.

Ligaments stabilize the knee by controlling:

- lateral and medial flexion in the frontal plane;
- anterior and posterior translation in the sagittal plane;
- medial and lateral rotation in the horizontal plane.

In extension

- All ligaments are fully taut, and the knee is perfectly stable as a consequence.

In flexion

- The posterior cruciate ligament tightens, irrespective of the degree of rotation. This is why there is no abnormal backward pull in knee flexion.
- The medial collateral ligament remains taut, which is why there is no laxity of the medial compartment of the knee in flexion.
- The lateral collateral ligament relaxes, producing physiological laxity of the lateral compartment when the knee is flexed.
- The anterior cruciate ligament is somewhat slack because its insertion on

the external condyle is located slightly behind the axis of knee flexion and extension. A slight forward sliding occurs when the knee is in flexion.

Flexion and lateral rotation

When lateral tibial rotation is added to the flexed knee, the medial collateral ligament tightens, as does the lateral collateral ligament. At the same time, the anterior cruciate ligament slackens off. This setup makes it easy to understand that a forced twisting of the knee during lateral rotation overstretches the lateral and medial ligaments first; it strains the anterior cruciate ligament secondarily.

Flexion and medial rotation

When medial tibial rotation is transmitted to the flexed knee, the lateral collateral ligament slackens off, whereas the anterior cruciate ligament tightens. In this scenario a knee sprained during medial rotation impacts the anterior cruciate ligament first.

Knee kinematics

The medial and lateral tibiofemoral compartments of the knee joint have differential motions. Each femoral condyle has a different curvature radius. In the sagittal plane, the tibial glenoid cavity of the medial compartment is concave, and the medial meniscus is not very mobile. Condylar displacement is minimal. In the sagittal plane, the tibial glenoid cavity of the lateral compartment appears convex, and the lateral meniscus is quite mobile. Condylar displacement is considerable.

Automatic rotation

Taken together these factors produce automatic rotation:

- Flexion is accompanied by medial rotation of the tibia on the femur.
- Extension occurs conjointly with lateral rotation of the tibia on the femur.

12.2.2 Stability

Unfavorable conditions

The knee joint operates under tremendous mechanical demand. Working conditions at the knee are clearly worse than at the hip:

- Knee joint surfaces are incongruent.
- The joint is very superficial and is not enclosed by a thick muscular sleeve as is the hip.
- The motor muscle tendons terminate close to the center of joint movement, which reduces torque and stabilizing ability.

"There is no other joint in the human body on which locomotion imposes a heavier load or puts more to the test. The construction of a joint, as exposed to mechanical stress with so little security provision, has surely been a tall order, even for the ingenuity of nature (Steindler 1995).

Enormous loads

Considerable compression forces are imposed on the joint surfaces of the knee with every step and strain generated by the lower extremity. The knee supports tremendous load during everyday activities:

- ascending stairs: 4.4 times body weight;
- descending stairs: 6 times body weight, or 30% more than stair climbing.

When even modest load forces are added, it is easy to see how some professional athletic activities are more damaging than others. The knee is not made to withstand heavy loads for long. Synovitis often results from overload.

Solutions

Ligamentous system

As the knee cannot be entirely stabilized by the powerful periarticular muscles, a complex arrangement of ligaments counters significant biomechanical demand in two ways:

- Passive stabilization is provided by strong capsuloligamentous connective tissue fibers.
- Active stabilization is provided by motor control muscles, particularly the powerful extensors. Muscle tone is regulated as a function of information provided by the ligament system, which is very well equipped with mechanoreceptors.

Muscle activity

Muscles are what give the knee power and sturdiness. Under physiological conditions, muscle actions are protective of the ligament system.

Menisci

Boney architecture contributes very little to knee stability and joint integrity. Joint surfaces make contact at only a few points. Menisci help to keep the knees steady by filling in the gaps. The knee is provided with medial and lateral menisci in the form of triangular fibrocartilages wedged between the tibia and the fibula.

Stabilizers

The crescent-shaped discs contribute to passive stability by their physical presence.

Fluid mobilizers

The meniscus can be pictured like a brush that distributes and mixes lubricating synovial fluid film at the interior of the knee.

Movement guides

Menisci can also be considered as joints guiding the motion of the femur on the tibia. They protect the flexed knee from excessive tensional forces. This is particularly important in the medial compartment, where the posterior horn of the medial meniscus resists lateral rotation of the tibia.

Cushioning and pressure distribution

When the knee is extended, the menisci spread load by increasing congruity of the articulation. In their absence, joint surfaces become vulnerable to intolerable strain peaks. This phenomenon is more marked on the lateral side of the knee. Pressure distribution requires that the meniscus be under proper tension (Fig. 12.5).

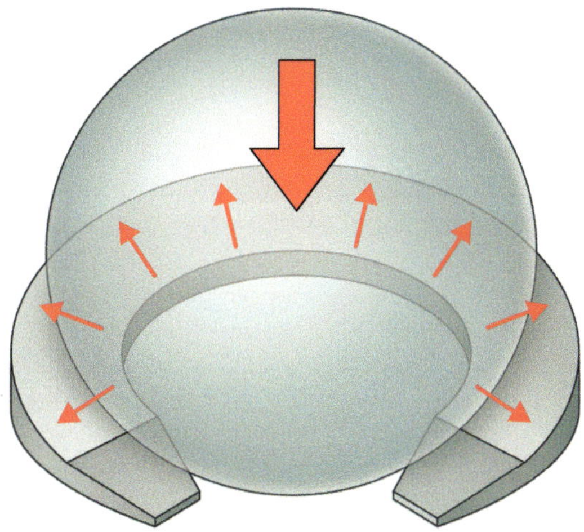

Fig. 12.5 Meniscal pressure distribution.

Peripheral knee defenses

Various capsuloligamentous elements are organized into a structural and coherent unit that constitutes peripheral knee defense (Kapandji 2011).

Three principle structures

Peripheral knee defense is provided by three main elements:
- tibial collateral ligament;
- fibular collateral ligament;
- posterior capsulofibrous complex.

Four accessory formations

There are four fibrotendinous nappes of unequal strength and importance.

Posterior medial fibrotendinous nappe

This is the most important sheet, sometimes referred to as the posterior lateral angle, although the concept is more surgical than anatomical.

This posterior medial fibrotendinous nappe

lies behind the tibial collateral ligament constituted by:

- the most posterior fibers of the tibial collateral ligament;
- the medial border of the medial condylar shell;
- two expansions of the semimembranosus tendon:
  - the reflected tendon that extends across the medial infraglenoid margin;
  - the meniscal expansion that affixes on the posterior periphery of the medial meniscus.

Posterior lateral fibrotendinous nappe

This formation is distinctly less powerful than its medial counterpart. Here the lateral meniscus is separated from the capsule and the fibular collateral ligament to allow passage of the popliteal tendon that attaches to the lateral condyle. This tendon sends a meniscal expansion that anchors to the posterior part of the lateral meniscus. The fibrous reinforcement is completed by the short fibular collateral ligament that constitutes the lateral pillar of the arched popliteal ligament and the lateral border of the lateral condylar shell.

Anterior lateral nappe

This sheet is formed by the iliotibial tract that sends an expansion to the lateral border of the patella. Direct and cruciate expansions of the quadricipital tendon contribute to it.

Anterior medial nappe

The anterior medial fibrotendinous formation is constituted by the direct and cruciate expansions of the quadricipital tendon, reinforced by the expansion of the sartorius muscle tendon that attaches to the medial border of the patella.

Muscle balance

In the sagittal plane

The quadriceps and gastrocnemius work together to give the knee balanced stability.

In the frontal plane

Medially, the knee is stabilized by the semimembranosus together with the muscles of the superficial goose's foot: the sartorius, gracilis, and semitendinosus. This arrangement counters valgus stress that might injure the medial collateral ligament.

From the lateral side, the iliotibial band can be considered the terminal tendon of the gluteal deltoid. It provides dynamic stability of the lateral compartment and counters varus tendencies.

On the posterior lateral side are two muscles:

- popliteus, whose actions are very peculiar;
- biceps femoris, whose powerful tendon attaches to the fibular head, doubling up the fibular collateral ligament.

On the transverse plane

The obliquity of the patellar tendon (biggest tendon in the body) protects the knee from transverse movement by locking the joint in extension.

Knee locking

Among knee muscles, the quadriceps is certainly the largest. Knee stability would not exist without it. Muscle power and coordination possibilities allow the knee to compensate for even major ligamentous breakdown. Quadriceps contraction provides the knee-locking mechanism that is essential to standing.

On this note, remember that both the semimembranosus, through its connections with the medial meniscus, and the tibial collateral ligament play influential proprioceptive roles.

Knee extension

In extension, the knee has good stability in the frontal and sagittal planes, thanks to tightened ligaments on either side (medial and lateral collaterals) and in the center (anterior and posterior cruciates). As the central line of gravity falls in front of the joint, however, there is a natural tendency for the knee to hyperextend. This action puts tension on the condylar shells that are supposed to stabilize the knee passively in the sagittal plane.

Patellar alignment

The patellar tendon is oblique caudally, laterally, and posteriorly. Quadriceps contraction pulls the knee into extension and draws the tibia anteriorly. The "Q," or quadriceps angle, represents the pull of the quadriceps relative to the axis of the patellar tendon.

Tracking of the patella through the femoral trochlea occurs because:

- the patellar tendon is oblique;
- the patella placement raises the patellar tendon off the end of the femur, increasing the lever arm of the quadriceps;
- transverse fibers of vastus medialis and rectus femoris are located more caudally than laterally.

Note that the patellar tendon is situated more laterally in women. About 75% of patellar syndromes afflict females.

12.2.3 Sensory motor function

Knee stability: a postural kinetic activity

The knee joint is capable of instantaneously analyzing masses of proprioceptive data that reach it, and all without relaxing for a second. The anatomical elements that constitute its peripheral defense system are very rich in mechanoreceptors. They function as veritable strain gauges.

All mechanical stretch demands made by posture or movement stimulate proprioceptive receptors to relay information to the brain. In return, the central nervous system modifies muscle contractions that assist the peripheral defenses of the knee, providing indispensable help to the ligaments and passive structures.

Joint receptors

Mechanoreceptors and free nerve endings are located in various joint structures. Their goal is to provide sensory information to the central nervous system as to relative joint angle, rates of movement, and mechanical stresses acting on joints (Fox et al. 1984).

The number of joint receptors at the knee have been particularly well researched. Numerous studies confirm their presence, particularly in the anterior cruciate ligament and the medial meniscus. Located here are the classic mechanorecepors: Pacini and Raffini corpuscles, Golgi tendon organs, and free nerve endings. These mechanoreceptors fall into two divisions: rapid acting and slow acting.

Rapidly adapting receptors

These receptors are best at adapting to rapidly changing signals. Pacini corpuscles are part of this group and are usually located in accessory joint tissues. After a stimulus appears, even if it is long-lasting, influx is decreased and extinguished in a few milliseconds. Their main function is the detection of sudden movements, acceleration at the start of a movement, or deceleration at the end of a movement.

Slowly adapting receptors

These receptors are best at detecting long, continuous signals. They continue to provide awareness as long as a stimulus is present. Ruffini corpuscles and Golgi tendon organs are in this category. Ligaments and joint capsules are the domain of Ruffini corpuscles. They are best at detecting slow movement, and they provide instantaneous signals about joint position.

Sensory pathways

Direct neurofibers link mechanoreceptors to spinal ganglions and posterior spinal nerve roots. This proprioceptive data is conducted along myelinated axons that have an elevated conduction speed.

Bipolar information

Stimuli collected by joint receptors have two main functions: protection and information.

Protection

Proprioceptive awareness is important for every joint in the body. The innate sense of the relationship of body parts with one another via sensory input protects the joints. The joint unit must maintain cohesion and harmonious interplay in the midst of the various disturbances that the body might be subject to as a whole.

Information

General sensory information is gathered from the body and reaches the central nervous system by way of conscious sensory pathways. Somatosensory impulses are transmitted to the cerebral cortex to be analyzed and integrated. Data is memorized in the part of the brain attributed to the perceived part of the body. The mapping of body surfaces in the brain plays a fundamental role in the creation of body image and participates in the control of muscle tone and movements. With this information, voluntary motor activity can be initiated.

Motor control

Once reaching the medulla, information coming from the joint receptors can be exploited in several ways for the protection of the joint.

Short loop

Segmentary reflexes intervene at the medulla, between the sensory neurofibers and motor neurons.

Long loop

Polysynaptic reflexes are integrated at the suprasegmentary level, which is to say higher up in the central nervous system. At this level, input gathered from joint muscles, ligaments, and tendons is integrated together with information from other sources. All serve to inform the central nervous system about the position of the body in space and balance.

Proprioceptors and visual and vestibular senses all play a part in posture regulation.

12.2.4 Dynamic knee stability

The knee is a singular joint in so many ways. All therapists are keenly aware that the knee is complicated! Added to structural complication is functional complexity. This is why it takes so much time before a therapist achieves a decent percentage of good results with knee problems. One must learn to respect the knee. It is very susceptible and reacts immediately with pain and inflammation to any maneuver that is the least bit disrespectful of its complicated physiology.

In the ensuing paragraphs we look at knee sensitivity in the context of local mechanics that guided us to a new understanding of knee joint dysfunction.

The regulatory effect of joint sensitivity

A great deal has been written about the importance of joint sensitivity in terms of posturomotor regulation and the execution of knee movement. In effect, depending on the loop involved, it is only a matter of milliseconds once afferent influx reaches the central nervous system that motor impulses are generated for the protection of joints or posture. It is through this regulatory motor system, based on information acquired from peripheral receptors, that muscles counter joint distortion through perfectly synchronized contractions.

Muscle action is sometimes coordinated to provide for constraints anticipated by the cerebral cortex. All of this can only happen, however, on the condition that afferent messages are not erroneous and that they reach the CNS in a timely manner. Any disturbance or delay can cause maladapted protective muscle responses that leave the joint overexposed, with serious consequences for the ligament system.

A triple envelope of movement

J. David Blaha and Edward Wojtys (2006) developed an interesting concept of knee kinematics. In their model, ligaments are not first in line when it comes to providing joint stability. This runs a little against prevailing kinematics and classic biomechanics.

Their concept revisits the notion of the functional envelope (Dye 2008) based on load levels tolerable to a joint or to the musculoskeletal system. When the load quantity exceeds load tolerance, the joint's self-regulatory limit is breached and homeostasis is threatened.

The authors consider the knee to have three movement envelopes, as depicted in Fig. 12.6:

- The central part, in green, represents the sector where the knee moves without external constraint. For example, in open chain movement, knee mobility remains within this envelope.
- With the application of external forces, such as when the foot meets the ground, knee movement occurs in the next envelope corresponding to neuromuscular control. Within these limits, joint surfaces can glide, roll, rotate, or translate to accomplish joint movements. This movement envelope is governed by neuromuscular control, in which the cruciate ligaments play a determinant role as system informers. Neuromuscular reaction depends on the information provided by imbedded mechanoreceptors sensing mechanical pressure or distortion.
- Once the limits of the neuromuscular envelope have been reached, the cruciate ligaments come truly into play as "brake" ligaments. Their intrinsic toughness prevents further displacement of joint surfaces. At this juncture, any additional forces can lead to rupture of the cruciate ligaments. Within this last envelope, ligamentous lesions affect flexion, valgus, and lateral rotation, along with extension, varus, and medial rotation.

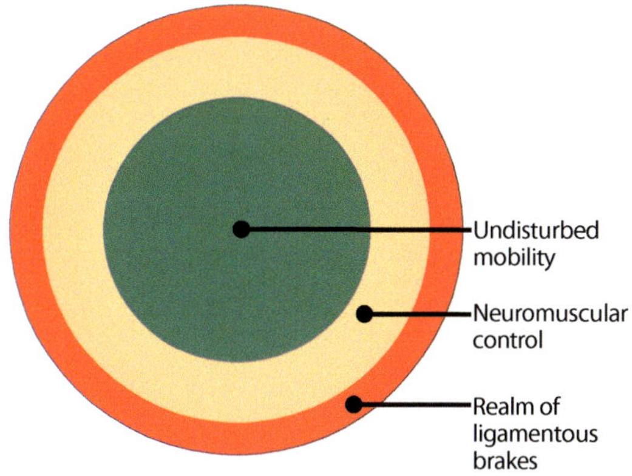

Fig. 12.6 The triple envelope of knee movement.

The patient and surgical reality

Patients very often complain of knee instability and are quick to tell you that their knee feels "loose." Surgeons only recognize objective instability, however, where abnormal movement tests reveal a ruptured ligament.

The triple envelope concept allows us to understand that what the patient experiences is often at odds with surgical interpretation because the two parties are not looking at the same envelope of limitation.

For the surgeon, the exam must allow him to decide whether surgery is warranted or not. In this conundrum, ligament rupture is a valid criterion for operation. On the other hand, what the patient undoubtedly experiences are the effects of defective neuromuscular control. Interaction between nerves and muscles can go wrong simply because of a distorted sense of position and movement. This imperfection can be the product of simple ligament scarring (following a sprain for example), capsular tension, or abnormal meniscal strain. In cases where surgery is of no help, our manipulative approach is very much indicated.

Our approach to the knee

Our knee techniques are able to detect fixations and mechanical problems of the structures that defend the knee. Even mild imbalances in tissues richly endowed with mechanoreceptors can distort joint information, changing the nature of knee movement. Dysfunctional nerves can produce the same result by slowing down or warping proprioceptive influx. Precise, well-executed manual techniques applied to key proprioceptive structures can often remedy the situation.

In our experience, the techniques presented in the next chapter optimize sensory motor control of the knee. They improve the homeostatic load envelope, to use Dye's terminology.

Elements of diagnosis

13

13.1 KNEE EXAMINATION

13.1.1 Knee morphotypes (Fig. 13.1)

The joint is examined while the patient is standing, knees straight, patellas facing forward. There are three morphotypic variations:

- normal axis knee, where the medial malleoli and the femoral condyles touch;
- varum knee, where a separation is located between the femoral condyles;
- valgum knee, where the medial malleoli are some distance apart.

These gaps can be measured by intercondylar or intermalleolar distances in either

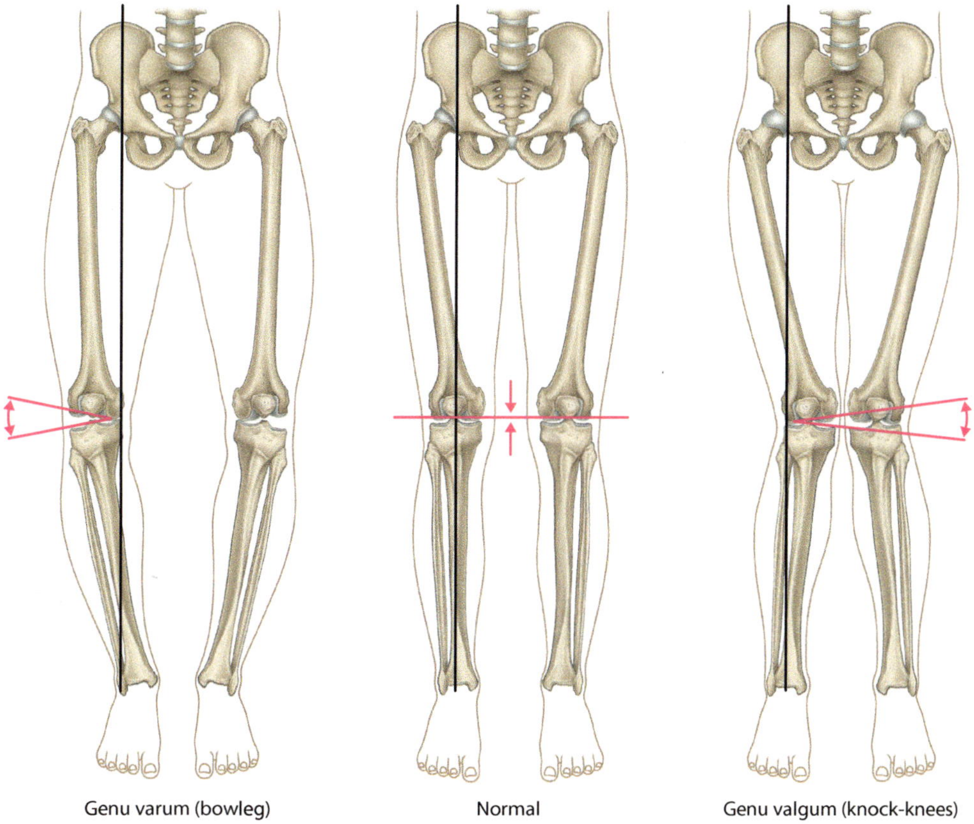

Fig. 13.1 Morphological knee types.

centimeters or finger widths. Hyperextension tends to exaggerate genu varum.

Note: Normal axis does not mean normal. A genu varum is not in itself pathological any more than a genu valgrum is defective. Morphotype simply gives you an idea of knee function and shows joint compartments that are naturally under more constraint. Knee morphotype is evaluated while the patient is standing, but it is interesting to note if it changes in non-weight-bearing.

13.1.2 Amyotrophy

While the subject is on his feet, take the opportunity to evaluate muscle tone in the standing position. Any amyotrophy of the quadriceps shows up as atrophy of vastus medialis. Examine vastus medialis to assess all the quadriceps muscles indirectly. Wasting quadriceps testifies to limited knee use. It can be quantified by measuring thigh perimeter.

13.1.3 Other elements of inspection

Take a moment to look for hematoma, signs of intra-articular swelling, and scars.

13.2 KNEE PALPATION

13.2.1 Principle boney landmarks

Femoral condyles

- Medial condyle: The anterior three-quarters of this bone is readily accessible just beneath the skin. One can clearly follow the anterior and distal borders. A little deeper, the powerful adductor magnus inserts on the posterior medial condyle at the adductor magnus tubercle.
- Lateral condyle: The anterior and inferior borders are less prominent. Posteriorly, however, the lateral tuberosity is more apparent. It gives the proximal insertion of the lateral collateral ligament.

Tibial condyles

The proximal ephiphysis of the tibia is large and very broad transversely. The tibial plateau or superior articular surface forms two glenoid cavities. The following structures are easily accessible:

- the tibial tuberosity;
- the tibial crest;
- the medial tuberosity or medial condyle;
- the lateral tuberosity or lateral condyle.

Gerdy's tubercle or the infracondylar tubercle

This bump is palpable with the knee flexed. Landmark it using a finger width above the middle of a line joining the tibial tuberosity and the head of the fibula. Place your middle finger on the tibial tuberosity and your thumb on the fibular head. Your index finger will automatically land on Gerdy's tubercle.

The other way to find it is to trace a line between the summit of the patella and the fibular head. Gerdy's tubercle is located midway along this line. The tubercle is generally found a finger width below the femoral tibial joint line.

Fibular head

This bone protrudes with the knee flexed and the leg internally rotated.

Patella

The patella is easily mobilized in extension where the quadriceps are relaxed. It is impossible to mobilize when the knee is flexed. With static contraction of the quadriceps, the obliquely oriented patellar ligament pulls the patella superiorly and laterally. This tendency to move laterally is countered by the lateral side of the trochlear groove, thus buttressing dislocation.

Femorotibial joint space

When the knee is in extension, the femorotibial joint space is located at the top of the patella. When the knee is flexed, the joint space is situated a finger width below the summit of the patella. The line can be clearly palpated in the posterior region of the semiflexed knee.

13.2.2 Collateral ligaments

Lateral collateral ligament

A 90° flexed knee is the only position where the ligament is not covered by the biceps femoral tendon. Find the top of the fibular head and palpate above the biceps femoris tendon. Ascend toward the joint space. You will be able to palpate the middle section of the lateral collateral ligament from beneath fibers of the iliotibial band that are spread over the lateral surface of the tibia.

Proximal and distal parts of the ligament are more difficult to discern, as they are more or less masked by the fascia lata above and obscured by the biceps tendon below.

Medial collateral ligament

Palpate the most anterior part of the femorotibial joint space on either side of the patellar apex. The medial collateral ligament is located three finger widths behind the medial border of the patellar tendon. The proximal insertion of the ligament is located in the prolongation of the terminal tendon of the caudal fascicle of the adductor magnus. The medial collateral ligament is found in front of the anterior concavity and is formed by the distal muscle fibers of sartorius.

13.2.3 Noteworthy muscles

Global muscle topography at the popliteal level

The following muscles are found by palpating from posterior to anterior and from lateral to medial in line with the popliteal fossa:

- semitendinosus (the most visible and prominent);
- semimembranosus;
- gracilis;
- sartorius.

Pes anserinus

The distal insertion of the conjoined tendons that form the "goose's foot" is not at the level of the tibial tuberosity, as is generally imagined, but is lower. The tendons insert in front of the distal insertion of the medial collateral ligament. The three tendons are more or less indistinguishable on palpation. The sartorius tendon covers the semitendinosus and gracilis tendons. We can, however, discern serous bursae that underlie the different tendons.

Adductor magnus

The terminal adductor magnus tendon is palpable behind the vastus medialis above the medial femoral condyle. This powerful tendon inserts on the tubercle of the same name. Ask your patient to contract the quadriceps isometrically. This will display the border of vastus medialis. Palpate the adductor magnus tendon by following the posterior medial border of the vastus medialis, sinking your finger pads transversely toward the superior border of the medial condyle.

Gracilis

Palpate the gracilis in the same region, lower limb in semiflexion. Ask the patient to bend the knee and resist hip adduction.

Semimembranosus

This muscle terminates behind the medial condyle, where it divides into three tendons. You can palpate the muscle mass at the distal third of the thigh, slightly lateral of the semitendinosus. It is easier, however, to palpate medially at the semitendinosus tendon. Contact the direct tendon that lies more medially and deeper than the semitendinosus tendon, and follow it as far as the medial tibial condyle.

13.3 GENERAL KNEE EXAMINATION

In simple cases, the examination can be

done in any order. When confronted with more difficult situations, it is best to be systematic and logical. Systematic, because it is essential that nothing be omitted. This is not always easy in view of the wealth of signs and symptoms and shear diversity of knee problems. Logical, as it is easier to remember a method once you understand it. We make every effort to explain the significance of the various signs.

13.3.1 Look for swelling

It is always important to determine whether the knee is "dry" or if effusion is present. This is an important evaluation. As the knee is a superficial joint, effusion is fairly visible and palpable. There are two leading indicators by which you can confirm real and organic knee problems in a matter of seconds—through flexum contracture and through joint swelling.

The analgesic position: flexum

Progressive effusion causes the knee to enlarge. The so-called "position of maximal capacity" corresponds to the position of reduced fluid pressure sensation. The patient with joint effusion naturally adopts demiflexion because it is the least painful position. Significant flexum is readily apparent. Less obvious flexum requires manual detection.

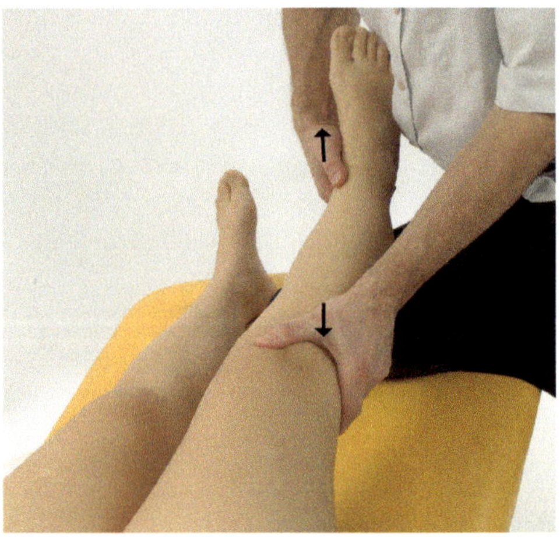

Fig. 13.2 Evaluating knee flexum.

Detecting flexum

The patient lies relaxed on his back. You use your palms to lift both heels about 10 cm off the table. This is the ideal position for discovering flexum. Alternately you can firmly place his feet against your belly or hand, and test the reducibility of the flexum by applying gentle pressure to the top of the knee (Fig. 13.2).

Joint swelling

Look for fluid in the knees by positioning your thumbs and last three fingers on either side of the patella. Squeeze the fluid toward the patella. Maintaining the pressure, tap the patella squarely with your index finger. The test is positive if the patella can be felt bouncing off the underlying femur and floating up like ice in a glass of water (Fig. 13.3).

It is important to note the time delay involved. If the swelling comes on within two hours of a trauma, it almost always signifies a hemarthrosis (bleeding into the joint space). The anterior cruciate ligament is frequently injured. Be alert for tibial eminence fractures as a variant of ACL ruptures, which tend not to present as typical fractures. Swelling that appears the next day is more likely a reactive hydrarthrosis (watery effusion into the joint cavity) and is less of a concern.

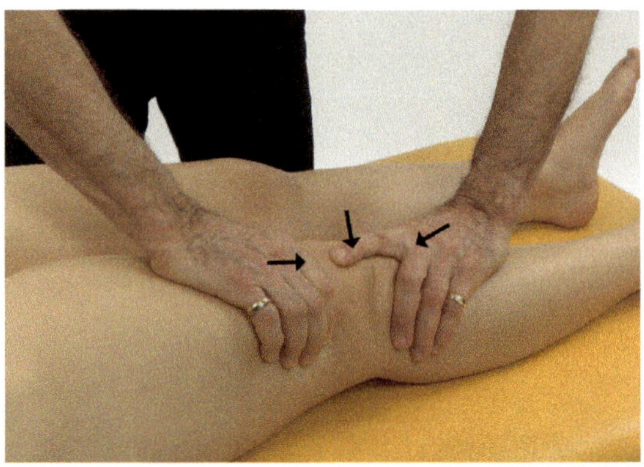

Fig. 13.3 Testing for patellar instability.

13.3.2 Testing flexion-extension

The subject is in decubitus. Your caudal hand grasps the instep of the foot, while your cranial hand is placed on the lower part of the popliteal fossa. Appreciate knee flexion and extension range. Move the knee gradually and without force. Note the distance between heel and buttock in maximal pain-free flexion. Evaluate the comparative freedom of extension or make a note of a flexum contracture.

13.3.3 Knee "auscultation"

While mobilizing the knee as outlined above, bring your ear close to the lateral surface of the joint and listen for noise. Alternatively you can place a stethoscope on different parts of the knee; even a normal knee will produce gliding noises. Abnormal sounds are clearly audible.

There are three categories of noise:

- Squeaking is likely to be intra-articular joint deposits. The sound can indicate microcrystals or the aftermath of hemarthrosis or hydarthrosis.
- Crackling often signifies meniscal or cartilaginous lesions. Cracking can be heard on chronically lax knees or following major meniscal tears.
- Crunching indicates the sudden gliding or abrupt passage of a ligament or tendon over a bone. This could indicate pathological exotosis, osteophytes, or abarticular elements.

Note: Noise is of no significance unless it can be reproduced by one or more knee movements.

13.3.4 Significance of painful points

Preamble

Generally speaking we try to not be blinded by pain in our work. Yet we recognize that the knee often shows us its lesions and dysfunctions. Searching out painful points can thus be a valid indicator, but the endeavor must satisfy at least two conditions:

- The therapist must avoid all forms of violent or aggressive palpation during the test. It is always possible to create pain, but the goal is not to provoke agony. The purpose of checking painful joints is to check the susceptibility of certain structures. The knee is a particularly worrisome joint for any patient, and it is of the utmost importance not to surprise or alarm them by sudden maneuvers or invasive palpation.
- Provoked pain is of no real value except to the extent it is familiar to the patient. Identifying the pain as "his pain" can be a useful indication.

Special note

- The anterior tibial tuberosity: Adolescents can develop epiphysitis accompanied by fragmentation within the epiphyseal ossification nucleus. Pressure on the anterior tibial tuberosity reproduces the patient's pain (Osgood-Schlatter disease).
- The patellar tendon: This is a common site of microtraumatic lesions linked to overdemand. Pain is local to the patellar tendon and is provoked by dysfunctional and repeated knee extension.
- Point of the patella: You rarely encounter epiphysitis of the point of the patella in adolescents.
- Medial edge of the patella: Palpation of the medial versant of the patella is sometimes painful and familiar to the patient. The syndrome is part of the painful patellar syndrome.
- Lateral edge of the patella: The examiner pushes the patella outward and palpates the cartilaginous and lateral surface of the patella. Femoropatellar dysplasias lead to lateral conflicts, which bring on lateral knee pain.

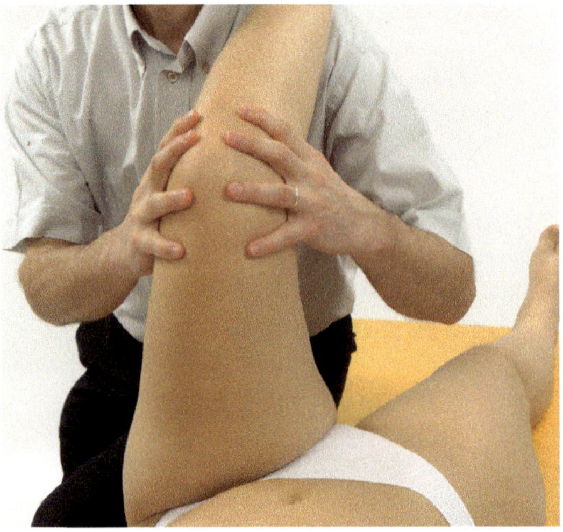

Fig. 13.4 Dynamic knee listening.

13.3.5 Dynamic knee listening (Fig. 13.4)

Listening gives you an idea of the location of mechanical knee problems. The patient is in decubitus. You sit on the table on the side of the evaluation, the patient's foot resting on your shoulder. Place your hands on either side of the knee by positioning your fingers in the following manner:

- Your index fingers should be placed on the superior and anterior parts of the medial and lateral tibial tuberosities.
- Your middle fingers are placed on either side of the patellar tendon on the femorotibial line facing that anterior part of the meniscus.
- Your ring fingers contact the anterior surface of the patella.
- Your little fingers are just above the proximal limit of the patella.
- Your thumbs rest behind the knee at the lower part of the popliteal fossa facing the joint line and the posterior part of the meniscus.

Ask the patient to flex and extend at the hip; allow the leg to remain relaxed on your shoulder the whole time. Knee bending and straightening are to be done without force, fairly slowly but amply, in order to avoid hurting the knee.

Palpate and compare the tension and texture of different tissues. Analyze their glide and deformation in the course of movement. Visualize the displacement and the movement of the boney joint pieces. Finally, allow your hands to follow the tissular listening (mechanical dialogue) that will pull you to the precise areas of conflict.

Compare your findings on the lateral and medial knee compartments. Any delay, loss of fluidity, or abnormal resistance to the movement should be suspect.

Next, make the same observations and comparisons in the sagittal plane. Feel for the movement to ascertain if it is regular and properly distributed among the various joint components. Any movement disturbance or lack of harmony are worthy of interest.

Listening is not a specific test. It indicates the mechanical sector that is transgressing the joint. The listening location is where you carry out precise tests that refine your diagnosis.

13.3.6 Femoropatellar joint tests

Patellar instability (Fig. 13.5)

Contact both patellar borders between your thumbs and index fingers so that you are able to observe the planes of the patella. Normally, there is little difference on the frontal plane of the knee, although physio-

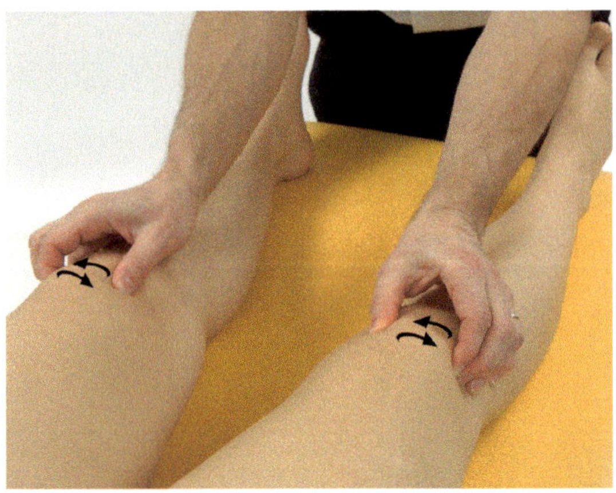

Fig. 13.5 Patellar toggling.

logically the patella is angled about 10°, tipping it laterally.

Next, delicately toggle the patella laterally and medially. Nudge the patellas to turn inwardly and then outwardly. Any disparity is called convergent or divergent patellar strabismus. Convergent strabismus is most commonly seen medically as part of painful patellar syndrome, while divergent strabismus tends to accompany patellar instability.

Femoropatellar joint translations tests (Fig. 13.6)

The patient is in decubitus, lower extremities in extension. Grasp the patella between your thumbs and index fingers and translate them laterally and medially. Physicians use this test to screen for hyperlaxities in patellar instability syndromes. Such hypermobile pathologies involve distension of periarticular soft tissues and are of little concern to us. These problems are not bothersome to the patient and are often just an innate outward appearance, which has nothing to do with function.

On the other hand, this is a useful test to feel for imbalances between the medial and lateral extensor retinacula and to assess femoropatellar and menisopatallar ligamentous tensions. Repeated lateral fixation of these elements creates hyperpressure on the patellar cartilage and can also destabilize meniscal play.

With the same hand hold, mobilize the patella up and down in a cephalocaudad direction. Appreciate the freedom and quality of movement in each direction. Normally, the movement is balanced in both directions. Fixations of the patellar tendon can thus be differentiated from those of the quadricipital tendon. Be alert for any perceptible or audible rustling sounds that signify injury to the femoropatellar joint surfaces.

Femoropatellar grinding test (Fig. 13.7)

Practice this test to appreciate the quality of patellar joint surfaces and the femoral trochlear groove. The patient is in decubitus, legs extended. Move the patella distally in the trochlear groove and ask the patient to contract his quadriceps to counter your mobilization. Patellar displacement should be smooth and streamlined.

Any irregularity of the joint surface manifests as palpable crepitation in the course of the movement. If the test is positive, the patient generally complains of knee pain or trouble. This type of cartilage damage gives pain in stair climbing and is relieved by sitting down. Chondromalacia of the patella, osteochondral lacunae, and degenerative changes of the trochlear groove can all cause pain on movement.

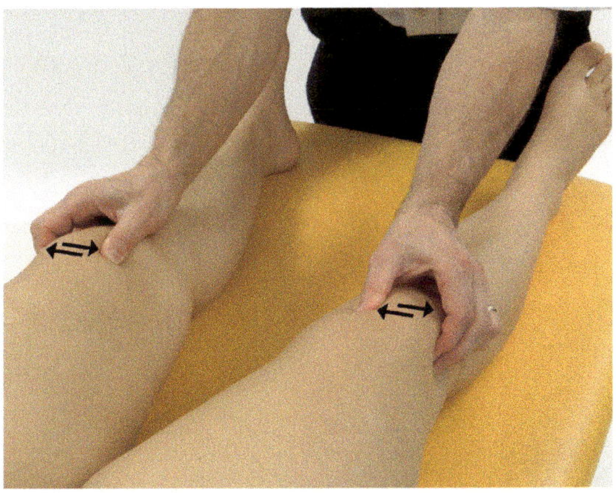

Fig. 13.6 Lateral translation of the patella.

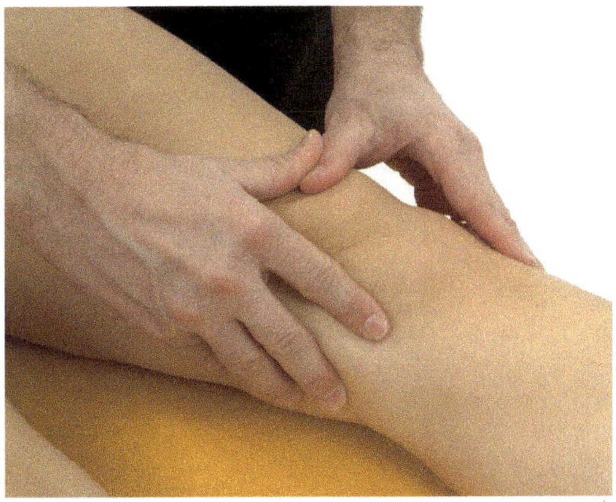

Fig. 13.7 Femoropatellar grinding test.

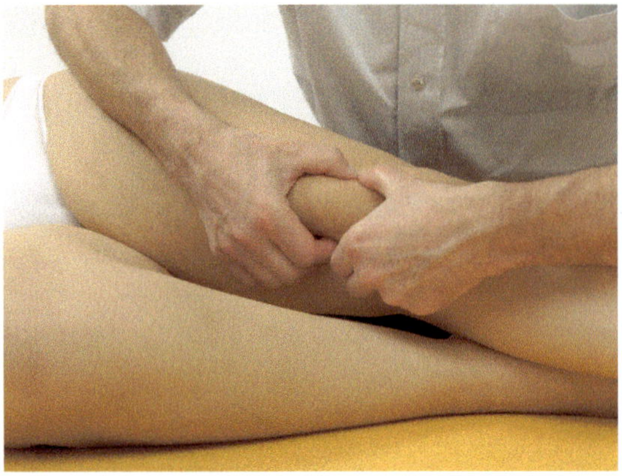

Fig. 13.8 Palpating to the posterior surface of the patella.

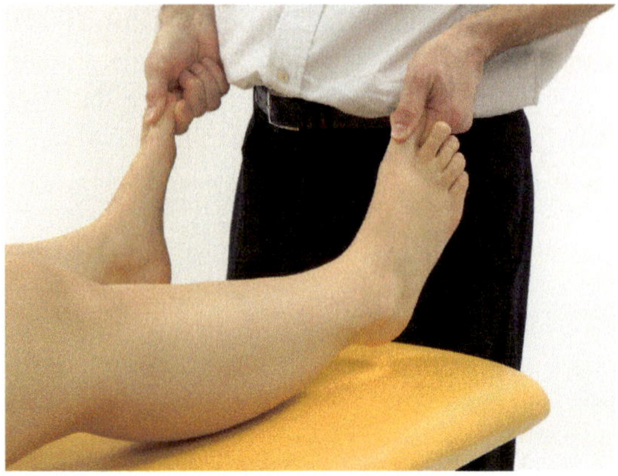

Fig. 13.9 Big toe sign.

Palpating the posterior surface of the patella (Fig. 13.8)

When the preceding test is suspicious of possible cartilage damage, it can be useful to palpate the posterior patella. This palpation is only possible with the knee in extension.

Push the patella medially to get a feel for the posterior surface of the lateral side, and move it inversely to test the medial side. You will find that it is usually easier to push the patella medially. This test can expose a cartilaginous defect on the posterior surface, or an irregular and hardened patellar edge, as can occur with osteoarthritis.

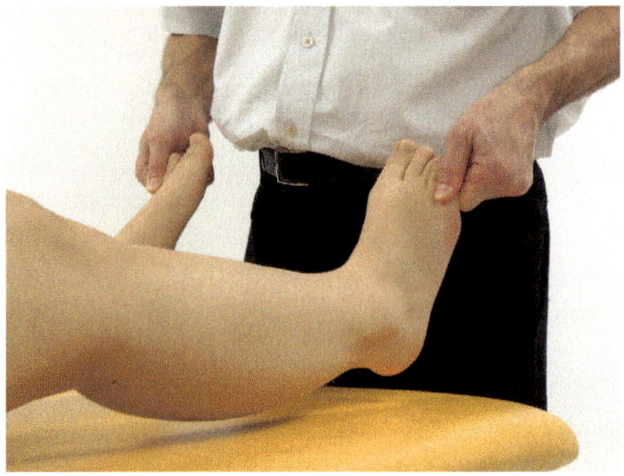

Fig. 13.10. Small toe sign.

13.3.7 Posterior knee tests (Figs. 13.9 and 13.10)

Testing the lateral and medial knee components is an easy test that helps to orient the clinical diagnosis. Lifting the foot by the little toe, then by the big toe, allows you to compare the responses of the right and left sides. Lift the foot by the little toe to evaluate the elasticity of the tissues of the posterior medial corner points of the knee. Lift the foot by the big toe to test the tissues at the posterior lateral corner points of the knee.

A difference in tension can be perceived as either a loss of elasticity or ligament laxity at the back of the knee. When posterior support structures are ruptured, the knee goes very clearly toward hyperextension.

Treatment of the active stabilizers

14

Active stabilizers act to restrain and maintain the knee in static or dynamic conditions. They are pivotal to joint cohesion and good proprioception. Considering the special way the knee fits together, it is important to be familiar with these muscles in order to manipulate them.

14.1 TOPOGRAPHY

These muscles are topographically enumerated below.

14.1.1 Medial (Fig. 14.1)

The semimembranosus is situated at the back and medial side of the thigh. Direct,

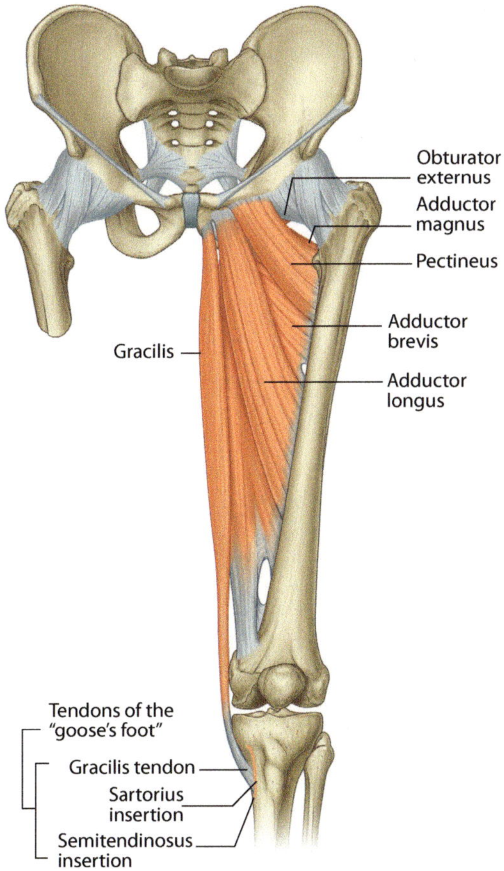

Fig. 14.1 Tendons of the "goose's foot."

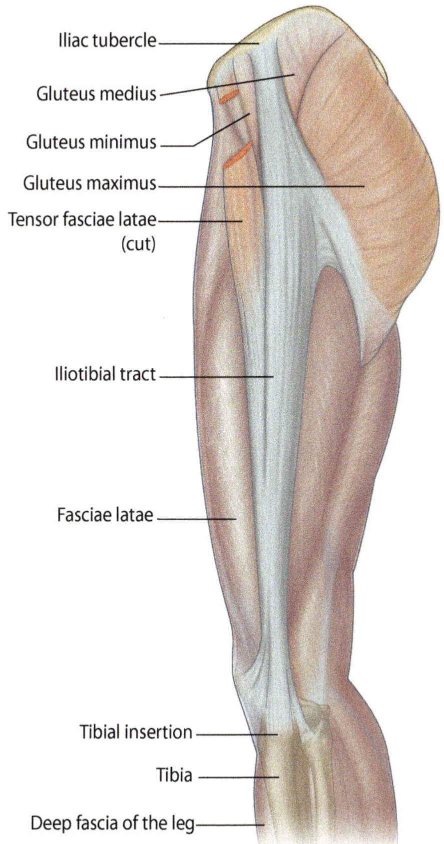

Fig. 14.2 Muscles of the lateral knee.

reflected, and recurrent tendinous expansions protect the posterior medial part of the knee. The conjoined tendons of the superficial pes anserinus resist valgus deformity and lateral rotation in the sartorius, gracilis, and semitendinosus.

14.1.2 Lateral (Fig. 14.2)

The popliteal muscle reinforces the fibular collateral ligament. The popliteal tendon is intracapsular, and it acts in concert with the biceps femoris and the iliotibial tract.

14.1.3 Anterior (Fig. 14.3)

The quadriceps is composed of:

- the rectus femoris;
- the vastus intermedius;
- the vastus medialis;
- the vastus lateralis.

Direct, indirect, cruciate, and arciform fibers blend with fibers of the sartorius and the iliotibial band. The quadriceps protect the anterior-posterior stability of the knee and hold the patella against the femur.

14.1.4 Posterior (Fig. 14.4)

The gastrocnemius arises cranially by a medial and a lateral head. It has powerful tendinous insertions that join the condylar shells. The gastrocnemius is a second component in sagittal knee protection. The lateral head is partially overlaid by the tendon of the biceps femoris. The medial head is partially overlaid by the semimembranosus and semitendinosus.

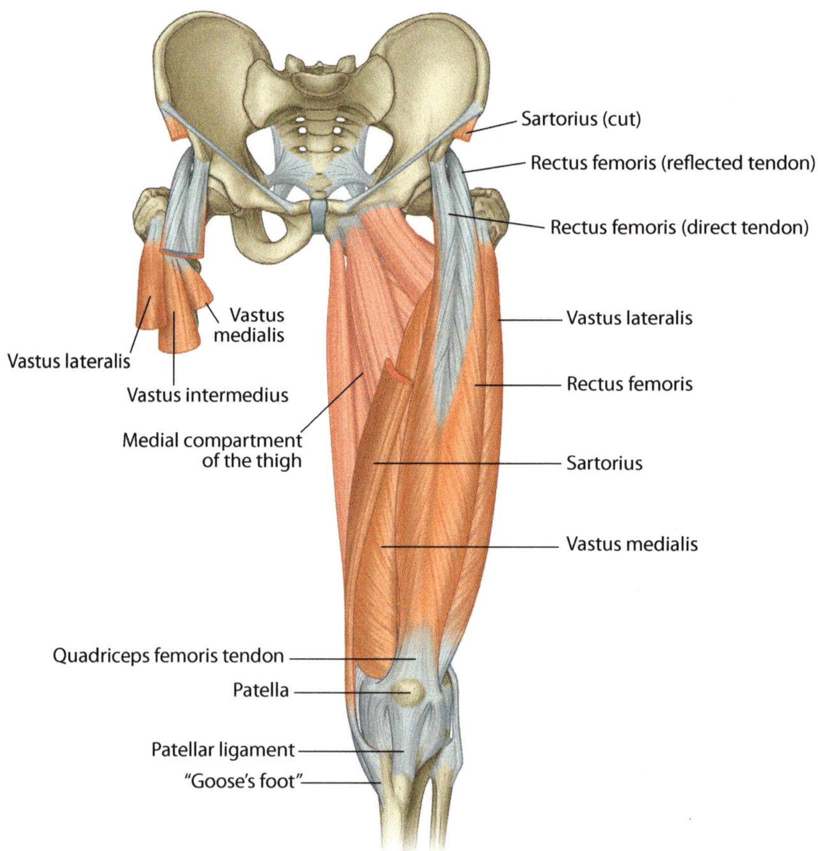

Fig. 14.3 Goose's foot.

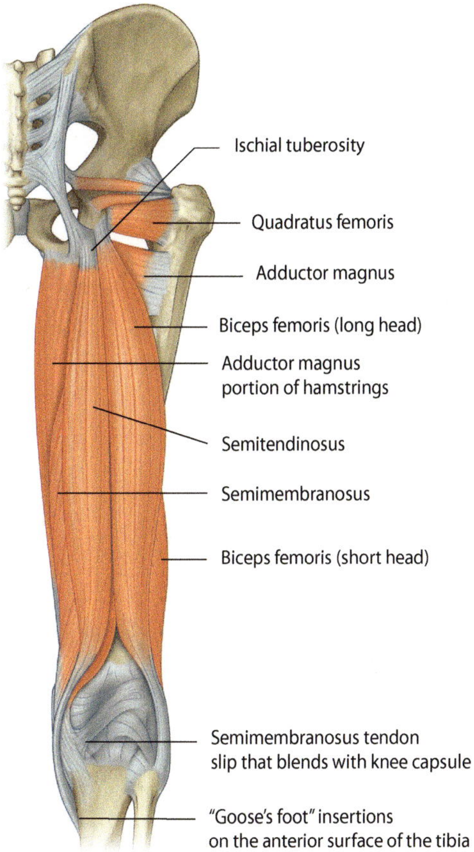

Fig. 14.4 Muscles of the posterior knee.

14.2 MUSCLES OF HIP-KNEE COORDINATION

This group of muscles coordinates hip and knee mobility. The muscles allow the knee a three-dimensional existence in space. They are the:

- sartorius;
- gracilis;
- semitendinosus;
- semimembranosus;
- tensor fasciae latae by way of the iliotibial tract;
- long head of biceps;
- quadriceps.

14.3 SUPERFICIAL "GOOSE'S FOOT" (PES ANSERINUS)

14.3.1 Review

Distal insertion of the pes anserinus

The conjoined tendons of the sartorius, semitendinosus, and gracilis insert as three prongs onto the tibia. We have already studied their relationship to the hip; here we look at the anatomy and treatment of their tibial insertions. The superficial pes anserinus is often victim to microruptures or adhesions that are detrimental to knee proprioception.

Termination (Fig. 14.5)

Distal insertion is on the anterior medial surface of the tibia. From anterior to posterior, the order of insertions is the sartorius, gracilis, and semitendinosus.

Serous bursa of the pes anserinus

The pes anserine bursa is interposed between the tibia and the ligament insertions. Tendonitis and bursitis often go together here. Anserine tendinobursitis syndrome is not easy to resolve.

Innervation

- Tibial nerve (L5–S2) for semimembranosus
- Obturator nerve, anterior branch (L2–L4) for gracilis
- Femoral nerve (L1–L3) for sartorius

It is apparent that the innervation of the pes anserinus derives from the lumbar and sacral plexus. Tendinitis and irritation at the pes anserinus can thus be referred pain of visceral origin. The likeliest organs involved are the kidneys, the intestine, and urogenital organs.

Vascular supply

- The perforating branches of the deep femoral artery

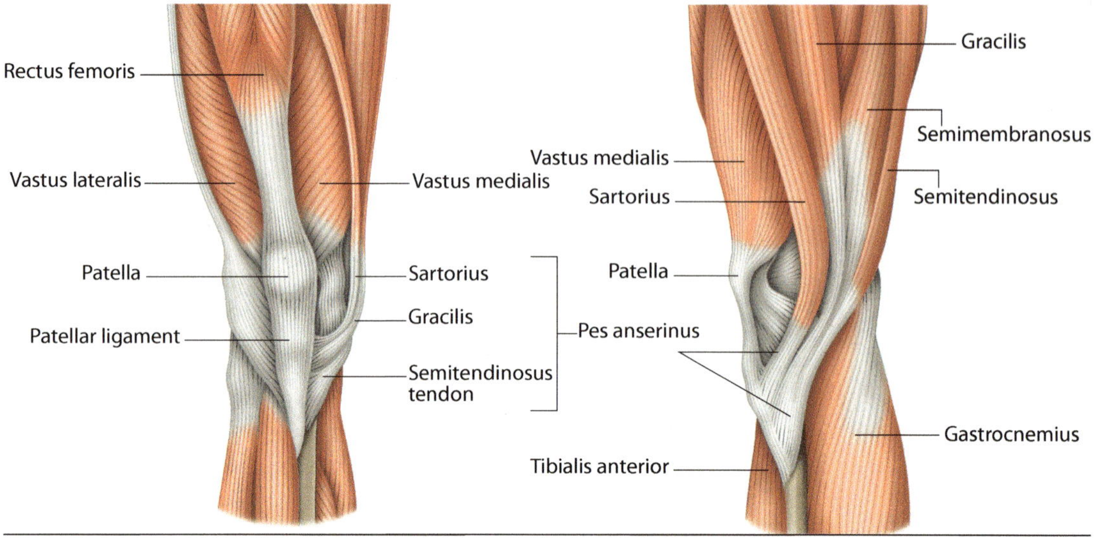

Fig. 14.5 Distal insertion of the superficial pes anserinus ("goose's foot").

Special note

- Sartorius exchanges fibers with the crural fascia

Role of the pes anserinus

The muscles of the pes anserinus protect the knee medially. They reinforce the medial collateral ligament and are a bulwark against twisting forces.

14.3.2 Techniques

The muscles of the superficial pes anserinus react very little to our manipulations, whereas their musculotendinous junctions and tibial insertions respond very well.

In lateral decubitus (Fig. 14.6)

The patient lies on the side of the leg in question, joint slightly flexed. You sit facing the knee. Glide your thumbs along the medial surface of the tibia, keeping in contact with the bone at the start. Check for any hardened and irregular areas on the tibial insertions. When tendinitis is present in addition to pain you will feel crepitation under your fingers. Treat the tendinous insertions with consecutive rounds of soft and progressive smoothing induction.

Next, move your two thumbs away from the medial posterior part of the tibia to follow the three tendons of the pes anserinum as far as their tibial insertion. Check to see that there are no adhesions between the tendons. It is a good sign if you can unstick them and separate them fairly easily upstream of their boney insertions.

Serous bursa (Fig. 14.7)

Still moving your thumbs from back to front, maintain a ventral stretch on the pes anserinus tendons for 12 seconds. Repeat

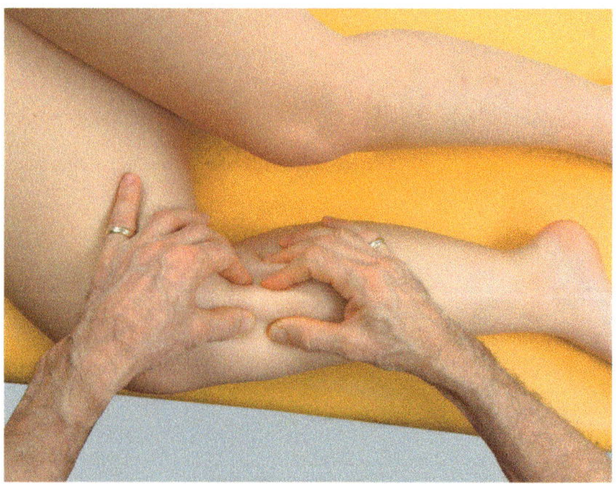

Fig. 14.6 Manipulation of the superficial pes anserinus.

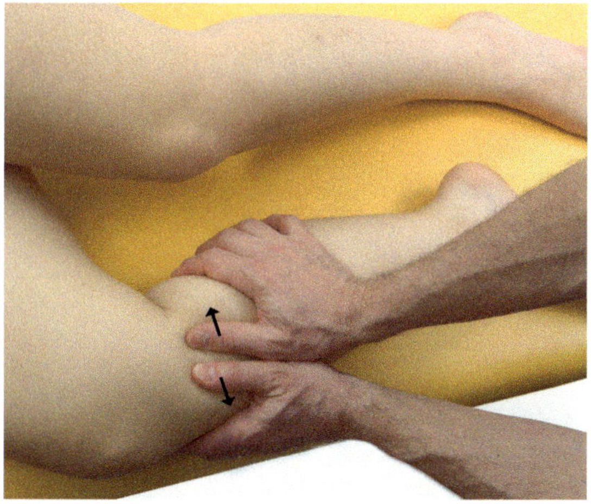

Fig. 14.7 Manipulation of the serous bursa deep to the pes anserinus tendons.

this several times. Come as close as you can to the tibial tendinous insertion. Spread the tendons and maintain the separation for 12 seconds. Repeat this stretch five or six times.

Decompression exerted around the serous bursa frees it of constraint, allowing it to regain its viscoelasticity. As a result, the bursa can once again produce good-quality serous fluid as well as effectively reabsorb it.

14.4 DEEP PES ANSERINUS

The pes anserinus profundus, or deep goose's foot, is constituted by the distal attachments of the semimembranosus tendon. This tendon plays a primordial role in knee stability and proprioception. The semimembranosus is closely linked to the medial collateral ligament, the medial meniscus, and the posterior capsule complex.

Refer to earlier paragraphs concerning each of these structures to understand the relevance of this muscle. It is certainly the most arduous part of the knee to know and to manipulate well. Curiously, therapists neglect it and tend to focus a little too much on the anterior part of the knee.

We have described the semimembranosus as it relates to the pelvis. Here we will consider its distal attachments.

14.4.1 Review

The semimembranosus tendon is deeply situated in the popliteal fossa. It is thus deeper and also more medial than the semitendinosus tendon (Fig. 14.8). The three

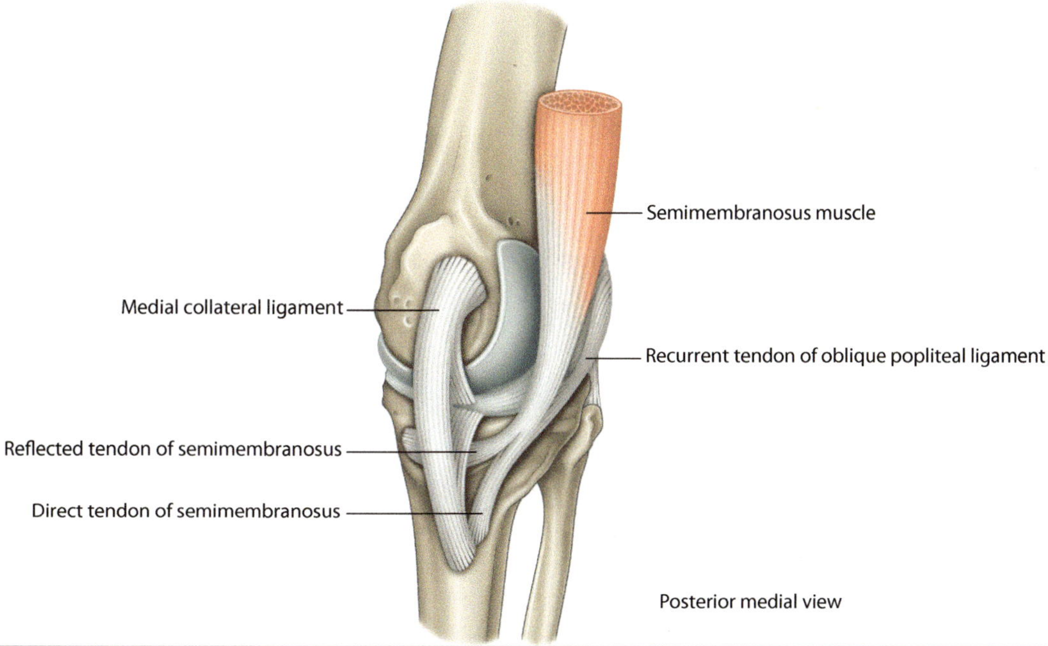

Fig. 14.8 Insertions of semimembranosus or the deep pes anserinus.

distal attachment zones of the semimembranosus form the pes anserinus profundus complex at the knee. They are:

- the popliteal fascia;
- the posterior surface of the capsule, where the insertion is called the oblique popliteal ligament;
- the medial condyle of the tibial epiphysis.

Direction and trajectory

The terminal part of the semimembranosus is vertical and turns medially. The muscle is more anterior, and is wider and broader than the semitendinosus.

Termination

The terminal insertion of the semimembranosus gives off certain fibrous expansions. One, of considerable size, passes upward and laterally to be inserted into the posterior lateral condyle of the femur, forming part of the oblique popliteal ligament of the knee-joint. A second is continued downward to the fascia which covers the popliteus muscle, while a few fibers join the tibial collateral ligament of the joint and the fascia of the leg.

Direct tendon

The direct tendon ends on the posterior surface of the medial tibial condyle. A few fibers insert on the medial border of the tibia, the popliteal aponeurosis, and the posterior part of the medial meniscus.

Reflected tendon

The reflected tendon attaches at right angles to the direct tendon then travels anteriorly and medially. It passes across the medial infraglenoid margin, which is a small hollow groove on the medial surface of the tibial condyle. It passes under the medial collateral ligament just beneath the femorotibial fibers, making it into a veritable reflexion pulley. It inserts onto the anterior part of the groove on the anterior surface of the medial tibial condyle.

Recurrent tendon

The recurrent tendon forms the oblique popliteal ligament. It passes proximally and laterally in the form of a broad triangular expansion. It attaches to the lateral condylar shell at the fabella (see "oblique popliteal ligament" in chapter 15) or the concentration of fascia that replace it.

Special Note

A serous bursa is evidence that you are dealing with a subtle gliding of movable parts subject to intense friction. Tendons, ligaments, capsule, synovial, and osseous attachments will be affected.

14.4.2 Techniques

Manipulation of the terminal semimembranosus insertions is the cornerstone of all manual treatments of the musculocapsular connections of the knee. It is difficult to carry out, however, because the anatomy is deeply situated, and access is hindered by the gastrocnemius muscle.

Attachment landmarks

The distal attachments of the semimembranosus are fairly easy to landmark. When the knee is in extension, the direct tendon is situated in the inferior end of the semimembranosus muscle. When the knee is flexed to 90°, it goes around the reflected tendon to continue in the general direction of the main tendon.

Tibial attachment of the direct tendon in decubitus

The patient lies in the supine position with you sitting beside him on the table. His knee is flexed and his foot rests on your shoulder. Use one thumb to locate the insertion of the direct tendon on the posterior surface of the tibial condyle. Place the other thumb on the musculotendinous junction of the semimembranosus, close to the upper part of the popliteal crease.

Ask the patient to make small flexion-extension movements of the knee. This allows you to check the elasticity of the tendon and to discover any tensions or restrictions. Take advantage of these movements to perform stretching-induction maneuvers to areas of the direct tendon that you perceive to be restricted.

Meniscal attachment of semimembranosus in lateral decubitus

The patient lies in lateral decubitus on the treatment side, knee flexed to 90°. Place yourself in front of the patient in line with his tibia. With your two index fingers arranged in parallel and back to back, penetrate the space between the posterior joint line of the knee and the semimembranosus tendon.

Ask the patient to glide his foot along the table, alternately flexing and extending the knee, using very small movements. Take advantage of these movements to infiltrate your fingers between the semimembranosus and the posterior part of the medial meniscus. Release any tensions you feel by separation-induction maneuvers.

The meniscal attachment of the semimembranosus is a powerful guide to the posterior part of the medial meniscus. Manipulating it is of the greatest importance in dysfunctions that affect the posterior horn. Treating it alone is sometimes enough to restore meniscal mobility.

The same approach can be used to release the connections between the direct tendon and the popliteal aponeurosis.

Oblique popliteal ligament

For didactic reasons, we have treated the anatomy of this ligament separately from the posterior capsular complex. The arcuate popliteal ligament constitutes the third semimembranosus insertion slip. It courses from the head of the fibula over the popliteus, inserting first on the fabella or aponeurotic capsular condensation of fibers and then merging with the oblique popliteal ligament.

Tibial attachment of the reflected tendon in lateral decubitus (Fig. 14.9)

By way of the reflected tendon, the semimembranosus is one of the very rare muscles that passes under a ligament before inserting onto a bone. It runs beneath the tibial collateral ligament under the tibiofemoral fibers. Tension in one always influences the other. Consequently, their manipulation cannot be dissociated.

Place yourself in front of your patient, who lies on the side of the knee involved. Moving from posterior to anterior, begin by closely following the semimembranosus tendon in the groove of the medial infraglenoid margin. Then carefully explore the interlacing fibers between the tibial collateral ligament and the semimembranosus tendon. Treat any hardened fibers with smoothing-induction. This section of the semimembranosus is very important for the tibial collateral ligament. Any fixations here can disturb its proprioceptive informational role.

14.5 BICEPS FEMORIS (FIG. 14.10)

14.5.1 Review

The role of this muscle is to transmit tensions to and from the lesser pelvis and the

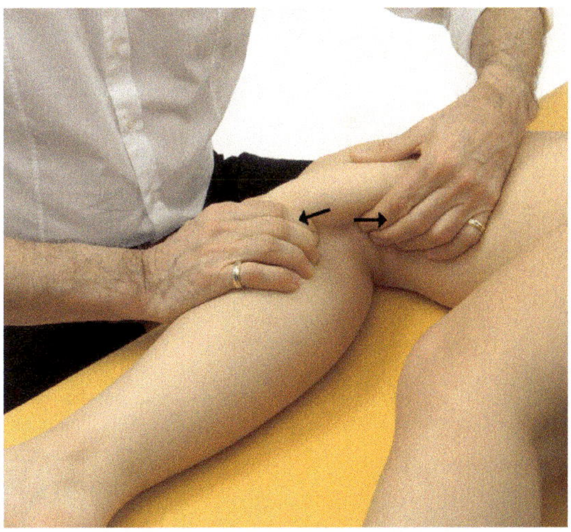

Fig. 14.9 Tibial attachment of the semimembranosus reflected tendon.

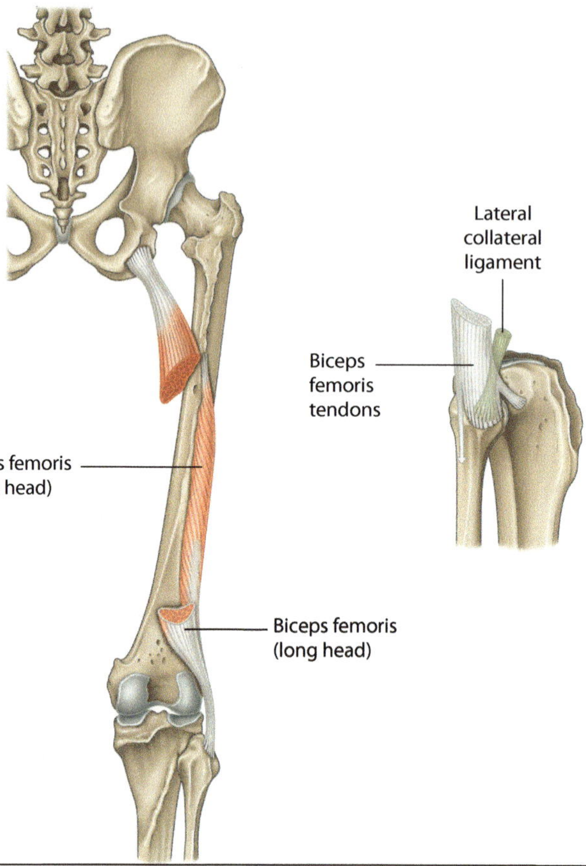

Fig. 14.10 Biceps femoris.

lower extremities. Its cranial insertion at the ischium is not very reflexogenic, and manipulating it offers little result. By contrast, the caudal part of the muscle, particularly its musculotendinous junction, offers dividends to the patient when you manipulate it.

Origin

The muscle has two heads of origin:

- Long head
  - Ischial tuberosity of the coxal bone
  - A tendon in common with semitendinosus

The long head forms the most lateral part of the hamstrings. It exchanges fibers with the sacrotuberous ligament, whereby the pelvis is linked to the knee.

- Short head
  - Lateral lip of the linea aspera, below the gluteus maximus and between the adductor magnus and vastus lateralis
  - Lateral intermuscular septum

Direction

- Vertical and longitudinal: follows and crosses the sciatic nerve

Termination

- Cranial end of the fibula, lateral in relation to the fibular collateral ligament (between the biceps femoris and the collateral fibular ligaments is a serous bursa)
- Lateral tibial condyle
- Crural aponeurosis (hamstring fascia)
- Tibiofibular capsule with which it exchanges fibers

Innervation

- Tibial nerve for the long head (L5–S2)
- Common fibular nerve for the short head (S1–S2)

This innervation shows that biceps femoris is dependent on the lesser pelvis, not only mechanically through the sacrotuberous ligament but also by way of fibers issuing from the sacral plexus.

Vascular supply

- Perforating branches of the deep femoral artery

Actions

- The long head retroverts (posteriorly rotates) the pelvis.
- Both heads affect flexion of the knee and lateral rotation (when the knee is flexed). Biceps femoris is the only muscle that can laterally rotate the leg at the knee joint.

Special note

The distal insertion envelops the fibular collateral ligament from which it is separated by a serous bursa. It functions as a capsule tensor together with the popliteus. It shares fibers with the sacrotuberous ligament and is proximal to the semitendinosus and semimembranosus.

14.5.2 Techniques

It is difficult to separate manipulation of the distal biceps femoris from treatment of the fibular collateral ligament. We are always acting on both.

In lateral decubitus (Fig. 14.11)

The patient lies on the side opposite the knee to be treated. You place one thumb on the insertion of the fibular head and two fingers of the other hand at the musculotendinous junction at the interior thigh. Move the tendinous insertion in lateral and medial flexion, as if you were playing the string of a bass violin. Locate any small irregularities on the fibular insertion. Remember that there is a bursa between the fibular collateral ligament and biceps femoris. Using the index and thumbs of both hands, mobilize the muscle on the ligament.

Because the biceps femoris is a lateral rotator, fixations can be easier to feel by including some medial rotation of the tibia.

Clinical application

Fixation of the proximal tibiofibular joint is rarely causal but occurs secondary to:

- pelvic problems—vesico-utero-annexial, prostate, cecum, or sigmoid related;
- foot problems—compensation.

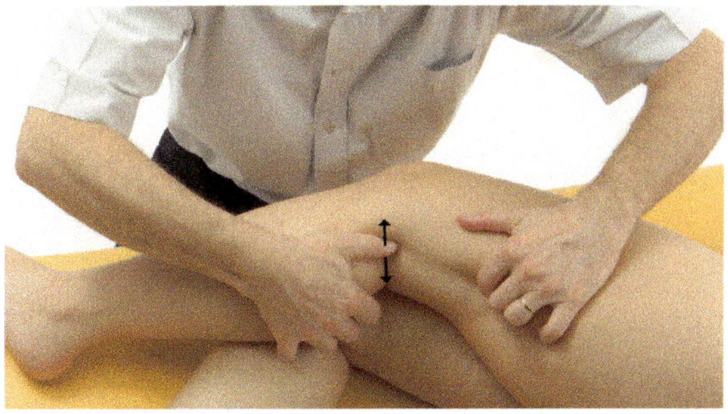

Fig. 14.11 Biceps femoris in lateral decubitus.

Separation-induction of the hamstrings in decubitus (Fig. 14.12)

The patient lies on the table, knee flexed, with his foot resting on your shoulder. Place both thumbs above the gastrocnemius muscles in the triangle formed by the biceps, semitendinosus, and semimembranosus muscles. Direct your thumbs as high as possible cranially against their musculotendinous junction and proceed with a spreading-induction.

14.6 GASTROCNEMIUS (FIG. 14.13)

We are astonished at the frequency of microruptures at the cephalad part of the gastrocnemius. This part of the muscle is closely connected to the knee capsule and is very sensitive to physical trauma. The muscle

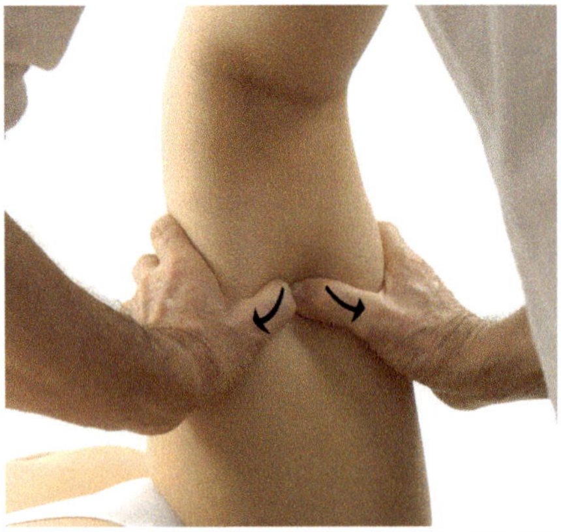

Fig. 14.12 Separation induction of the hamstrings in decubitus.

body itself is particularly vulnerable with respect to chemical and metabolic assaults such as gout, chondrocalcinosis, and microlithiasis (urinary stones), which can all make it more fragile.

14.6.1 Review

The gastrocnemius runs from two heads, a medial and a lateral.

Origin

- Femoral condyles
- Joint capsule
- Medial head arising slightly caudally and behind the adductor magnus tubercle
- Lateral head, which contributes fibers to soleus

14.6.2 Termination

- Calcaneal tuberosity, which forms the Achilles tendon together with the soleus and plantaris

14.6.3 Innervation

- Tibial nerve (S1–S2)

14.6.4 Vascular supply

- Branches of the popliteal artery

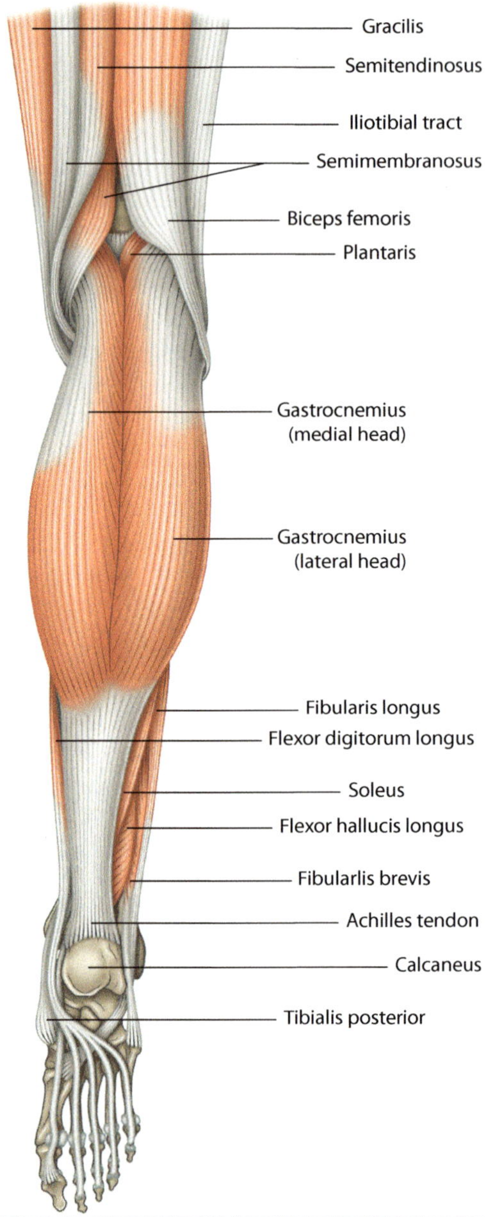

Fig. 14.13 Gastrocnemius.

14.6.5 Characteristics

- Medial head
  - The medial head attaches to the adductor tubercle. It sends fibers directly or by way of interposing fascia to the adductor magnus and to the tibial collateral ligament.

- It covers the semimembranosus tendon.
- The medial gastrocnemius subtendinosus bursa allows the muscle to glide on structures anteriorly adjacent to it.

• Lateral head
- The lateral head is the thinner and shorter of the paired lateral and medial bellies.
- The fibrocartilage formation called the fabella is embedded in the tendon behind the lateral condyle of the femur. When the fabella is absent, a connective tissue forms in its place, which feels hardened and dense. To locate the fabella, the first step is to separate the biceps tendon. The fabella is found on the anterior gliding surface of the lateral gastrocnemius, where it merges with the oblique and arcuate popliteal ligaments. The inconstant fabella, or fabella analog, is a key zone for manipulation of the posterior capsule.

14.6.6 Techniques

In decubitus (Fig. 14.14)

Rest the patient's foot on your thorax or shoulder. Direct just one thumb or both on top of each other toward the lateral part of the medial gastrocnemius in order to come as close as possible to the paired boney insertions. The goal of the technique is to spread the insertions transversely from each other. Try to go as deeply as possible to meet the capsular fibers. Move the knee into flexion and extension to better stretch and release the fibers.

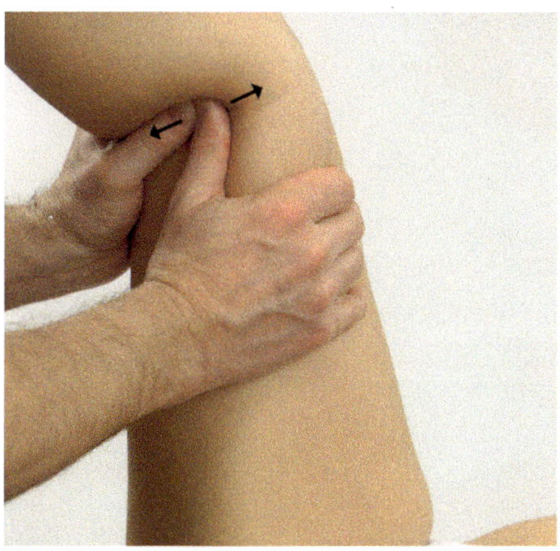

Fig. 14.14 Gastrocnemius in decubitus.

Special note

On the medial head, think of freeing all the fibers that attach to the adductor tubercle. On the lateral head, locate the fabella first to release the fibrous tissues that merge with it.

14.7 POPLITEUS (FIG. 14.15)

The popliteus rotates the tibia inward to allow the knee to unlock when walking, and it slightly rotates the femur to lock the knee joint in place when in full extension. This active knee ligament is also a capsule tensor. The popliteus attaches to the lateral meniscus.

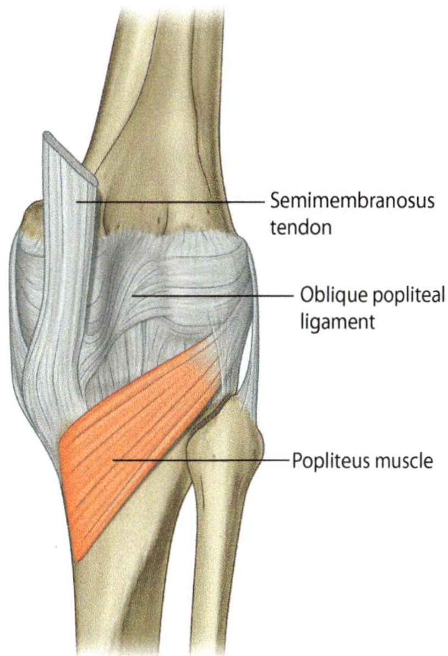

Fig. 14.15 Popliteus.

14.7.1 Review

Origin

- Lateral femoral epicondyle
- Within the deep surface of the capsule

Direction

- Distal and medial

Termination

- Posterior surface of the tibia
- Superior 25% of popliteus joins fibers at outer margins of lateral meniscus.
- Fibers sent to semimembranosus

Characteristics

- The popliteus is important to proprioception.
- The popliteus is intracapsular proximally and extracapsular distally.
- The popliteal recess is between the popliteus muscle and the knee joint.
- The muscle tendon passes in the osteofibrous tunnel formed by the arcuate popliteal ligament that arches over it.
- It stabilizes the dorsal knee region.

Actions on the knee

- The popliteus is a knee extensor lying behind the joint (Kapandji 2011).
- It medially rotates the femur.

Actions on the lateral meniscus

- The popliteus pulls the convex part dorsally during flexion, thus preventing entrapment.
- It provides a lateral femoral rotary component in flexion.
- It could be described as a "joint muscle" that locks the knee against excessive rotation.

The popliteus acts on the lateral compartment of the knee synergistically with the way the semimembranosus acts on the medial compartment. Working together these muscles help to balance the two posterior knee joint angles.

14.7.2 Techniques

In lateral decubitus (Fig. 14.16)

The patient lies on the side opposite the knee to be treated. Position yourself facing him. Place one thumb as near to the femoral popliteal attachment as possible. Immediately under your thumb you will meet the lateral gastrocnemius muscle and the arcuate popliteal ligament. To avoid these structures, place one of your thumbs on the inside of the lateral gastrocnemius muscle and the arcuate popliteal ligament to push them laterally. Place your other thumb on the muscle body and draw both thumbs in a medial and oblique direction toward the tibia. Mobilize the muscle fibers longitudinally and also transversely.

In decubitus (Fig. 14.17)

The foot of the flexed knee to be treated rests on your shoulder or on your thorax. Perform the same technique as described above. One thumb pushes back on the lateral gastrocnemius and the arcuate popliteal ligament such that you are on the popliteal surface of these structures. Place the other thumb on the body of the muscle and move the knee in flexion-extension and medial rotation. Differentiate the lateral gastrocnemius fibers from the arcuate popliteal ligament. Mobilize the popliteal muscle, alternately inclining it laterally and medially.

14.8 ILIOTIBIAL TRACT

The iliotibial tract is a longitudinal fibrous reinforcement of the fascia lata. This band contributes to knee stability and assists proprioception. We have already studied its thigh component as it relates to the hip and the coxofemoral joint. This section deals with the band's tibial attachments and their effect on the knee (Fig. 14.18).

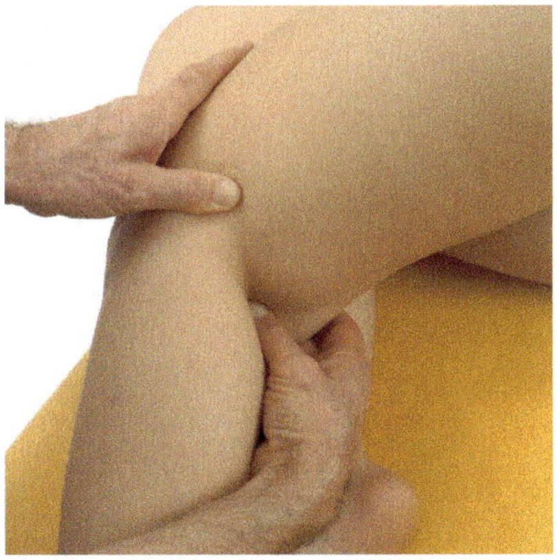

Fig. 14.16 Popliteus in lateral decubitus.

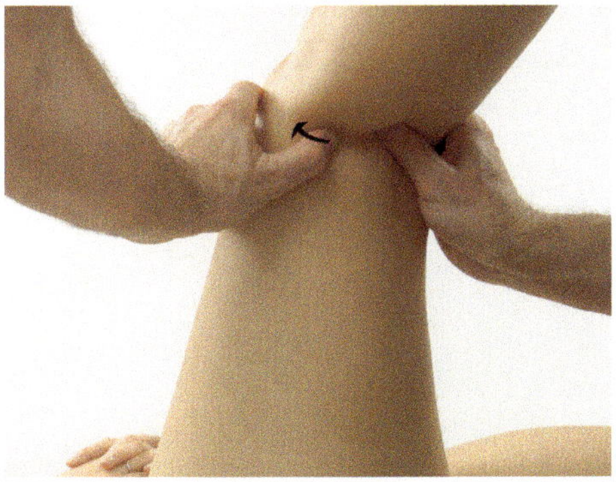

Fig. 14.17 Popliteus in decubitus.

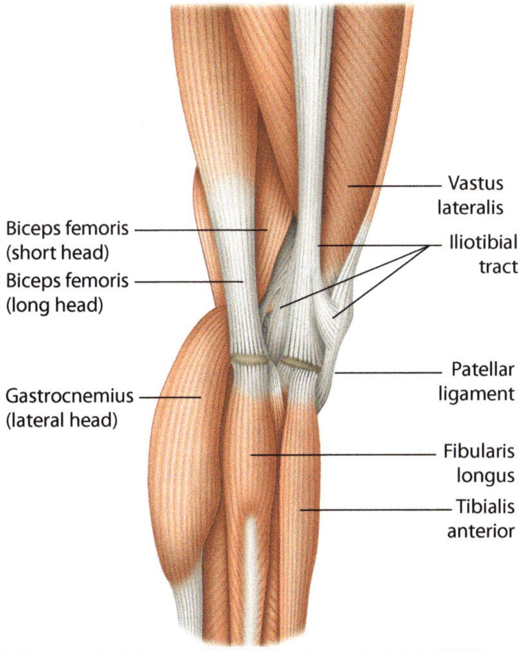

Fig. 14.18 Tibial attachment of the iliotibial band.

14.8.1 Review

Origin

- Borders the gluteus medius and gluteus minimus
- Merges with tensor fasciae latae at the lateral surface of the femur
- Shares fibers with the fascia covering the gluteus maximus

Direction

- Vertical caudally and slightly posterior

Termination

- On the lateral tibial condyle (Gerdy's tubercle)
- Fibular head
- Contributes fibers to:
  - the femoral and crural fascia;
  - the lateral border of the patella;
  - the sartorius, rectus femoris, and vastus lateralis;
  - the lateral patellar retinaculum.

Actions

- Passively braces the hip and knee laterally
- Provides ease and stability in single leg stance (developed with bipedal stance to allow us to stand vertically without muscle exertion)
- Helps stabilize the femoral head

Innervation

- Femoral nerve
- Lateral femoral cutaneous nerve (whose perforating branches are very effective to manipulate, as we shall see)

Characteristics

- Medially it is thin and merges with the fibrous expansion of the sartorius.
- Laterally it forms a thick fibrous sheath that makes up the largest component of the tensor fasciae latae.
- It is often incriminated in femoral patellar syndromes.

14.8.2 Techniques

The perforating nerves of the iliotibial tract in decubitus (Fig. 14.19)

Place yourself to the side of the treatment knee, which is slightly flexed. Search for small perforating branches of the lateral femoral cutaneous nerve, which are often surrounded by small fascial rings that we are able to release.

Glide your thumb along the lateral surface of the femur looking for an area that is sensitive, hardened, and dimpled. There can be several of these zones, but the most distinct nerve is often found mid-thigh. Before releasing the nerve as it pierces the IT band, release the fascial ring around it. Place your thumbs either side of the sensitive nerve and open the ring using induction. Most of the time, just opening the surrounding fascia is enough to make the sensitivity vanish. If the nerve remains sensitive, contact it lightly and treat it with induction.

The distal insertions in lateral decubitus (Fig. 14.20)

The patient lies on the side opposite the treatment knee, which is somewhat flexed. Place one thumb a little above the knee and the other on the lateral condyle of the tibia. Attempt to spread the iliotibial band insertions working in induction, while the patient slowly flexes and extends the knee.

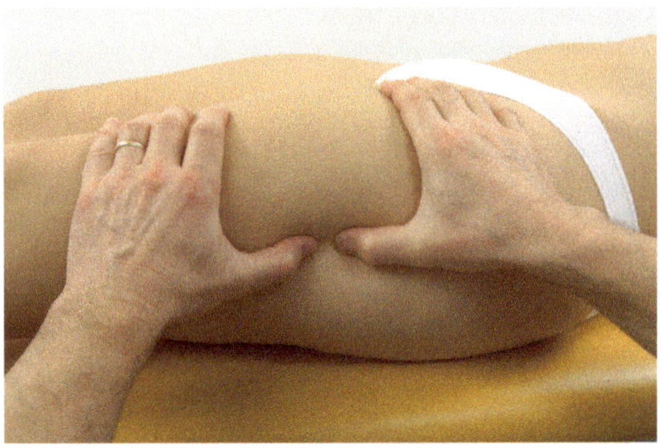

Fig. 14.19 Perforant nerves of the iliotibial tract.

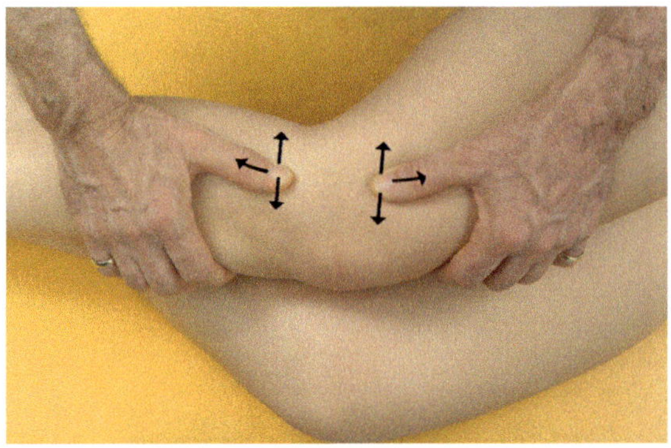

Fig. 14.20 Iliotibial tract in lateral decubitus.

Treatment of the passive stabilizers

15

15.1 ANTERIOR CAPSULOLIGAMENTOUS ELEMENTS

15.1.1 Adipose ligament (Fig. 15.1)

Constitution

Early anatomists such as Leo Tustut described an adipose ligament that, strictly speaking, does not exist. This fatty formation is of interest nonetheless.

The anterior part of the knee's synovial membrane is intimately related to a fatty mass called the infrapatellar fat body. This "ligament" separates and isolates the patella from the patellar tendon. Synovial membrane fringes called alar folds are located on either side of the fatty cushion below the patella. These are the infrapatellar synovial folds.

Roles

Fat, in general, serves a number of physiological functions:

- storage;
- stabilization;
- gliding;
- cushioning;
- proprioception;
- hormonal influence on some parts of the body.

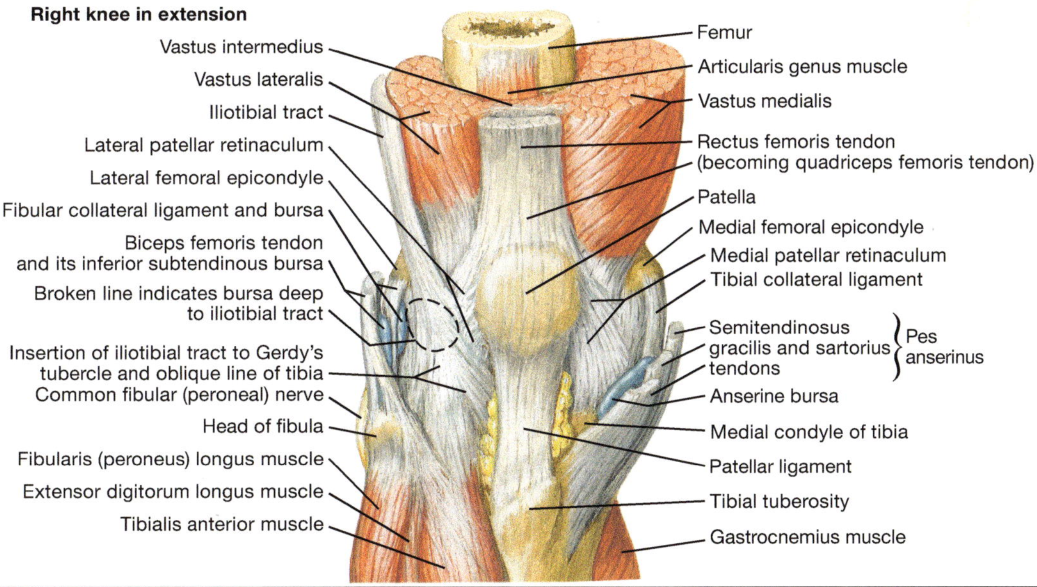

Fig. 15.1 Adipose ligament of the knee. (After Netter, Frank H. YEAR. Atlas of Human Anatomy. 3rd edition, 489. Used with permission of the editor.)

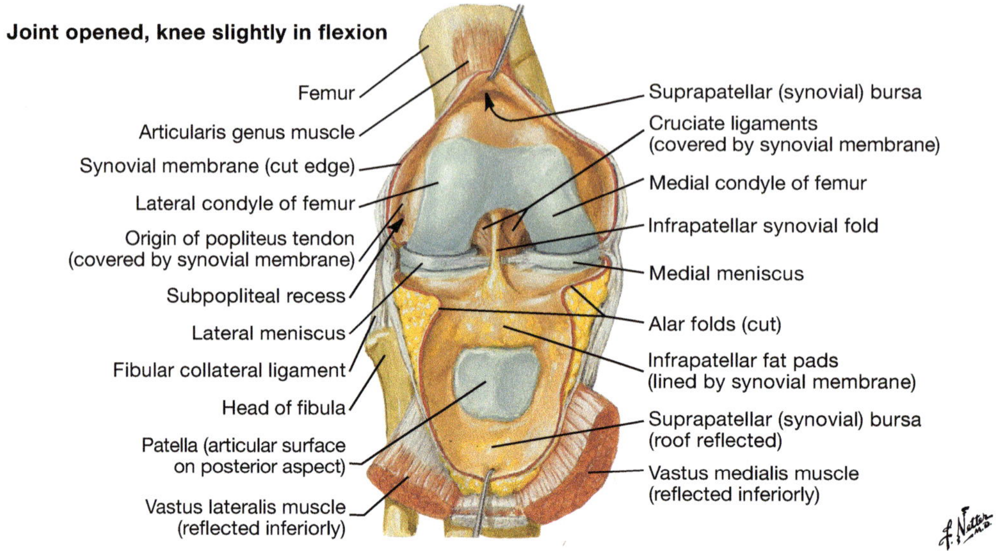

Fig. 15.2 Retinaculum of the knee. (After Netter, Frank H. 2002. Atlas of Human Anatomy. 3rd edition, 489. Used with permission of the editor.)

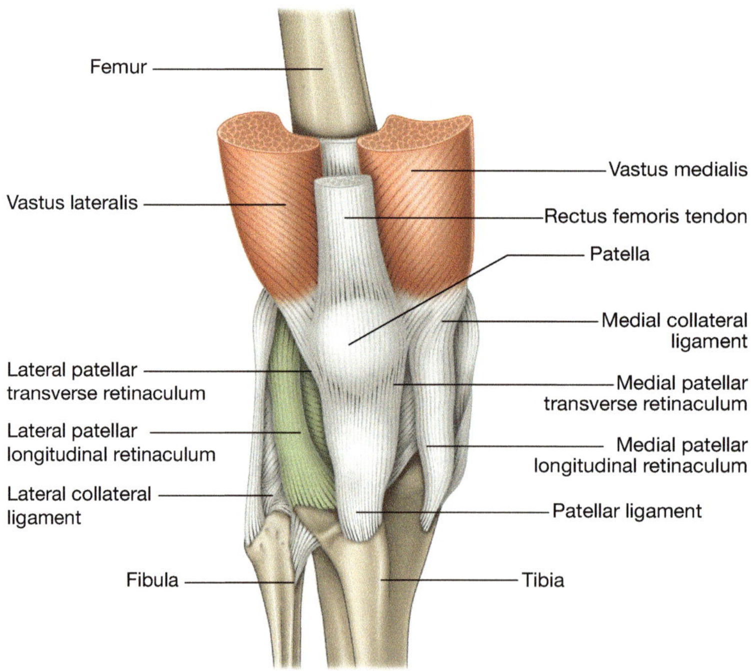

Fig. 15.3 Organization of the lateral retinaculum fibers.

While the adipose ligament is a ligament in name only, it primarily fulfills the cushioning and proprioceptive function.

Shock absorption

Infrapatellar fat cushions and distributes mechanical strain by guaranteeing the "attack angle" of the patellar tendon.

Mechanoreceptor

A slender, elongated cord-like extension of the infrapatellar fat pad is often found at its intercondylar part in front of the joint space. Fatty pads in the vicinity of joints are very rich in mechanoreceptors. Any abnormal tension, unequal fatty distribution, or pressure change, creates distorted neural impulses that are integrated centrally and adversely influence motor loops.

Retinacula (Fig. 15.2)

Fibrous bands called retinacula insert on either side of the patellar ligament and the quadriceps tendon. There also is a lateral retinaculum and a larger medial band that consists of a transverse and longitudinal retinaculum.

15.1.2 Lateral retinaculum (Fig. 15.3)

Origin

It is derived from fibers of the vastus lateralis, rectus femoris, and iliotibial tract.

Terminations

The lateral retinaculum inserts on the lateral part of the tibial tuberosity and tensor fasciae latae. It exchanges fibers with the tibiofibular capsule.

15.1.3 Medial retinaculum (Fig. 15.4)

The medial band is the more important of the pair. Note that the most important structures for stabilizing the knee are generally medial structures such as the collateral tibial ligament, the medial meniscus, the vastus medialis, and muscles of the pes anserinus.

Origin

The medial retinaculum is composed of fascia layers from the vastus medialis and fibers issuing from the medial epicondyle. It also attaches to the adductor tubercle, whose importance derives from the fact that many

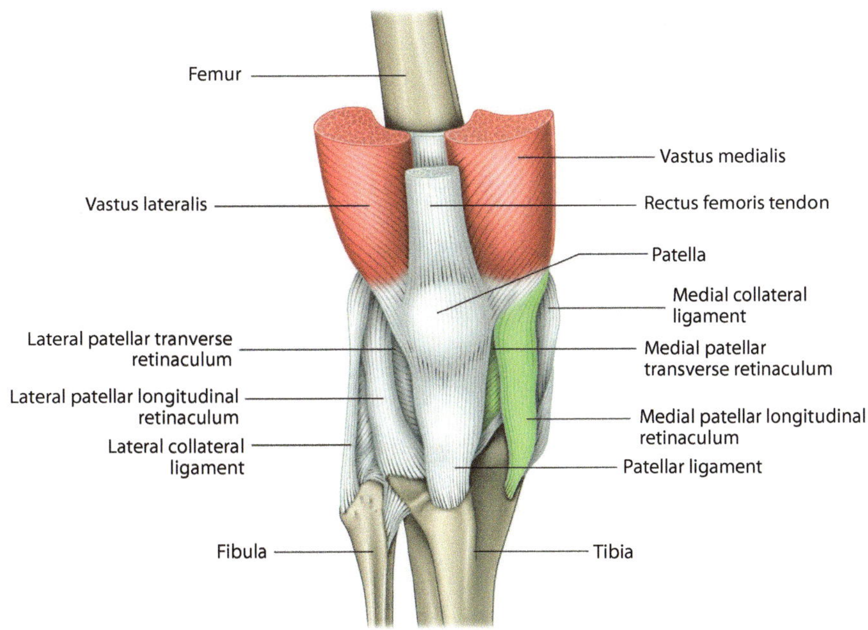

Fig. 15.4 Organization of the medial retinaculum fibers.

structures attach to it and exchange fibers among each other.

Termination

Fibrous bands terminate on the tibia between the patellar ligament and the tibial collateral ligament. Some retinacular fibers merge with the tibial collateral ligament.

15.1.4 Patellar wings (Fig. 15.5)

Patellar wings are formed by the external patellar retinaculum together with cruciate arciform fibers arranged like a laterally reinforced knee brace. It receives fibers from the fascia lata, sartorius, and vastus muscles.

The oblique fibers of the vastus medialis are of special importance in retaining lateral patellar displacement. The patellar wings are treated following the same directions as for the retinaculum.

Special note

Remember that the knee is very much a neurological joint. Its stability depends on perfect musculoligamentous coordination. Knee manipulation demands finesse and subtlety. It is a question of knowing how to interpret small dysfunctions that we can turn to good use with our hands. It is not a question of centimeters but rather millimeters!

15.1.5 Techniques

Lateral retinaculum in decubitus (Fig. 15.6)

Place your fingers on either side of the quadriceps tendon, the patellar ligament, and the corresponding lateral surface of the patella. Begin by moving the lateral retinacular fibers laterally as far as the fibular collateral ligament. Next, draw the quadriceps tendon and patellar ligament medially to better contact the retinacular fibers. Lastly, mobilize the tendon and ligament laterally, searching out microadhesions and microruptures. We are mainly after a proprioceptive benefit here. Alternate a dozen lateral and medial movements and complete the maneuver with induction.

Lateral retinaculum in lateral decubitus (Fig. 15.7)

The patient rests on the side of the knee to be manipulated. You perform the same action as described above. Side lying allows better release of the deeper fibers that lay against the tibia and the tibiofibular joint capsule. Work your way from the cranial part of the patella to the head of the fibula.

Medial retinaculum in decubitus (Fig. 15.8)

Place your fingers on either side of the patellar tendon, encompassing the patellar ligament and the medial retinaculum. Move the patellar ligament and patellar tendon fibers from side to side. Look to separate them from the vastus medialis and the tibial collateral ligament. Pay special attention to the insertion zone of the adductor tubercle located on the medial epicondyle.

Medial retinaculum in decubitus (Fig. 15.9)

The subject lies on the side of the knee in question. This position affords you deeper access. Proceed as outlined for in decubitus.

Adipose ligament in decubitus

Position yourself near the end of the table with the patient's leg on your shoulder. Place the index fingers and middle fingers of both your hands on either side of the patellar tendon.

Test

Using your trunk to create the movement, gently straighten the knee toward full extension. Along the way, compress the adipose ligament against the intercondylar femoral groove. The fat pad should isolate the patella from the patellar tendon. Make a mental note of how the fatty pad moves on either side of the patella. In the normal knee, defor-

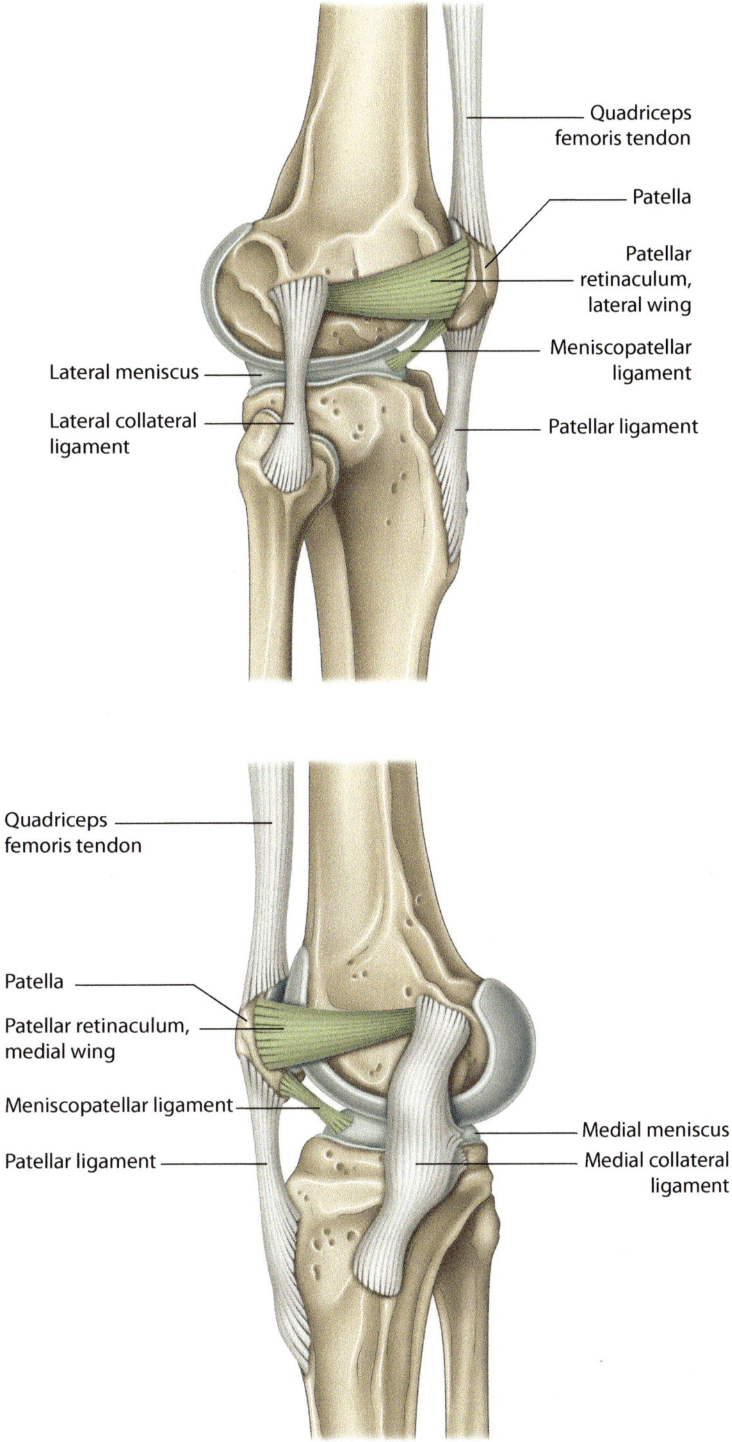

Fig. 15.5 Patellar wings.

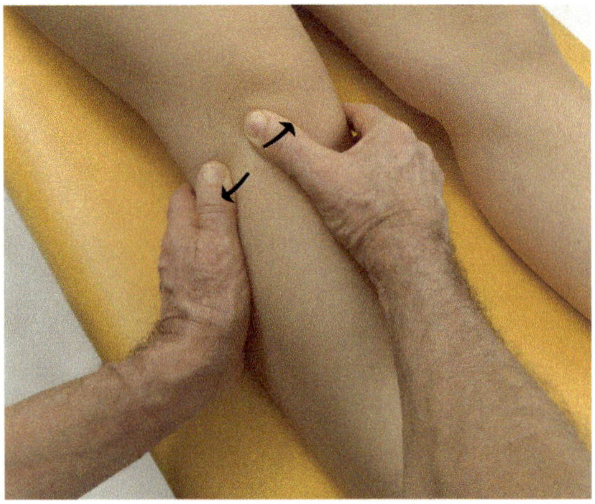

Fig. 15.6 Lateral retinaculum in decubitus.

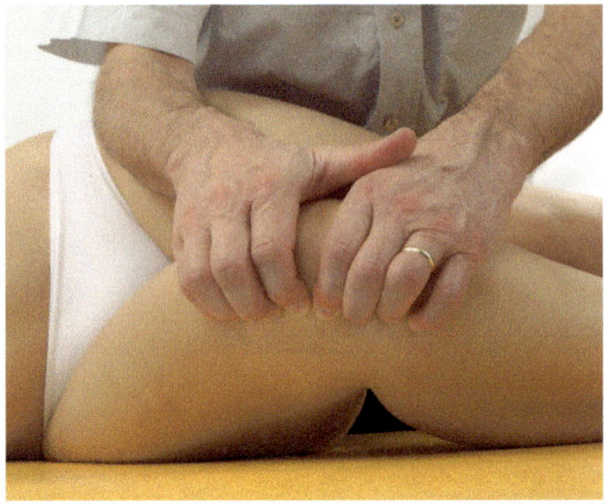

Fig. 15.7 Lateral retinaculum in lateral decubitus.

mation is balanced. If it is not, the disparity must be corrected; otherwise it becomes an underlying cause of patellar tendon strain.

Correction

Keeping the hands in the same position as the test, compress the adipose ligament and the fatty mass between your fingers. Move the knee into extension; as you do, follow the listening with induction. Repeat three or four times before re-testing. If your maneuver is successful, the fat body will recover its symmetrical deformation on both sides of the patellar tendon.

15.2 TIBIAL COLLATERAL LIGAMENT (FIG. 15.10)

15.2.1 Review

This is the most complex of the two collateral ligaments. It is injured 20 times more often than the fibular collateral band. Manipulating the tibial collateral ligament demands finesse. It is triangular in shape and is formed from the capsule.

Origin

The medial epicondyle of the femur, immediately below the adductor tubercle, is an

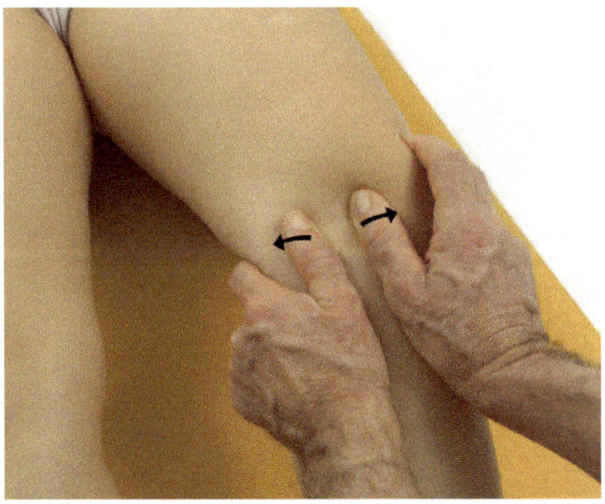

Fig. 15.8 Medial retinaculum in decubitus.

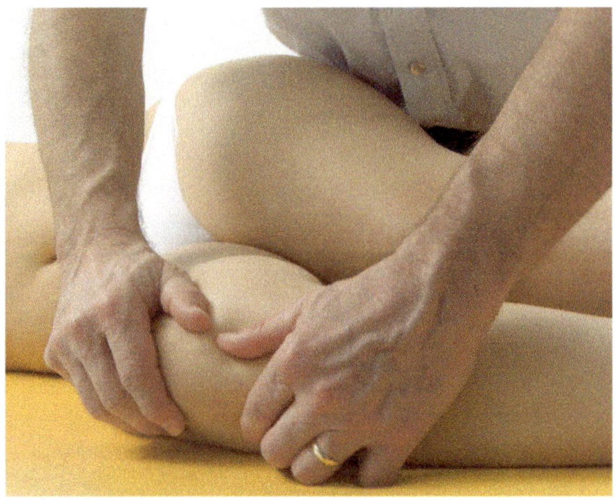

Fig. 15.9 Medial retinaculum in lateral decubitus.

important knee landmark. Also at this level are attachments of:

- the plantaris;
- the medial gastrocnemius;
- the adductor magnus (forms the walls of the adductor hiatus);
- the medial retinaculum.

Direction

- Anterior caudal and slightly lateral

Dimensions

- Width: 1, 2, or even 2.5 cm
- Length: 8–12 cm

Planes (Fig. 15.11)

While narrow cranially, it widens over the meniscus, where it divides into a superficial and a deep plane.

Superficial plane

Femorotibial fibers form the superficial plane. Anterior longitudinal fibers are longer and extend from the medial femoral epicondyle to the medial border of the tibia.

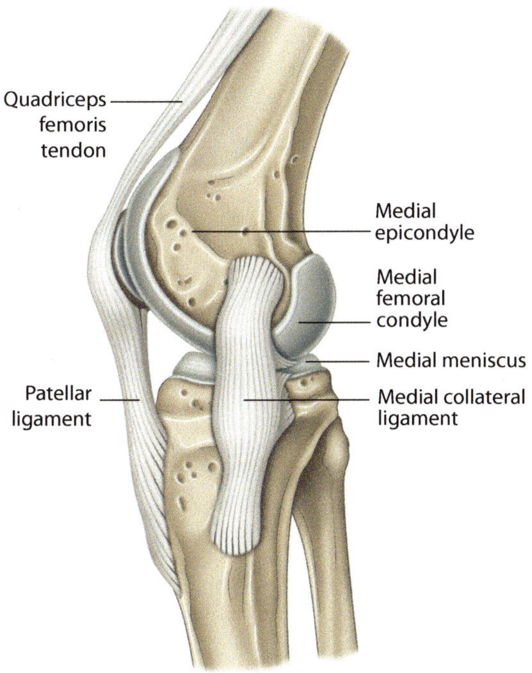

Fig. 15.10 Medial or tibial collateral ligament.

Deep plane

Here we find femoromeniscal fibers and tibiomeniscal fibers. Short posterior and proximal fibers fuse the collateral ligament to the medial meniscus. Posterior and distal fibers attach the medial meniscus to the tibia.

Termination

- Medial surface of the tibia
- Attaches deeply to the proximal quarter of the superficial pes anserinus

Special note

The ligament is fused to the medial meniscus; this is why knee sprains tend to involve the medial meniscus, almost as a matter of course. As it is partially covered by the superficial pes anserinus, comprehensive ligament treatment includes manipulation of the caudal insertions of the sartorius, semitendinosus, and gracilis.

The ligament crosses over the reflected semimembranosus tendon, implying that treatment of the medial collateral ligament must also include the various caudal insertions of the semimembranosus. The reflected tendon curves as it passes beneath the medial collateral ligament, retaining this curvature during knee extension. Note that the tendon straightens out in knee flexion.

Keep in mind, we have observed that the adductor tubercle serves as the insertion of several muscles and fascia. Explore this tubercle well, as any abnormal fibrous attachment tensions can alter proprioception. The same applies to the pes anserinus, where you often discover microtears or microadhesions on the boney muscular insertions. Recalcitrant tendinitis can easily arise here.

15.2.2 Techniques

In lateral decubitus

Femorotibial fibers (Fig. 15.12)

Position yourself before the patient, who is lying on the side of the knee to be treated, leg slightly flexed. Place one thumb on the

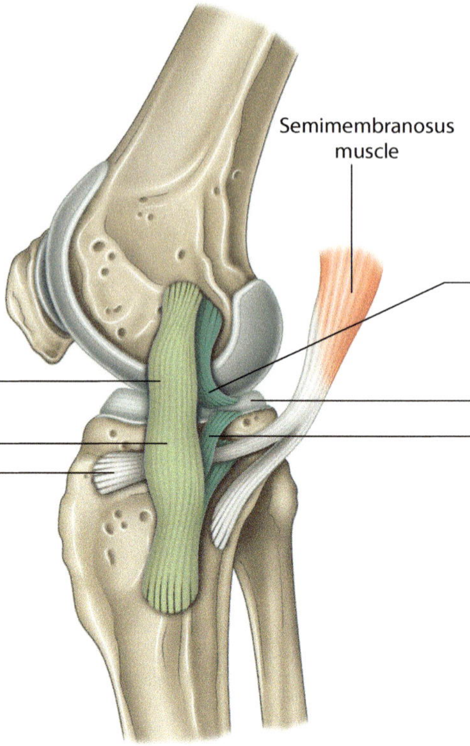

Fig. 15.11 Two planes of the tibial collateral ligament.

medial epicondyle, immediately below the adductor tubercle. Place your other thumb on the tibial insertion of the MCL.

Glide your thumbs in searching for microirregularities that you work in smoothing-induction. Hunt longitudinally and transversely through fibers of the tibial collateral ligament. Fixing the cranial and caudal parts of the ligament between your thumbs, ask the patient to flex and extend his knee. In extension you will feel the fibers tense. Accentuate this tension in order to reduce ligament fibrosis and to free the especially subtle mechanoreceptors located here.

Femoromeniscal fibers (Fig. 15.13)

Direct your fingers from the femoral insertion of the tibial collateral to the medial meniscus. While any true division is somewhat of a contrivance, fibers can nevertheless be separated methodically and minutely. Remember that the knee is a neurological joint where precision counts. High-leverage or heavy-handed maneuvers are ineffective and irritating.

Proceed along the edge of the tibia plateau as far as the medial meniscus, softening any irregular ligamentous zones. You will be surprised by the number of small irregularities you come across.

Tibiomeniscal fibers (Fig. 15.14)

First differentiate fibers of the reflected semimembranosus tendon, located at the caudal part of the meniscotibial segment of the tibial collateral ligament. Apply the same techniques as for the other parts of the ligament.

Adductor tubercle (Fig. 15.15)

Several structures attach to the tubercle. It is useful to differentiate their fibers to better inform the delicate and subtle proprioceptive system at the medial surface of the knee.

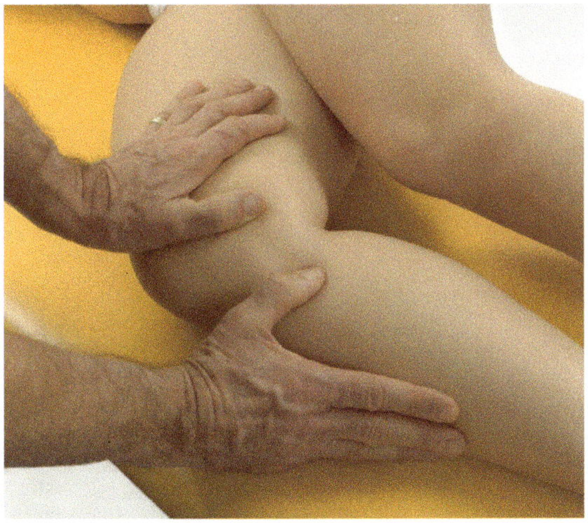

Fig. 15.12 Femorotibial fibers of the medial collateral ligament.

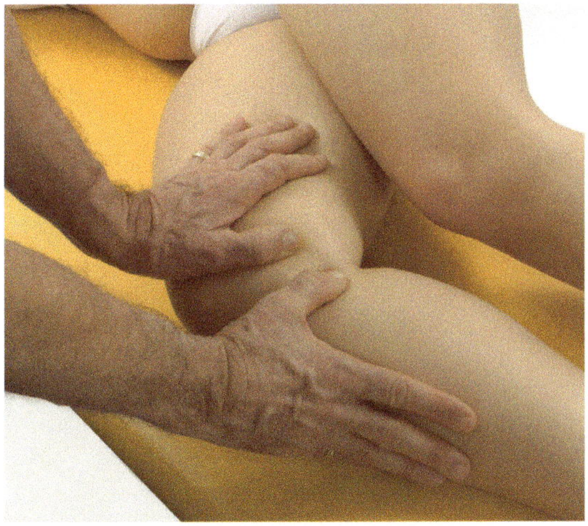

Fig. 15.13 Femoromeniscal fibers of the medial collateral ligament.

Attached to the adductor tubercle are:

- the adductor magnus;
- the medial collateral ligament;
- the capsule of the knee;
- the medial retinaculum;
- the vastus medialis (more or less directly);
- the medial gastrocnemius.

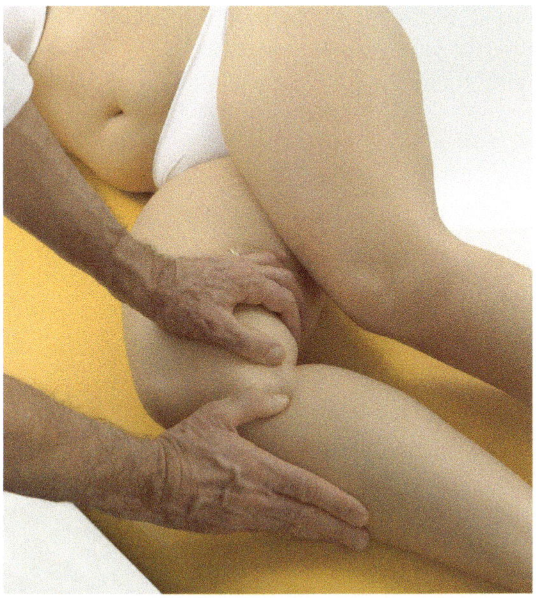

Fig. 15.14 Tibiomeniscal fibers of the medial collateral ligament.

15.3 FIBULAR COLLATERAL LIGAMENT (FIG. 15.16)

15.3.1 Review

This band is totally different from the tibial collateral ligament in structure and arrangement. It attaches neither to the lateral meniscus nor to the capsule.

Origin

- Posterior caudal part of the lateral femoral condyle

Direction

- Oblique caudal, posterior, and slightly medial

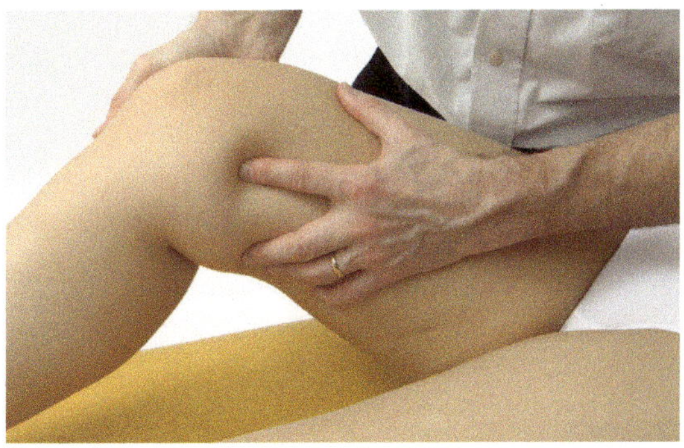

Fig. 15.15 Adductor tubercle location.

- Four centimeters long, making it much shorter than its medial counterpart

Termination

- Head of the fibula on its posterior lateral slope
- The greater part of its lateral surface covered by the biceps tendon

Characteristics

- Round
- Runs about 1 cm distant from the joint capsule
- Has no direct contact with the capsule or the lateral meniscus
- Covered by the popliteus tendon
- Situated laterally to the arcuate popliteal ligament
- Reinforced by biceps femoris and the iliotibial tract
- Stronger than the medial collateral ligament

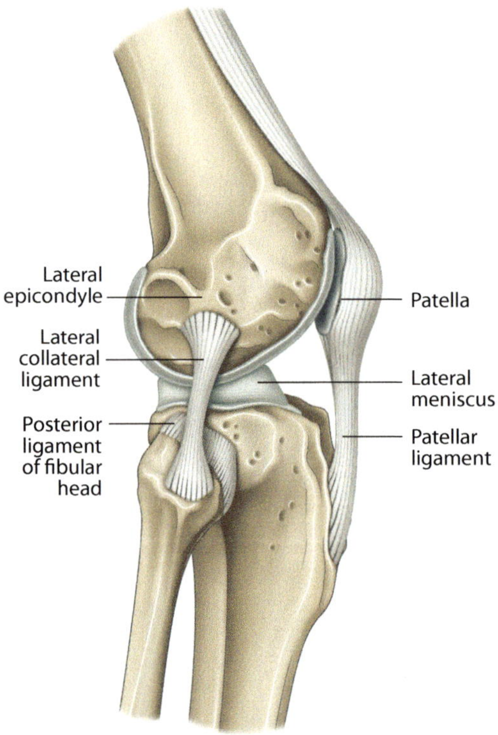

Fig. 15.16 Lateral collateral or fibular ligament.

Extensibility and mobility

- The lateral collateral ligament is taut when the knee joint is in extension and during lateral rotation.
- It relaxes more quickly in flexion than does the medial collateral ligament. This allows it to free up the lateral part of the knee, permitting automatic medial rotation during knee flexion.

Remember that in extension both collateral ligaments tighten, along with the anterior portion of the anterior cruciate ligament.

15.3.2 Techniques

In lateral decubitus (Fig. 15.17)

The patient lies on the side opposite the affected knee. Approach this technique by placing yourself either in front of or behind the patient.

Technique for the insertions

Place one thumb on the lateral femoral epicondyle and the other on the head of the femur. Search methodically for rough spots, first on the tendinous insertions at the bone and next along the course of the ligament itself. Work in induction either statically or by asking the patient to move the leg in slight flexion and extension during the treatment.

Clinical applications

Generally speaking, therapists pay less attention to the fibular collateral ligament than to its tibial analog. In tibial collateral ligament sprain, however, the tibia glides laterally, impacting the fibular collateral ligament, as well. In response, the fibular ligament "resends" the tibia in a medial direction. This is why it is always important to treat the lateral collateral ligament, even if it appears to be uninjured. The fibular collateral ligament receives the aftermath of mechanical forces from a forced twist to the opposite side. It thus merits reprogramming in the proprioceptive sense.

Technique for the body of the ligament (Fig. 15.18)

With the patient in the same position as above, ask him to flex and extend the knee in order to put the ligament on traction. Look for small lesional patches on the body of the ligament and treat with induction.

15.4 ANTERIOR CRUCIATE LIGAMENT (FIG. 15.19)

15.4.1 Review

This band is less powerful, less thick, and less vascularized than the posterior cruciate ligament.

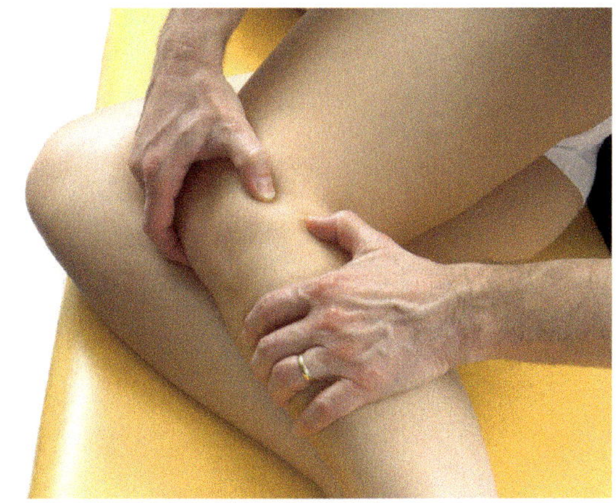

Fig. 15.17 Lateral collateral ligament in decubitus.

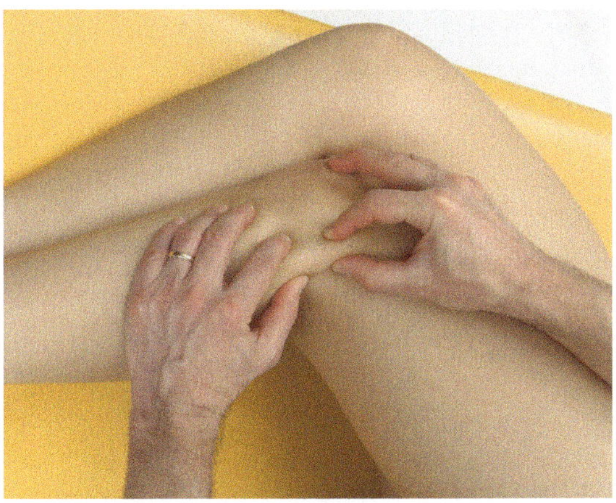

Fig. 15.18 18 Manipulation of the body of the lateral collateral ligament in lateral decubitus.

Origin

- Attaches to the anterior intercondylar area of the tibia, partly blended with the anterior horn of the meniscus

Direction

- Oblique cranial, posterior, and lateral

Termination

- Femoral attachment of ligament is on posterior cranial part of medial surface of the femoral condyle, at lateral surface of intercondylar notch

Mobility of the anterior cruciate ligament

In extension, the anterior part of the cruciate ligament is tight. In the last 10° of knee extension, the femur rotates 5° to lock the joint in place (locking rotation). This terminal rotation is made possible by:

- the shape of the medial condyle of the femur;
- the popliteal muscle action;
- the tension on the anterior cruciate ligament.

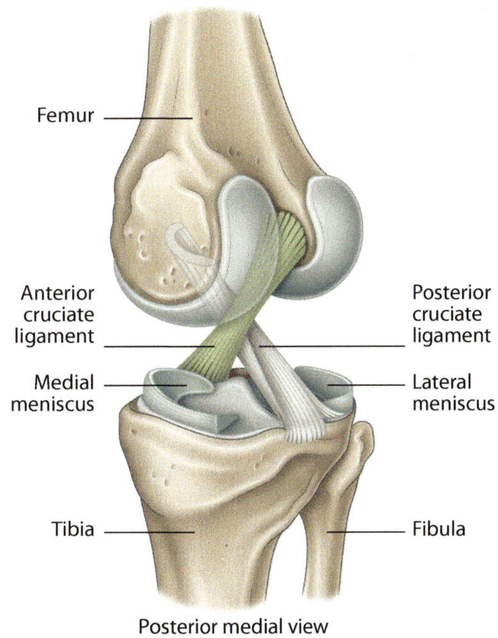

Fig. 15.19 Anterior cruciate ligament.

The two cruciate ligaments twist around each other slightly in the straight leg.

Locking rotation is accomplished by:

- lateral rotation of the tibia on the supporting leg;
- medial rotation of the coxofemoral joint.

In flexion, the cruciate ligaments twist around each other to impede excessive medial torsion. The anterior cruciate ligament slackens.

Special note

The obliquity of the cruciate ligaments in all knee positions means that one pair or a part of one pair is always under tension. The anterior cruciate ligament has rather weak vascularity, making it more fragile.

Role of the anterior cruciate ligament

- This ligament limits anterior to posterior displacement of the tibial plateau.
- It prevents excessive rotation during flexion.
- It inwardly rotates the femur when taut to allow the medial condyle to increase its joint surface and become more curved.
- It diminishes full extension to unlock the knee.
- The last 10° of extension obliges the knee to rotate 5°.
- The paired cruciate ligaments have partial synovial sheaths that contribute to lubrication by redistributing synovial fluid.
- The anterior cruciate ligament is less vascularized than its posterior counterpart, which factors in its fragility. It is also less robust.

15.4.2 Pathology

Our patients often say things like, "My knee just gave way." We have seen numerous patients whose cruciate ligament ruptured during a simple rotation movement, such as turning around to see someone.

In the aftermath of microtrauma, the anterior cruciate ligament thins to the point of frailty. The least suspected tension can rupture it because of its predisposed weakness and mediocre blood supply. In addition, the anterior cruciate ligament exchanges fibers with the anterior horn of the medial meniscus, meaning that the meniscus is implicated with every sprain. Add to this the fact that the medial meniscus receives fibers from the medial collateral ligament. A sprain of this collateral ligament destabilizes the anterior cruciate ligament.

Cruciate ligament pivot

The cruciate ligaments of the knee form a central system of attachment that stabilizes the inside of the joint, in contrast to the collateral ligaments, which stabilize the sides of the joint. The cruciate ligaments have a thickness a little less than one centimeter.

The lower extremity is distinguished from the upper extremity by its central system of bonding unions, which are:

- the ligament of the head of the femur;
- the cruciate ligaments of the knee;
- the talocalcaneal ligament of the subtalar joint.

Anterior cruciate ligament tears are among the most common knee injuries. Rare is the high-level athlete who has escaped a dreaded lesion of the anterior cruciate ligament.

Lachman test in decubitus (Fig. 15.20)

The patient rests the foot of the knee concerned on the table. You sit on the foot. This test is always performed on the table. Mobilize the anterior and posterior tibia with your hands placed on either side of the tibial plateau. We never do this test in a sudden manner. A progressive push and pull more than suffices to evaluate the cruciate ligaments.

Knee drawers (Fig. 15.21)

Anterior drawer

This test is positive when the tibia translates anteriorly more than 5° in relation to the femur, except in hypermobile subjects. Excessive anterior displacement of the tibia—

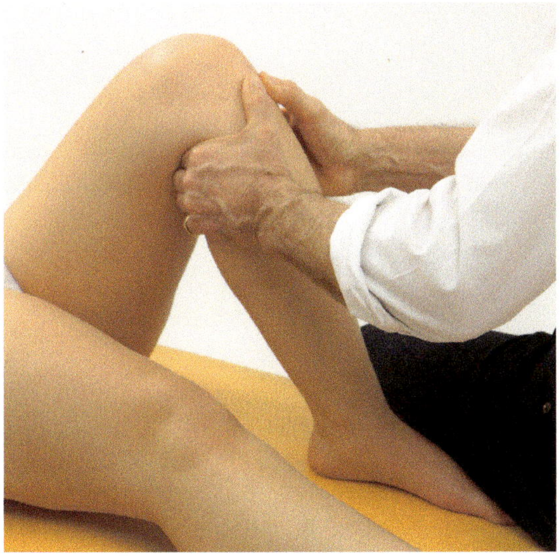

Fig. 15.20 Lachman test.

more than 5°—suggests a rupture of the anterior cruciate ligament.

Posterior drawer

In the same position, excessive posterior displacement of the tibia—more than 5°—indicates injury to the posterior cruciate ligament.

15.4.3 Techniques

The objective of our technique is never a question of reconstructing a ruptured ligament but of working to improve proprioceptive awareness. The test, like the manipulation, is best performed in the precise direction of the cruciate ligament insofar as the ligament is still intact.

Anterior cruciate ligament test

The patient is in decubitus, leg flexed, foot resting on the table. With both hands surrounding the tibial plateau, draw the plateau anteriorly and medially to put the ligament under tension. If the tibia comes forward excessively, the anterior cruciate ligament has a lesion.

Be careful with recent sprains. The draw test is negative because of the pain and edema at the knee, which stabilize the articulation. This false negative is a frequent

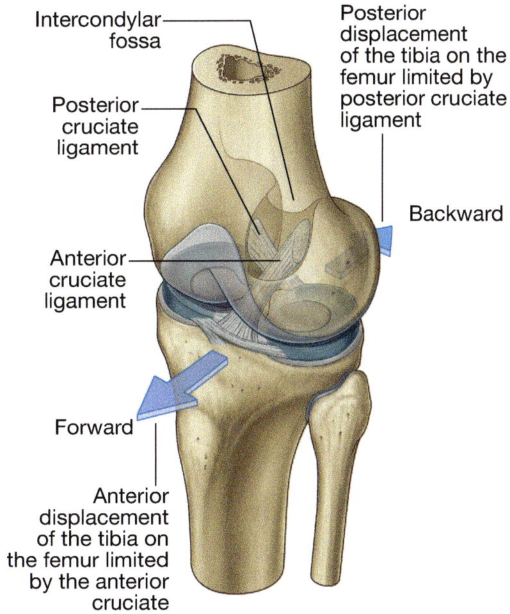

Fig. 15.21 Knee drawers.

diagnostic error. It is advisable to wait one month before doing a complete knee assessment.

Anterior cruciate ligament technique decubitus (Fig. 15.22)

The foot is flat on the table, knee up. Encompass the tibial plateau with both of your hands and perform several small anterior drawer movements. To be sure that you are on the cruciate ligament axis, draw the tibia in an anterior medial direction. Do this several times to stimulate the mechanoreceptors, and finish with a slow and progressive induction.

15.5 POSTERIOR CRUCIATE LIGAMENT (FIG. 15.23)

15.5.1 Review

The posterior cruciate ligament is the more powerful, thicker, better vascularized, and stronger of the two central ligaments. Its thickness approaches 3 cm.

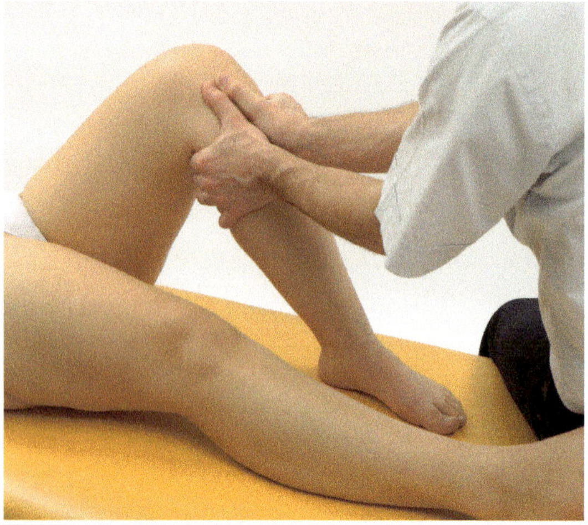

Fig. 15.22 Anterior cruciate ligament technique in decubitus.

Origin

- Lateral surface of the medial tibial condyle bordering the posterior intercondylar surface of the bone

Direction

- Oblique cranial, anterior, and medial, twisting into anteriomedial and latero-lateral fiber bundles

Termination

- Medial condyle of the femur in the intercondylar fossa at the anteriocranial part of the axial surface

Special note

It attaches to the posterior meniscofemoral ligament, which it serves to reinforce.

Meniscofemoral ligament (Fig. 15.24)

Origin

- Posterior horn of the lateral meniscus

Termination

- Anterior surface of the posterior cruciate ligament with which it affixes to the lateral surface of the lateral condyle

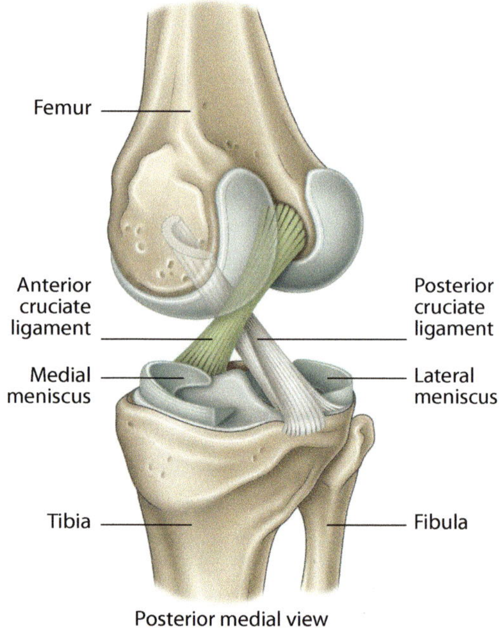

Fig. 15.23 Posterior cruciate ligament.

Function of the posterior cruciate ligament

When the knee is flexed in weight bearing, it prevents the femur from gliding forward on the tibial plateau. In walking downhill, it similarly resists anterior displacement of the femur on the tibial plateau. Recall that the strain on the knee when walking down stairs amounts to five to six times the body weight.

15.5.2 Technique

In procubitus (Fig. 15.25)

The patient lies prone with the leg flexed. The manipulation essentially pushes the tibia in a posterior direction. To accomplish this, place the palm of one hand against the proximal border of the tibia near the tibial tuberosity. With the other hand, stabilize the flexed knee. Stretch the tibia along its axis, flexing it somewhat. Work in induction.

Effectiveness of our ligament techniques

While we have no formal proof of the effectiveness of our ligament techniques, we

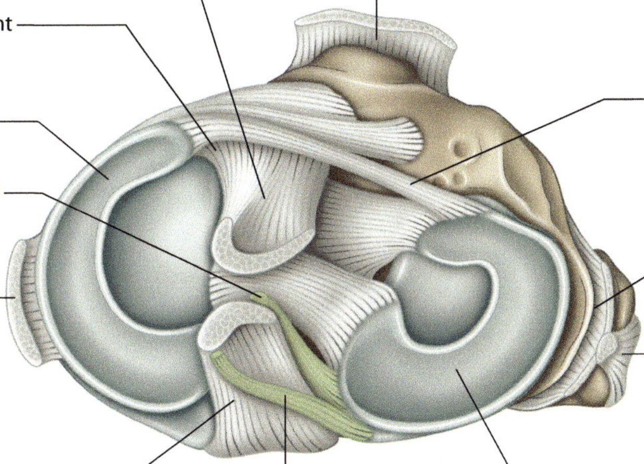

Fig. 15.24 Meniscofemoral ligament.

have empirically witnessed their result on many patients. Improvements that have sometimes been spectacular have encouraged us to persevere along this path.

We have already stressed that the knee is a neurological joint. Our goal is to restore proprioception to every soft tissue component. We believe that our actions influence the established proprioceptive loop that connects ligaments with stabilizing muscle action. In the past few years much research has been done globally on the subject of proprioceptive feedback loops.

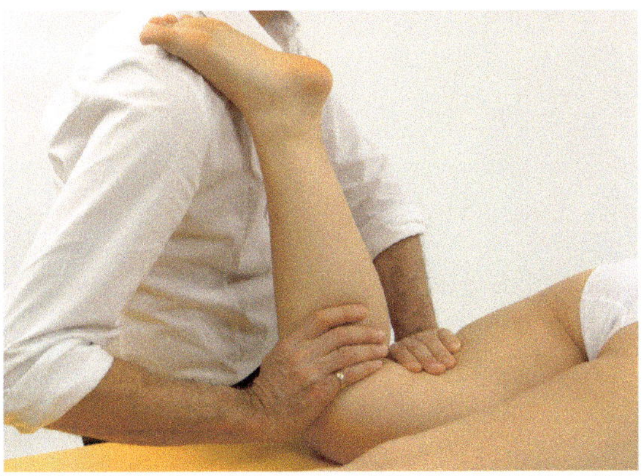

Fig. 15.25 Posterior cruciate ligament technique in procubitus.

It would be illusionary to think we might obtain good results using our techniques on completely ruptured ligaments. This being said, there are a good many instances where partial tears or their aftermaths have responded to our techniques. Patients have reported improved sensation coming from the joint, and they tell us that the knee feels better. Some who have suffered longtime instability, a feeling of being off kilter, and have endured frequent falls as a result, tell us they no longer suffer sprains or have the feeling that their knee might give way.

To quantify and objectify a therapeutic action requires a tremendous amount of clinical study with trial carried out according to precise methodology. This demands not only a huge amount of energy but, above all, time! Should we wait for such "scientific" proof before we use certain new techniques? This course might well be necessary for the administration of certain pharmaceutical substances or for innovative surgical techniques. It seems to us, however, that techniques such as ours, which have negligible iatrogenic potential, can wait a bit on this step.

Among the many problems that arise in the pursuit of research in the emerging field of osteopathy is the role of the technical operator. For a study to be valid, it must not only respect a solid methodology, but the practitioners that take part in the study must also be chosen for their skilled level of practice. They must have put these techniques to use for some time and have significant clinical experiences.

Under these conditions, if an operator is experimenting with a new technique, this means by definition that he is using it for perhaps the first time. In truth, a practitioner must have substantial and convincing clinical experience with any technique for it to be of value. This presupposes that he has not waited on scientific proof before he begins the study! Herein lies the paradox of administering such research.

15.6 POSTERIOR CAPSULAR COMPLEX

A heterogeneous array of anatomy provides posterior strength to the knee. The posterior capsular complex is frequently injured in extension trauma to the knee. The various component tissues often carry a lasting mark of injury. Precision requires a good understanding of anatomy basics.

15.6.1 Condylar shells

Constitution

These structures are thickenings of capsular fibers. Spherical in shape, their anterior surfaces mold over the femoral condyles, producing their concave shell-like shape. The posterior surface relates to the medial and lateral heads of the gastrocnemius muscle. The lateral shell is thicker and denser than its medial counterpart. We find the fabella at this level.

Expansions

The condylar shells connect to attachments of:

- the oblique popliteal ligament;
- the arcuate popliteal ligament;
- the gastrocnemius muscle, specifically the lateral head where the fabella is found.

15.6.2 Fabella (Fig. 15.26)

The fabella, "little bean," is a small sesamoid bone embedded in the thickened aponeurosis of the lateral head of the gastrocnemius muscle, behind the lateral femoral condyle. When the fabella is absent, you feel a fibrous body where thickened capsular fibers blend with the aponeurosis of the lateral head of the gastrocnemius muscle.

Why is this structure of interest? The fabella is an important landmark because fibers of the lateral head of the gastrocnemius arise from the articular capsule of the knee. The fabella, or the aponeurotic capsular reinforcement that replaces the fabella, therefore functions as a witness to capsular tensions. It also registers oblique and arcuate popliteal ligamentous stress.

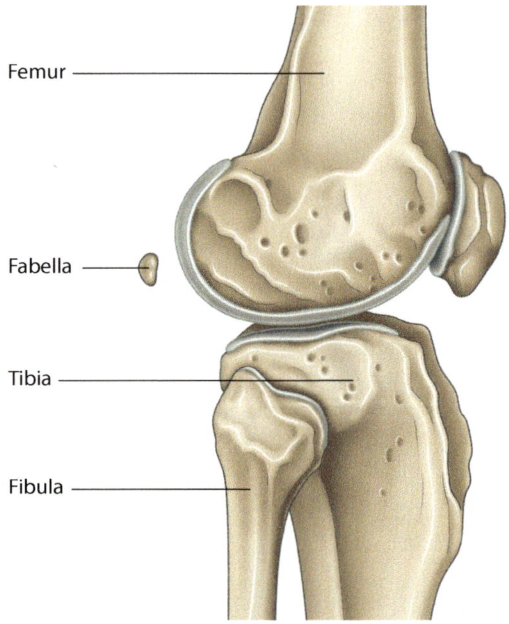

Fig. 15.26 Fabella location.

15.6.3 Arcuate popliteal ligament (Fig. 15.27)

The arcuate popliteal ligament terminates on the fabella, which is why we describe it below.

Origin

- Apex of the fibula

Direction

- Cranial, with some fibers more medial

Termination

- Arches over the proximal popliteus muscle tendon insertion
- Condylar shell and the fabella
- Lateral part of the oblique popliteal ligament with which it exchanges fibers
- Anterior part of the lateral head of the gastrocnemius muscle

15.6.4 Oblique popliteal ligament (Fig. 15.28)

This flat, fibrous band is both a ligament and the recurrent termination of the semimembranosus muscle. It inserts onto the capsule as a broad triangular expansion.

Origin

- Lateral side of the semimembranosus muscle

Direction

- Fans out cranially and laterally

Termination

- Condylar shell and fabella

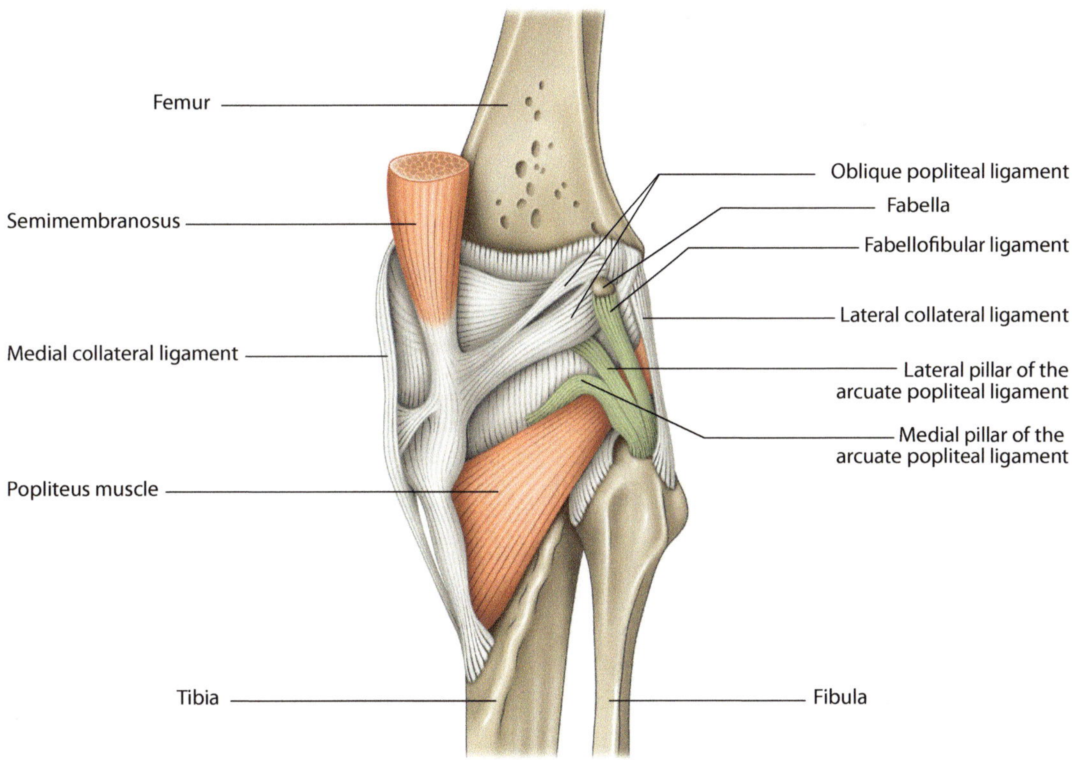

Fig. 15.27 Arcuate popliteal ligament.

15.6.5 Techniques

Opening the popliteal space

Before embarking on posterior capsular manipulation, it is best to first spread open the diamond-shaped popliteal space.

Borders and contents

- Laterally and cranially: biceps femoris
- Laterally and caudally: lateral head of gastrocnemius
- Medially and cranially: semimembranosus and semitendinosus
- Medially and caudally: medial head of gastrocnemius

On the floor of the space is the popliteal fossa, which is the main conduit for the tibial nerve laterally. Medially it transmits the popliteal artery and vein.

Rigidity of the diamond-shaped space

In the aftermath of trauma or knee arthrosis, muscles of the popliteal space have a tendency to become rigid and close the space. This in turn irritates the tibial and common fibular nerves and compresses the vascular structures passing through it. The patient feels tingling, sometimes even pain, in the leg due to this neurovascular compression.

The popliteal space should be spread open preliminarily to all deeper manipulations of the posterior knee, whether structural, neural, or vascular.

Popliteal space in procubitus (Fig. 15.29)

The patient lies prone on the table. First, have both your thumbs maintain spreading-induction of the biceps, semitendinosus, and semimembranosus muscles. Next, spread the heads of the gastrocnemius. Alterna-

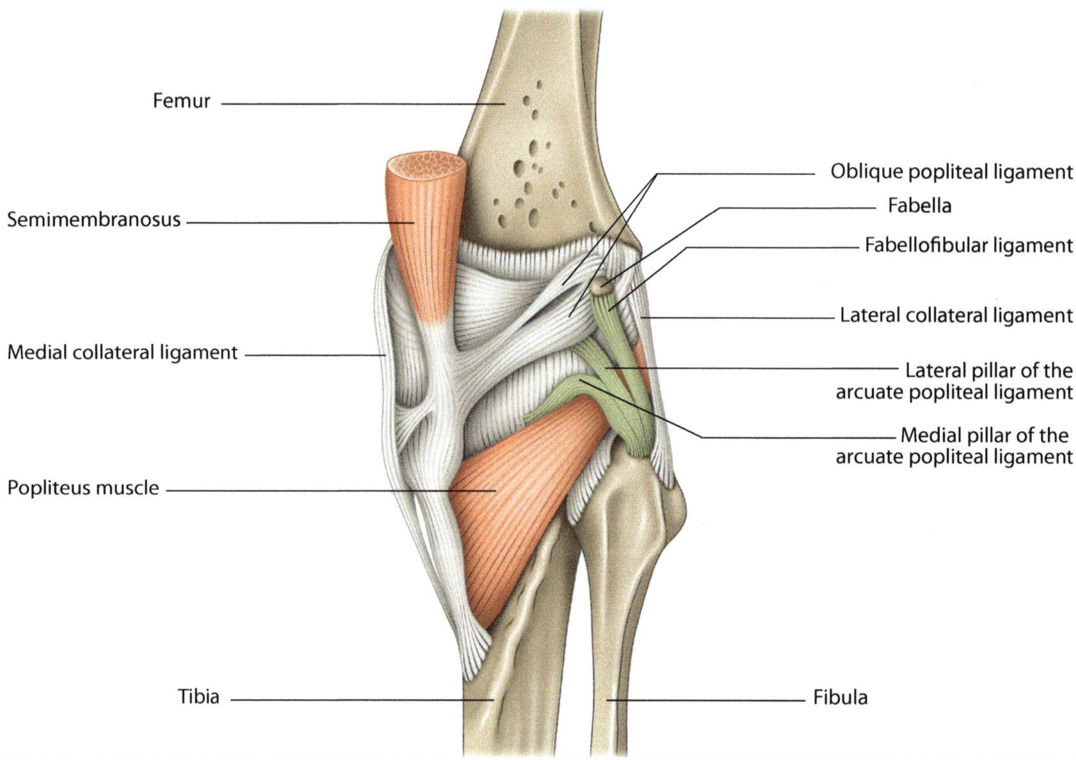

Fig. 15.28 Oblique popliteal ligament.

tively, this opening maneuver can be done working the back of the knee in supine, with the patient's foot on your shoulder.

Oblique popliteal ligament in lateral decubitus (Fig. 15.30)

Place yourself in front of the patient, who is lying on the side of the knee in question. Have him place the slightly flexed knee in front of the straighter leg. Begin with your index fingers on the lateral part of the knee at the level of the fabella or the area of concentration of the aponeurotic capsular fibers. Draw your fingers in the direction of the semimembranosus attachment toward the medial part of the tibia. Stretch the oblique popliteal ligament transversely from lateral to medial and from medial to lateral. Do this several times. Next, mobilize the tendon longitudinally from cranial to caudal and from caudal to cranial.

Always finish the technique with induction. This maneuver brings the gastrocnemius into this technique, as well. Mobilize your fingers in between the two muscle heads to be sure to affect the capsule.

Note: This technique can also be done with the patient lying on the opposite side.

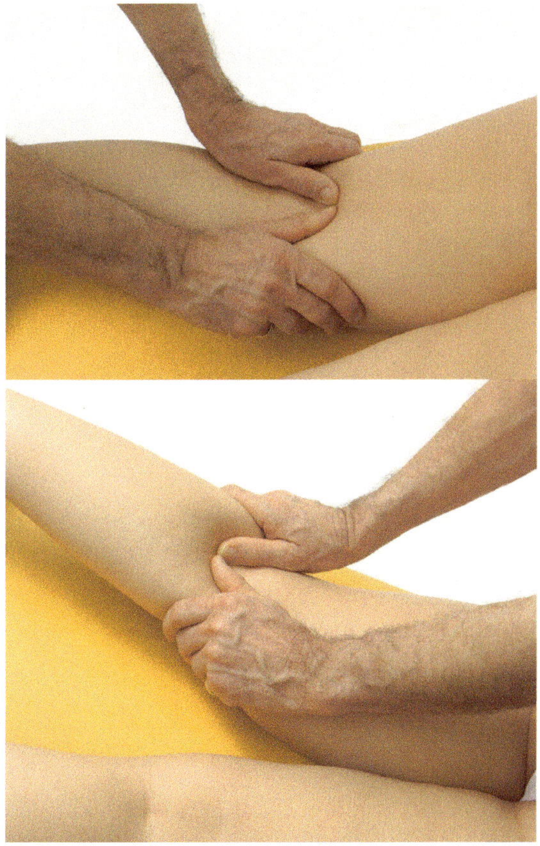

Fig. 15.29 Opening the diamond-shaped popliteal fossa.

Popliteal cysts or Baker's cysts

In medicine it is often said that popliteal cysts are due to inflammation of the serous bursa of the muscles of the popliteal pit. While this is partly true, we believe that quite often the synovial problem has a mechanical origin, either on account of an activity or because it is hormonally induced in perimenopause.

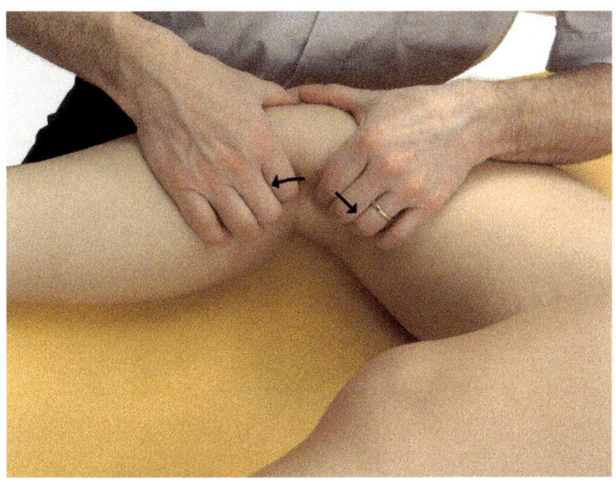

Fig. 15.30 Oblique popliteal ligament in later decubitus.

Arcuate popliteal ligament in lateral decubitus (Fig. 15.31)

The patient lies on the side opposite the knee concerned. To clearly differentiate the arcuate popliteal ligament from the fibular collateral ligament, ask the patient to flex the knee. Both the fibular collateral ligament and the biceps femoris ligament move more laterally when the knee is bent. With your thumb and index finger, start at the apex of the head of the fibula to meet the fabella or the aponeurotic capsular counterpart. Work the fibers transversely until you feel the initial tensions release.

Fibular head (Fig. 15.32)

This is another zone well worth familiarizing yourself with in order to better inform the proprioceptive system of the knee. Numerous mechanical influences reflective of a system of adaptations for the lower extremity are concentrated here. Examination of the fibular head is often rich in diagnostic as well therapeutic value.

The attachments of the fibular head are:

- the collateral fibular ligament;
- the arcuate popliteal ligament;
- the tibiofibular capsule;
- the biceps femoris;
- the extensor digitorum longus muscle;
- the interosseous membrane;
- the lateral retinaculum;
- the common fibular nerve that winds around the fibular head.

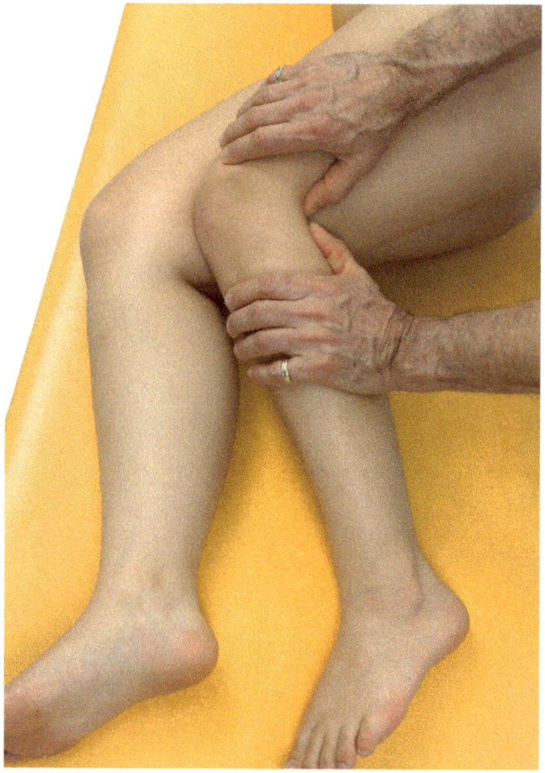

Fig. 15.31 Arcuate popliteal ligament in lateral decubitus.

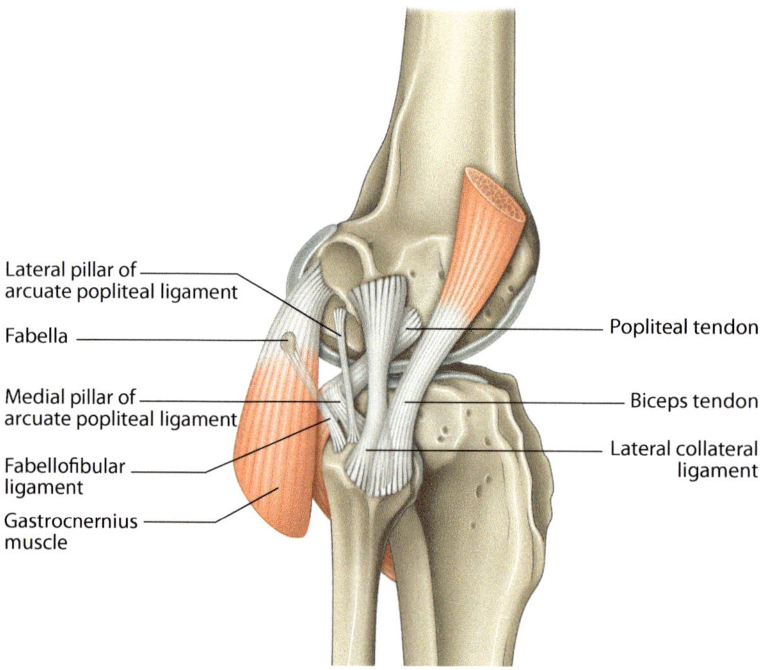

Fig. 15.32 Insertions on head of the fibula.

Treatment of the gliding apparatus

16

16.1 ARTICULAR MUSCLE OF THE KNEE (FIG. 16.1A AND B)

16.1.2 Review

Insertions

- The articular muscle of the knee is a small muscle annexed to the vastus intermedius of the quadriceps. The quadriceps inserts at the junction of the two proximal thirds and the distal third of the femur on the anterior and lateral surfaces of the bone.
- Situated behind the rectus femoris, the articular muscle is distinctly separate from the vastus lateralis but less distinct from the vastus medialis.
- Some fibers attach to the anterior surface of the capsule.
- It terminates on the capsulosynovial subquadricipital cul-de-sac and the suprapatellar bursa.

Functions

The articular muscle of the knee elevates the capsule and prevents capsular folds from being pinched during extension of the leg. It tenses the subpatellar synovial bursa. When the muscle becomes fibrosed, synovial fluid circulation is compromised. Some-

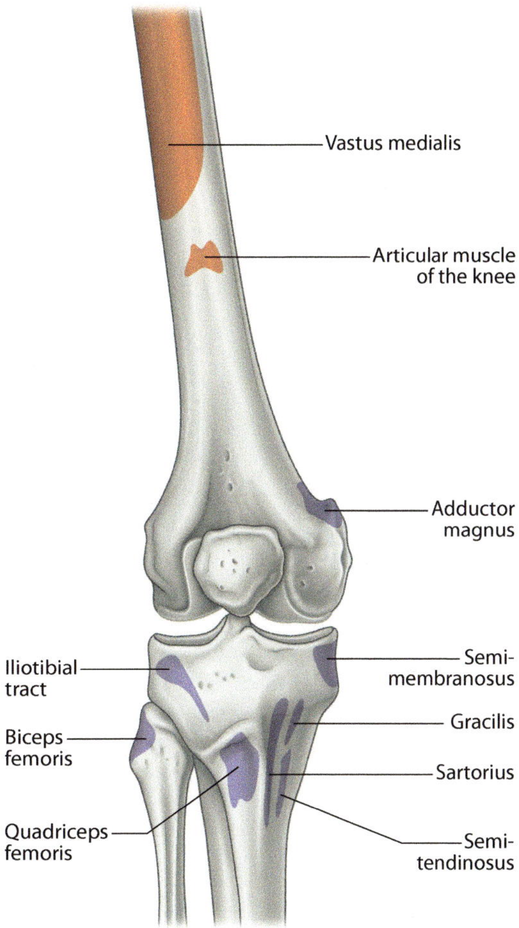

Fig. 16.1A Articular muscle of the knee.

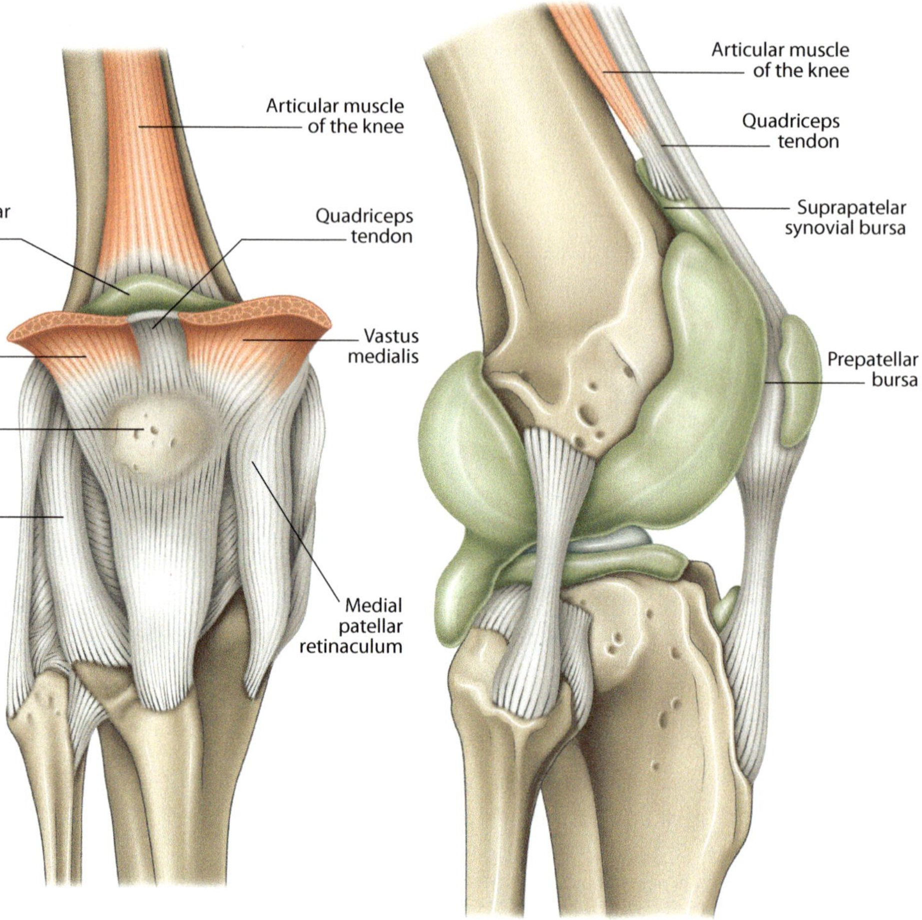

Fig. 16.1B Articular muscle of the knee.

times resorption is insufficient; other times, production is inadequate. Either way, the outcome is quantitative and qualitative synovial fluid disturbance. Manipulation of this small muscle garners good results, notably in cases of synovitis.

16.1.2 Techniques

In decubitus (Fig. 16.2)

The patient rests his hands on his abdomen. You position yourself at the height of the knee concerned. Direct your thumbs under the vastus lateralis, very close to the patellar tendon, in a medial direction.

Next, direct your thumbs under the vastus medialis, very near the patellar tendon, in a lateral direction. You will immediately feel the articular muscle exchange more muscle fibers with the vastus medialis.

Finally, mobilize the articular muscle side to side, being careful to keep the thumbs and fingers against the femur. As you mobilize, you want to disengage the articular muscle from the anterior surface of the femur, finishing with induction.

In lateral decubitus (Fig. 16.3)

The patient rests by turning onto the medial and lateral side of the treatment knee. Proceed as in decubitus above. The

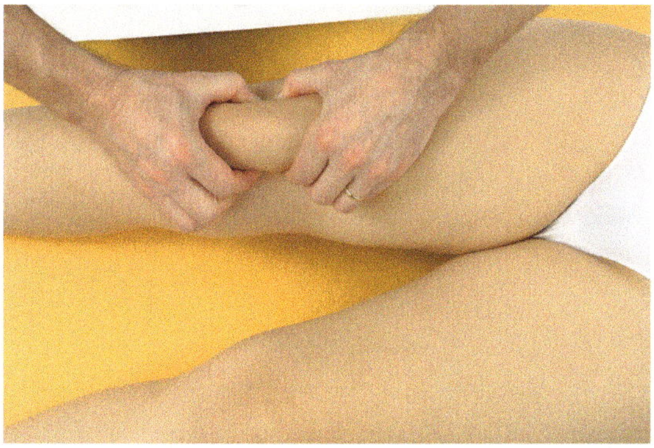

Fig. 16.2 Articular muscle of the knee in decubitus.

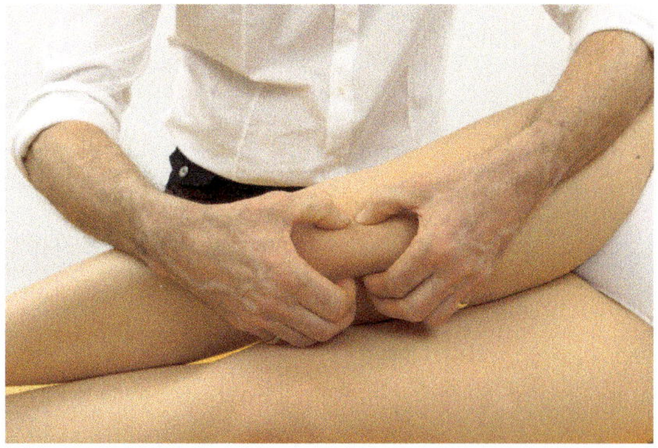

Fig. 16.3 Articular muscle of the knee in lateral decubitus.

side-lying position permits a deeper access to the underneath of the articular muscle. It is not always easy to move this muscle on the femur, especially with chronic knee pain where the muscle is firmly flattened against, if not adhered to, the bone.

Indications

These techniques are recommended:

- after knee surgery;
- following direct or indirect knee trauma;
- synovitis;
- musculocapsulo-synovial fibrosis and thickening;
- proprioception deficits;
- difficulty bending the knee.

Comment

Since the articular muscle has a close relationship with the vastus medialis, mediolateral mobilization is naturally more difficult to perform. You must be a little more insistent in your maneuver.

16.2 MENISCI

16.2.1 Review

Structure (Fig. 16.4)

- Menisci of the knee are lamina composed of collagen-rich connective tissue embedded in cartilaginous cells, especially at the interior.
- Menisci are not cartilage, strictly speaking.

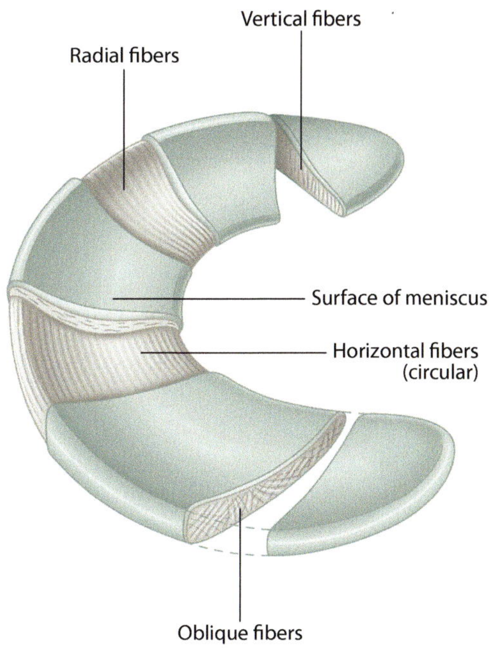

Fig. 16.4 Fibrillar structure of the meniscus.

- The strongest fibers follow the peripheral contour of the meniscus.
- Thinner fibers run toward the center.

Form

- The lateral meniscus is nearly circular. Shaped like an O, it is broader and shorter.
- The medial meniscus is semicircular. In the form of a C, it is narrower and longer.

Attachments

- Their peripheral margins adhere to the capsule.
- Menisci are firmly attached at their ends (horns) to the tibia; toward the center they are unattached and more mobile.
- The attachments terminate at the intercondylar eminence.
- The two meniscopatellar ligaments can destabilize both menisci in the event of a patellar problem.

Meniscal attachments (Fig. 16.5)

- To the tibia, the anterior horns attach to the intercondylar area.
- To the patella, meniscopatellar ligaments run from the peripheral surface of the meniscus to the lateral border of the patella.
- To the femur, the meniscofemoral ligament runs from the posterior horn of the lateral meniscus to the posterior cruciate ligament and the intercondylar fossa.
- To each other, the transverse ligament joins the anterior edges of the menisci.

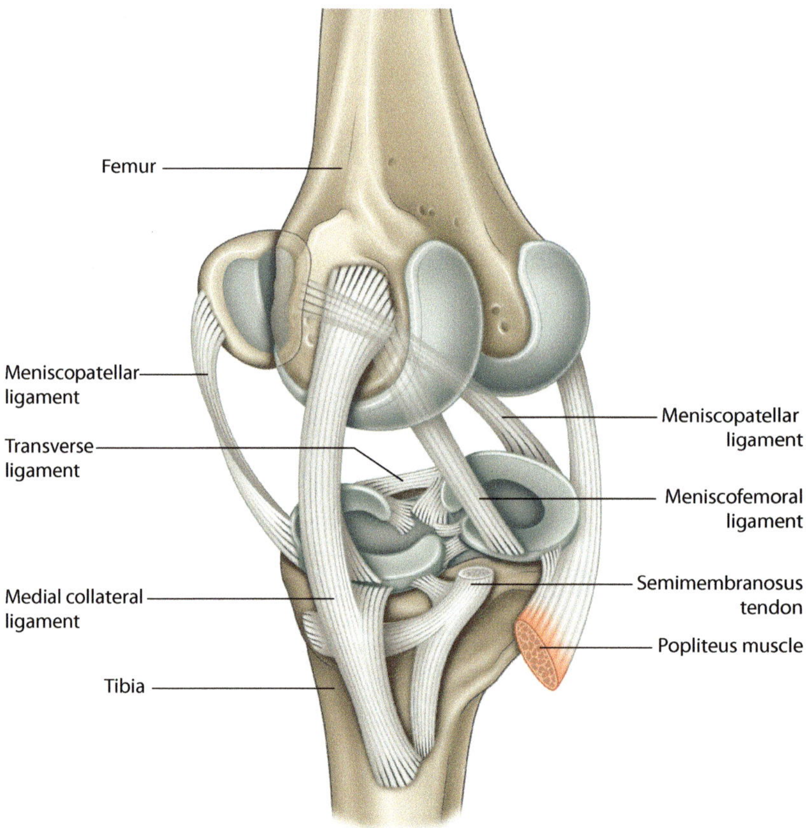

Fig. 16.5 Meniscal attachments.

- To the capsule, the menisci attach by their peripheral surface.
- To the muscles:
  – the lateral meniscus attaches to the popliteus and biceps femoris;
  – the lateral meniscus attaches to the semimembranosus.

Directly accessible attachments are:

- the meniscopatellar ligaments;
- the transverse ligament;
- the capsulomeniscal attachments (coronary ligaments);
- the popliteus muscle (partial accessibility);
- the semimembranosus.

Constitution (Fig. 16.6)

The meniscus has two parts:

- an inner zone: thin and easily torn in trauma;
- a peripheral part: strong, adhered to the capsule.

Surgeons avoid removing the peripheral part in consideration of the meniscal role in distributing compressive forces at the knee.

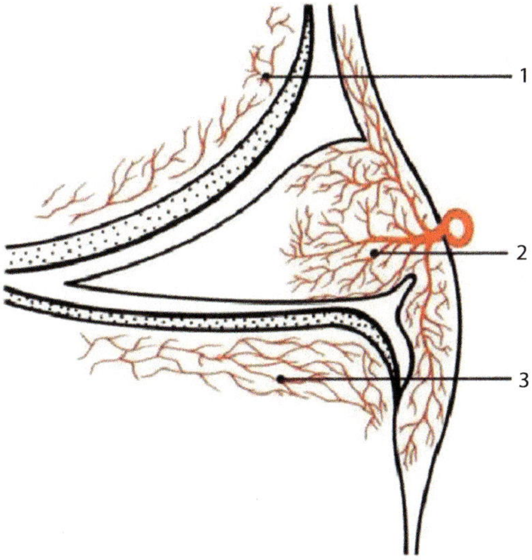

Fig. 16.6 Vascularization of the meniscus.
1- subchondral femoral vessels.
2-meniscal vessels in the outer part of meniscus.
3-subchondral tibial vessels.

Sixty-six percent of the periphery of the meniscus and horns of the meniscus possess baroreceptors and nociceptors.

Intrameniscal capsular sector

This part is thicker. Circular fibers form the coronary ligaments that connect the meniscus to the tibial condyles.

Vascularization (Fig. 16.7)

It has been known since the works of Steven P. Arnoczky (1982) that the meniscus is partially vascularized. At birth the meniscus is entirely vascularized. In the course of childhood, an avascular zone develops at the inner meniscus and progresses toward the periphery. By the second decade of life, all but the outer third of the meniscus becomes devoid of vascularization.

This progressive loss of blood supply is the result of knee movements and load bearing. Meniscal peripheries are supplied by capillary vessels arising from the fibrous capsule that penetrate up to 15%–20% of the meniscus, leaving the inner regions avascular.

The lateral meniscus is avascular adjacent to the popliteal hiatus. The meniscal horns are well supplied starting from their osseous insertions.

Innervation

The anterior and posterior horns are richly innervated, compared to the remainder of the meniscus. Most nerves are associated

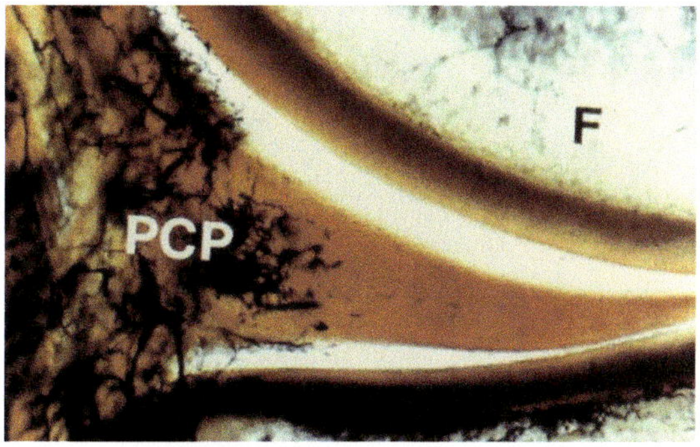

Fig. 16.7 Meniscal vascularization. PCP = meniscal wall; F = femur (After Arnoczky. 2003. Beaufils. Teaching conferences SOFCOT, p. 71.)

with vessels. Many nerves are found at the outer third of the meniscus. The presence of mechanoreceptors in the meniscus suggests that these lamina play a sensory role for the knee and provide proprioceptive feedback to the joint. It has been demonstrated that proprioception can be disturbed by an isolated meniscal lesion and restored after partial meniscal resection (Jerosch et al. 1996).

Transverse ligament of the knee (Fig. 16.8)

This intermeniscal ligament connects the two menisci anteriorly. Ligament dimensions are 3–4 mm wide and 4–5 cm long. It is always essential to check both menisci, even if examinations and symptoms suggest only a medial meniscal lesion.

16.2.2 Lateral meniscus (Fig. 16.9)

While the lateral meniscus is injured 20 times less often than its medial counterpart, it is nevertheless always a good idea to mobilize it whenever the medial one is injured. Remember that the two menisci are linked by their transverse ligament.

Characteristics

- It has greater mobility than the medial meniscus because it does not adhere to the fibular collateral ligament.
- It is twice as mobile as the medial meniscus (12 mm vs. 6 mm).
- It is nearly circular.
- It is protected by freedom of movement that reduces mechanical demand.
- It is drawn posteriorly in knee flexion.
- Its sagittal insertions are close to one another.
- It is uniform in breadth.
- In the front, it attaches anteriorly to the tibial eminence and to the anterior cruciate ligament.
- In the back, it attaches on the medial tibial tubercle in the fossa separating the intercodylar eminences.
- It sends a fibrous fascicle from the posterior horn to the posterior cruciate ligament, which then joins the medial condyle. This point is the anterior meniscofemoral ligament, which is in front of the posterior cruciate ligament.

Reinforcements

The lateral meniscus receives fibers from the popliteus and biceps femoris muscles. The popliteus runs between the meniscus and the capsule. Its muscular fibers draw the posterior convex part of the meniscus posteriorly during flexion of the tibia; the

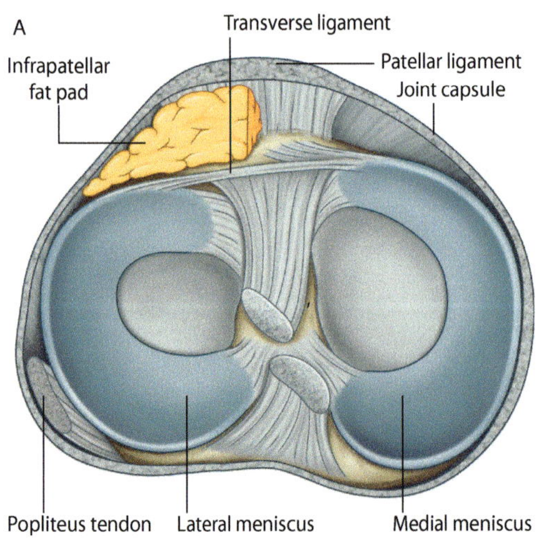

Fig. 16.8 Transverse ligament of the knee.

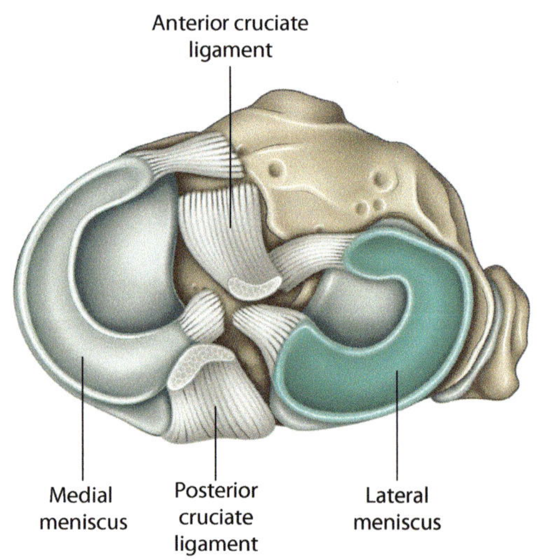

Fig. 16.9 Lateral meniscus.

fibers also produce a slight lateral rotation of the femur. Cephalad fibers of the popliteus are active in locking the knee. They turn the femur slightly laterally before placing the foot. Popliteus contraction during knee flexion pulls the lateral meniscus posteriorly out of harm's way, avoiding entrapment within the joint space.

Remember that the posterior horn of the lateral meniscus blends with fibers from the posterior cruciate ligament.

Etiopathology

The lateral meniscus is implicated in medial collateral ligament sprains. Injury commonly occurs when the foot is planted and the knee is semiflexed and twists laterally. It is also damaged in a posterior tackle, when the weight of the body forcibly rotates the femur medially with the leg in abduction. The medial collateral ligament is usually injured at the same time as the medial meniscus.

16.2.3 Medial meniscus (Fig. 16.10)

Characteristics

- It is semicircular in shape.
- It adheres to the tibial collateral ligament, although its attachments are weaker than those of the lateral meniscus.
- Its insertions are fairly distant from one another.
- It is particularly wider posteriorly and altogether broader than its lateral counterpart.
- Its comparatively thinner anterior horn attaches to the tibial plateau.
- It is less mobile than the lateral meniscus because it is firmly attached to the tibial collateral ligament.
- It is displaced most by lateral rotation.
- It is relaxed most by internal rotation.
- In flexion, it may shift 5–6 mm.
- Its anterior-posterior insertions are some distance apart.
- It is stretched and under maximal traction in lateral rotation.
- It is attached to the semimembranosus muscle.
- Manipulation of the medial meniscus automatically involves the tibial collateral ligament.
- This medial fibrocartilage is 20 times more frequently injured than the lateral meniscus because it is relatively fixed and has a weak anterior horn.
- The anterior horn lies in front of the anterior cruciate ligament.
- The anterior attachment blends with the anterior cruciate ligament.
- The joint capsule adheres more firmly to the medial meniscus.
- Its attachments are weaker than the bonds of the lateral meniscus.

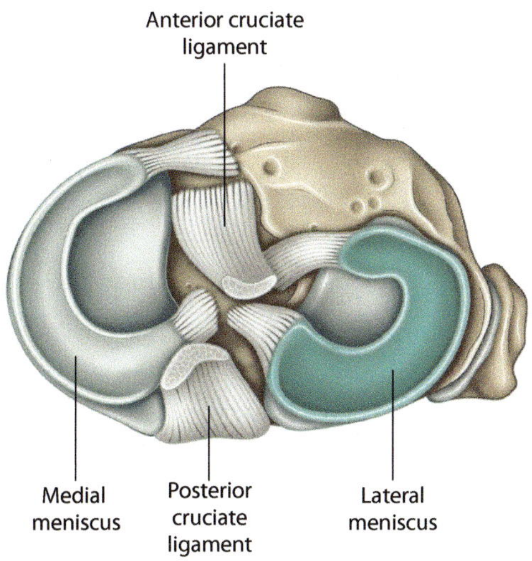

Fig. 16.10 Medial meniscus.

16.2.4 Meniscal physiology

Reduction of femorotibial joint constraint

The menisci are dynamic structures that transmit 50%–70% of compressive forces coming across the knee during weight bearing (Beaufils et al. 2010) (Fig. 16.11).

Load transmission, friction reduction, and shock absorption are the principle functions of the menisci. Menisci improve the

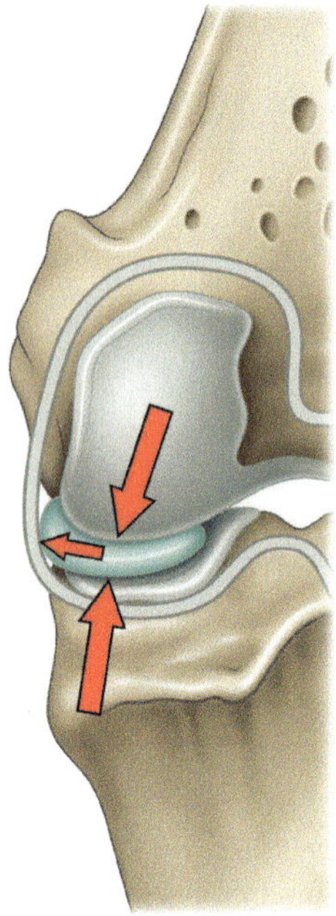

Fig. 16.11 Meniscal and capsular constraints.

nutrition and lubrication of the articular cartilage. Along the same lines, fluid transmission between menisci and the joint cavity helps to spread forces by improving resiliency. When the joint is unloaded, the rubbery menisci fill with water like a sponge. Inversely, the fibrocartilages discharge water during axial weight bearing.

Diminishing joint pressures

The menisci serve to increase stability by improving joint contact and diminishing unilateral pressure. They protect the cartilage against premature wear and tear.

Lubrication role

Menisci plasticity and movement facilitate joint lubrication. They evenly distribute synovial fluid and improve the entire joint surface lubrication. They subdivide the joint into gliding divisions: a suprameniscal level and an inframeniscal level.

Improved joint congruence

The wedge-shaped menisci are able to increase the contact between the tibial and fibular articular surfaces considerably. They give stability to the knee in axial rotation.

Proprioceptive information

The menisci are richly innervated, especially at the peripheral horns. Menisci provide proprioceptive feedback that is vital to dynamic stability of the knee.

Deformation and mobility (Fig. 16.12)

Mobility is what allows the meniscus to provide joint congruity and to transfer load over the knee joint in various knee positions. During flexion-extension of the knee, the lateral meniscus slides as much as 10 mm in the sagittal plane, while the medial meniscus moves about 5 mm. Meniscal tissue deforms in the process. The anterior horns deform more than the posterior horns. During flexion the meniscus deforms toward the back; in extension it reshapes.

16.2.5 Meniscal dysfunction

The concept of meniscal dysfunction is very different from the notion of meniscal lesion. Meniscal dysfunction does not imply a structural problem. Only meniscal kinetics are affected in dysfunction. Very often meniscal motions go out of sync with femorotibial joint movements.

The causes of dysfunction are multiple and varied:

- A wrong move can send the meniscus into a movement barrier, where it is excluded from normal joint play.
- Abnormal meniscopatellar or tibial collateral ligament tension can disturb meniscal dynamics in certain mobility ranges.
- Tensions or spasms of the muscles, such as the semimembranosus or popliteus, can exchange fibers with the meniscus.

The concept of meniscal dysfunction is a

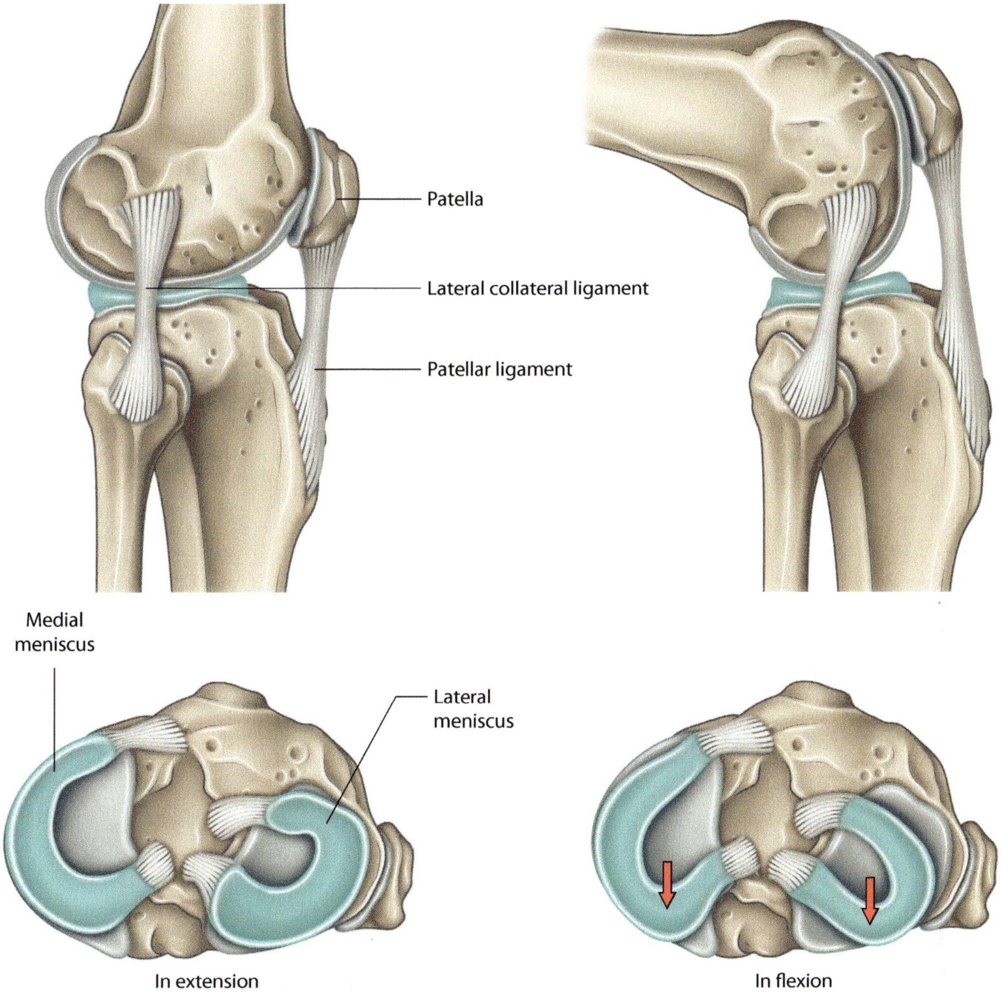

Fig. 16.12 Meniscal mobility and deformability. (After Beaufils, Teaching conferences SOFCOT, 2003, p.71.)

perfect illustration of the distinctive osteopathic concept. What differentiates osteopathy from many other manual medicine disciplines is that what matters most is not a joint components' position but rather its capacity for movement.

In manual diagnosis, an osteopath tracks structures whose mobility is defective. Osteopathic treatment seeks neither to reposition nor to replace anything. In the eyes of a true osteopath, the only consideration is the restoration of movement.

This is exactly what occurs in meniscal dysfunction, where defective kinetics do not depend on a structural lesion or misalignment of the meniscus or joint.

16.2.6 Meniscal lesion evaluation—clinical context

A meniscal tear can happen at any age. Classically there is an identifiable episode underlying the complaint. Generally, meniscus injury is caused by twisting or turning quickly with the foot planted and flexed to about 20°, the tibia in lateral rotation and the femur in medial rotation. This accident is typical of young football players. The forced twist causes other ligamentous lesions such as medial collateral ligament or anterior cruciate ligament injury.

At the other end of the spectrum, patients of a "ripe old age" can suffer degenerative meniscal tears just by getting up suddenly from a squat or by putting the knee through an awkward twist getting up from a chair. The patient experiences a pop together with severe pain. The meniscus finds itself impinged by the medial condyle, and it can be either crushed or torn. Longitudinal tears in the axis of the meniscus are known as "bucket handle" tears. When a released meniscal fragment moves between the condyle and the tibia, it blocks full extension of the knee joint. The patient experiences cracking associated with severe pain.

Symptoms

Meniscal lesions are very common. Clinically, pain, joint swelling, and joint blockage are the usual symptoms.

Blockage is the critical symptom to understand, as misinterpretation gives rise to a number of diagnostic errors. It is necessary to distinguish and even contrast types of blockages.

Meniscal blockage or true blockage: The patient finds it impossible to fully extend the knee, and lasting extension is impossible (passive flexum). This signifies that a mechanical obstacle is preventing complete extension. This can be a strip of meniscus in the intercondylar notch, a foreign body, or a bit of the anterior cruciate ligament interposed between the joint surfaces. In this case the patient walks on tiptoes.

Blocked knee or pseudo blockage: What many patients interpret as true blockage is simply functional blockage of the knee in flexion and extension. This type of friction disappears once weight is transferred to the other knee, and it is not long-lasting. Usually some sort of knee cartilage change is responsible for this fleeting hitch.

Looking for signs of a meniscal lesion

Many of the tests described below are standard medical examinations. We include them here because it is important to be familiar with what they signify. Most of the time, symptoms quickly suggest meniscal lesions.

Medical diagnosis is based on questioning and comparative clinical examination of both knees. Manual testing must be done with care. As anyone with knee problems can tell you, forceful testing can be traumatic. Our preferred way is to test the knee with the patient's knee resting on our shoulder.

Very often the injured knee exhibits:

- flexion contracture;
- meniscal blockage;
- hydrarthrosis, which is common but not constant;
- pain on direct palpation of the medial or lateral meniscus;
- other signs of meniscal damage with specific tests (McMurray's test, Cooper-Apley grind test, etc.).

Looking for meniscal blockage (Genety's sign) (Fig. 16.13)

Testing is performed in procubitus, the lower leg off the table with the knees extended naturally. Observe the height of the two heels; this will reveal even a slight flexum.

On the side of the restriction, try to slowly bring the heel toward the floor. In the case of meniscal blockage, pain is triggered immediately and you feel a strong elastic resistance under your hands. A positive

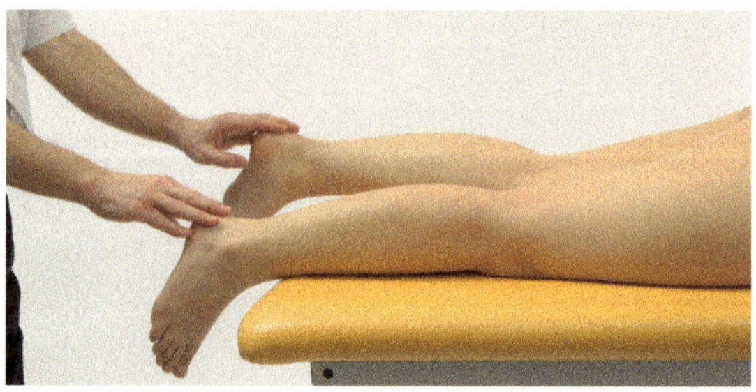

Fig. 16.13 Looking for Genety's sign.

Genety's sign usually reveals a lesion of the anterior horn of the meniscus.

Provoked pain

Meniscal pain on pressure is elicited with the patient in decubitus, his knee flexed to 90°, foot flat on the table. Move your thumb or index finger from front to back along the joint line. The painful point on the medial meniscus is usually located immediately facing or just behind the medial collateral ligament. Anterior pain can be found in the anterior femorotibial fossa (see Steinmann's sign below). Lateral meniscal pain can be awakened along the lateral joint space when you evaluate along its joint line.

Tenderness displacement test

Pain that changes with knee position constitutes Steinmann's sign.

- A positive test is indicated if tenderness moves posteriorly toward the medial collateral ligament with increasing flexion.
- A positive test is indicated if tenderness moves anteriorly toward the femorotibial fossa with increased extension.

With degenerative arthritis of the knee, pain remains topographically unchanged.

Meniscal pain provoked by mobilization

The femoral condyles naturally compress the meniscus as it moves back and forth during flexion and extension. The posterior horn is compressed during flexion. The anterior horn is compressed during extension.

Tenderness of the anterior horn is discovered by placing a finger in the anterior joint space while the patient progressively extends the knee. Pain provoked under these conditions constitutes the "meniscus cry." Tibial rotation causes the posterior horns to move/come forward. Medial pain occurs during lateral rotation (MP in LR), and lateral pain comes on during medial rotation (LP on MR).

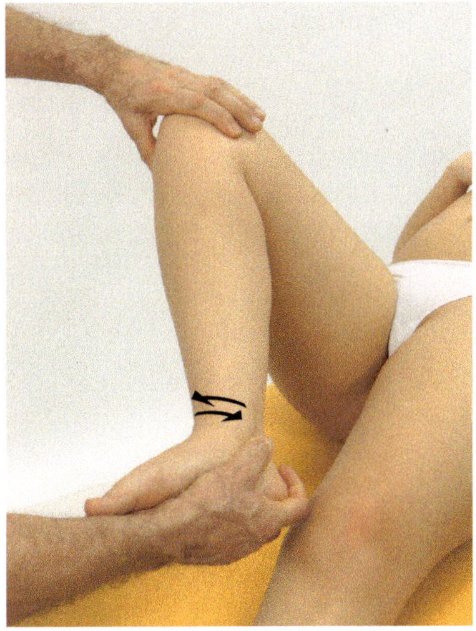

Fig. 16.14 McMurray's test.

Duck-walking test

The inability to "walk like a duck" is a sign of a meniscal problem. The medial meniscus comes under maximal tension when the leg is laterally rotated.

McMurray's test (Fig. 16.14)

This test evaluates the knee for meniscus injury. The patient is in decubitus, with the knee to be tested fully flexed. Grasp the sole of the foot with one hand and contact the medial or lateral aspects of the tibiofibular joint with the other hand.

To test the lateral meniscus, palpate the posterior lateral joint line while extending the knee and internally rotating the tibia. A valgus stress is also applied.

To test the medial meniscus, palpate the posterior medial joint line while extending the knee and externally rotating the tibia. A varus stress is also applied.

Compression of the lateral joint space impinges on the lateral meniscus, whereas compression of the medial joint space impinges on the medial meniscus. If pain is felt by the subject, or the examiner perceives

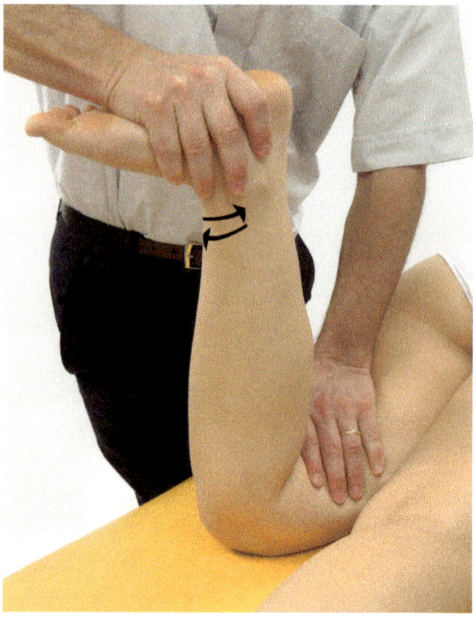

Fig. 16.15 Apley's grind test.

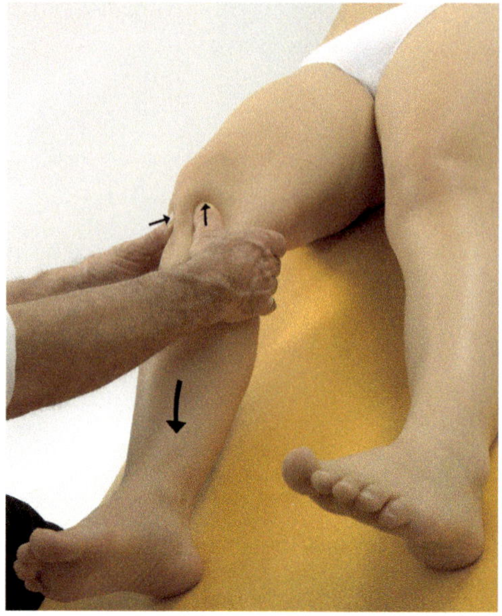

Fig. 16.16 Meniscal test in extension.

a palpatory or auditory intra-articular click, the test is considered positive.

Apley's compression test (Fig. 16.15)

The Apley compression test, or grind test, is performed in procubitus with the knee flexed to 90°. Gently stabilize the posterior aspect of the patient's thigh and lean on the plantar surface of the foot to compress the meniscus between the femur and the tibia. Medially and laterally rotate the tibia while maintaining joint compression.

Pain in the medial joint compartment suggests medial meniscus damage. Pain in the lateral compartment suggests a lateral meniscal problem.

This test is always accompanied by a counter test. Internal and external rotation without compression will not cause pain unless there is a peripheral ligamentous lesion. A medial collateral ligament sprain is likely.

Special note

A positive distraction test suggests benign or intermediate ligament injury. Apply axial traction to the leg by gently pulling the tibia away from the femur. Lateral tibial rotation solicits the medial and lateral collateral ligaments. Pain indicates a sprain. Distract the tibia from the femur as above. Medial rotation of the tibia solicits the anterior and posterior cruciate ligaments, which may be painful.

Lateral meniscal cyst

A cyst can appear on or near the lateral joint margin. A cyst will be perfectly obvious and palpable in semiflexion. The mass disappears in hyperflexion. It reappears as the knee is progressively extended, only to disappear again on full extension. Diagnosis is confirmed by arthroscopy or MRI.

16.2.7 Meniscal mobility tests

To the above tests we add our own meniscal examinations that allow us to uncover meniscal dysfunctions.

Meniscal mobility in extension, in decubitus—first method (Fig. 16.16)

The patient rests his foot on the table, knee slightly flexed. You place your two thumbs on either side of the patellar ligament. Glide your thumbs toward the cranial surface of the tibial plateau to come slightly behind it in an effort to reach the intra-articular aspect of the knee. Take a moment to evaluate the anterior meniscal tibial attachments.

Next, reposition your thumbs as closely as you can to the median axis of the tibia. At this point, the anterior horn of the meniscus interests us, as it is the most commonly injured.

Slowly and progressively bring the knee into extension, gliding the foot on the table. Do this as if your thumbs would like to gently enter the joint space. This test can also be practiced with the patient's foot on your shoulder. This position allows you to incorporate tibial rotation.

In case of a meniscal lesion

Under your medial thumb (more rarely your lateral thumb) you will feel a small, hardened, and sensitive zone that will not drop posteriorly in extension. The anterior horn butts against your thumb. Any forceful posteriorization of the tibia creates pain and must be absolutely avoided.

Mobility test in flexion (first modality) (Fig. 16.17)

In severe cases of meniscal injury, the patient must keep his knee semiflexed. Even tentative extension creates strong pain.

Pay attention to flexion!

In fresh meniscal injuries, synovial fluid often produces pressure. The knee becomes extremely painful, and any forceful flexion that increases intra-articular suppression must be avoided. As we noted earlier in chapter 13, fluid pressure can lead to false diagnosis in the case of a recent knee injury.

On the other hand, flexion tenses up numerous elements such as:

- the anterior capsule;
- the anterior synovial membrane;
- the retinaculum;
- the patellar tendon;
- the patellar ligament;
- the adipose ligament.

Manual approach

The manual articular approach has a subtlety that surpasses information provided by MRI and CT scans. Joint proprioception, particularly as it pertains to the knee, has a fine-tuned subtlety.

We emphasize once more that the knee is above all a "neurological joint." It is often implied that we do not speak the same language as our surgical friends. They have been known to challenge the capsular tensor role that certain muscles play, or even to contest the pathogenic effect of plica syndromes.

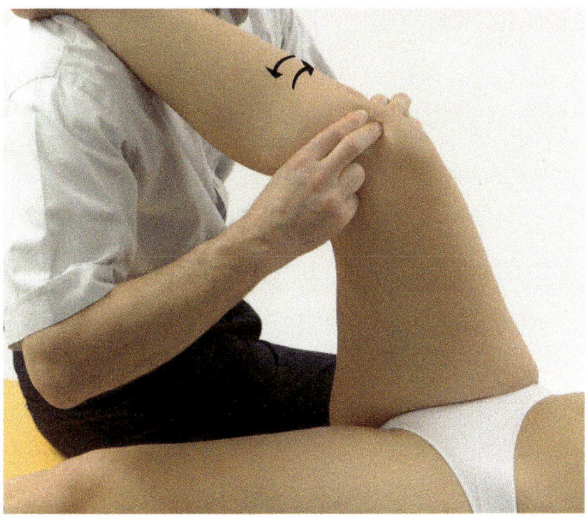

Fig. 16.17 Meniscal test in flexion.

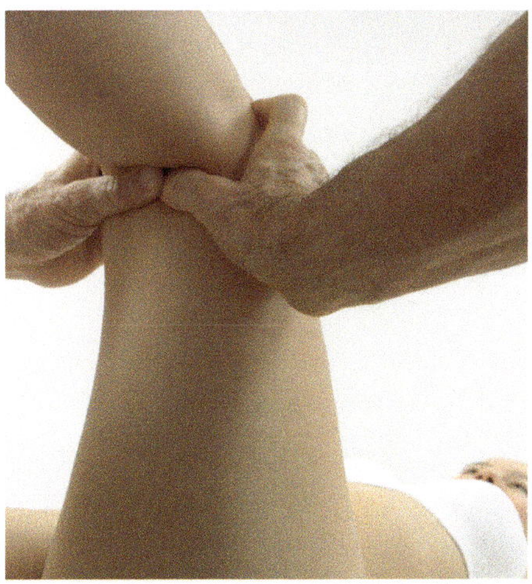

Fig. 16.18 Meniscal test in extension (second method.

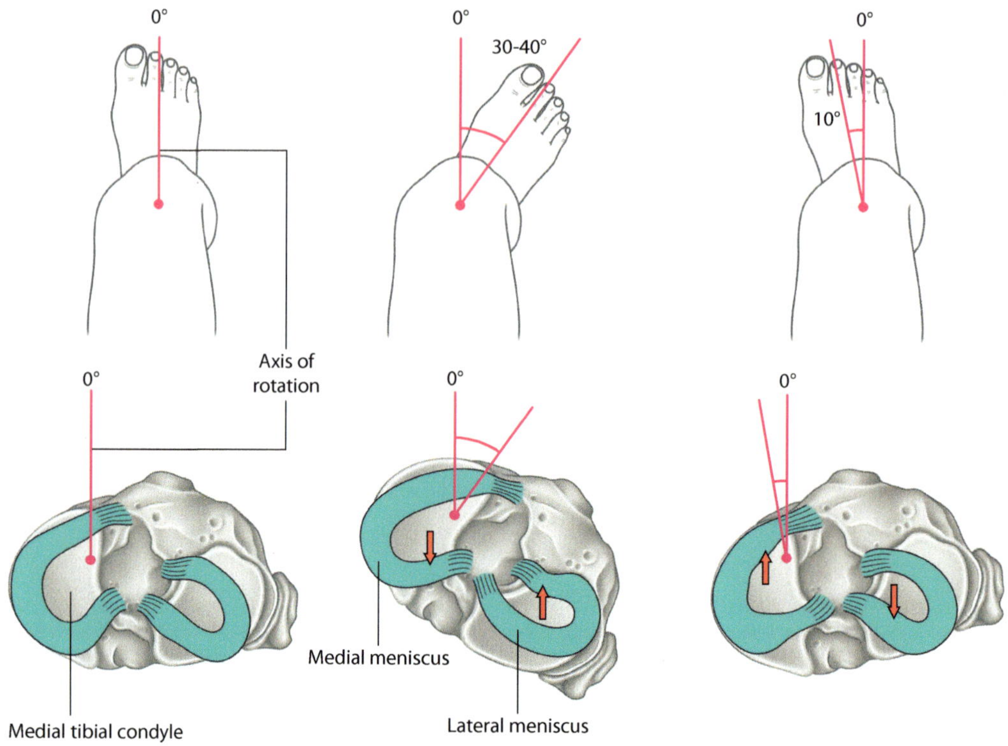

Fig. 16.19 Meniscal movement test in rotation.

We do not dispute the need for surgeries in the event of significant lesions. But manual therapy is less devastating to the knee and, in a great many cases, provides reliable reprogramming of the knee's mechanoreceptors, bringing functional improvement as a consequence.

Test of meniscal mobility in extension, in decubitus—second method (Fig. 16.18)

The patient lies on his back, foot resting on your shoulder. Place both thumbs against the posterior cranial border of the tibial plateau; the aim is to anteriorize it delicately. Allow your index fingers to rest lightly on the anterior part of the tibial plateau and play with flexion-extension of the knee. During both movements, appreciate the resistance of the anterior meniscal horn, which normally shifts posteriorly. When it remains fixed forward, there is a lesion. To increase meniscal tension, turn the tibia slightly laterally.

Test of meniscal mobility in rotation (Figs. 16.19 and 16.20)

The patient lies on his back with his foot on your shoulder, the knee flexed to 90°. Stand at the end of the exam table. Place your index fingers on the anterior joint space facing the anterior horns of both menisci. Place your thumbs in the popliteal crease on the posterior joint line facing the posterior horns. With the other fingers of both hands, stabilize the lateral and medial surfaces of the knee to keep it in line with its axis.

Ask the patient to rotate his knee slowly by moving his foot like a windshield wiper. With your thumbs on different parts of the joint space, feel alternating deformations linked to displacement and meniscal deformations.

Normally during medial rotation of the tibia, the anterior horn of the medial meniscus on the anterior surface of the joint shifts forward and "pushes" against the pad of your

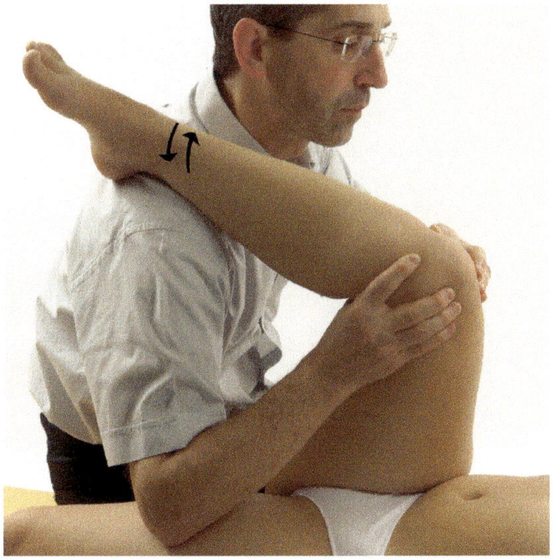

Fig. 16.20 Meniscal test in rotation.

index finger, while the lateral joint space "caves in" under your thumb. At the same time, in the popliteal crease, the posterior horn of the lateral meniscus moves posteriorly and pushes against the pad of your thumb, while the medial joint space caves in.

The opposite occurs with lateral rotation of the tibia. The posterior horn of the medial meniscus posteriorizes, and the anterior horn of the lateral meniscus anteriorizes.

Any disturbance in this movement scheme points to a meniscal mobility dysfunction, generally at the level of the meniscal horn, which seems excluded from the mechanism.

16.2.8 Techniques

Manipulation of meniscopatellar fibers

Fiber landmarks

Fibers of the patellar retinaculum, whose orientation is particular, sometimes go by the name meniscopatellar ligaments. Their organization is more consequential on the medial side of the patella. Their fixation is to be treated in problems of the medial meniscus.

After manipulating the medial patellar retinaculum, as we have shown earlier in this chapter, and before manipulating the medial meniscus itself, investigate the fibers of the meniscopatellar ligament.

These fibers run obliquely, distal, and posterior. On the knee in extension they run from the distal half of the patella to where the medial collateral ligament crosses the medial joint space. Search along this axis for excessive fiber tensions.

For both testing and treatment, you should vary their tension to individualize fibers.

Technique

The patient is in decubitus. Situate yourself at the side of the knee to be treated. With your thumbs, mobilize the patella laterally to medially. With your index fingers, feel the fiber tension. Mobilize the patella several times, altering the axis of the pressure slightly each time. This will help you find areas of reduced elasticity. Work these zones following the same principles as testing, performing stretch-induction maneuvers.

Quite apart from any mechanical strain placed on the meniscus by meniscopatellar fiber tension, the entire informational component of meniscal kinetics is affected when meniscopatellar ligaments lose elasticity. The precision of your maneuver plays on these two elements.

Manipulation of the transverse ligament in decubitus (Fig. 16.21)

Position yourself to the side of the knee in question and have the patient place his foot on your shoulder. Position either your index fingers or thumbs on either side of the patellar ligament and make small flexion-extension movements of the knee with your body. Progressively spread your fingers, entering deeper into the joint space.

Make small rotations of the knee medially and laterally to put the anterior meniscal horns on tension; then repress posteriorly with precaution.

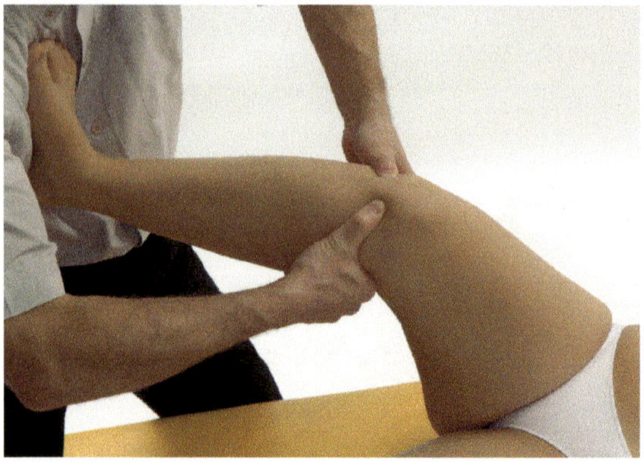

Fig. 16.21 Transverse ligament of the knee.

Manipulation of the medial meniscus (Fig. 16.22)

The patient remains in decubitus, knee flexed. This time, the foot of the knee concerned rests against the other leg. The lower limb is in moderated abduction and lateral rotation. Place your palm against the medial surface of the tibial plateau, and place your thumb on the anterior medial part of the joint space. Ask the patient to slowly flex and extend the knee in a controlled way, his foot maintaining contact with the outstretched leg.

This maneuver must allow the patient to recover extension a little bit at a time. The patient controls the movement. This way it is possible for him to bring his leg immediately into flexion in the event the movement becomes painful.

During the extension phase, lightly compress the posterior tibial plateau laterally, while softly subjugating the anterior horn of the meniscus posteriorly. This technique is painless and most effective. If you feel that the treatment has not produced the anticipated result, ask the patient to carry out the technique himself with a series of 12 or so repetitions.

It is important to allow the lower extremity to complete the natural range of adduction/medial rotation that automatically occurs when the foot follows down the contralateral leg into full extension.

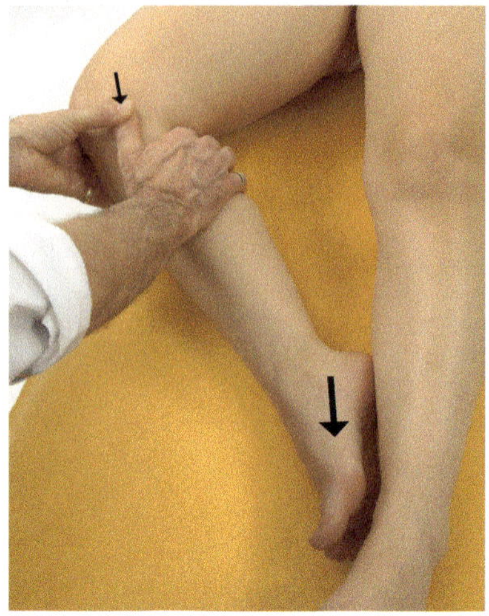

Fig. 16.22 Manipulation of the medial meniscus (first method).

Manipulation of the medial meniscus—second method (Fig. 16.23)

Perform the same maneuver as for the medial meniscus test, the patient's foot resting on your shoulder. At the end of the movement, as the leg is drawn progressively into extension, add an element of medial tibial rotation. All these mobilizations must be gentle, progressive, and painless.

Manipulation of the lateral meniscus (Fig. 16.24)

In the same position as for the medial meniscus test, begin the movement with the foot of the knee concerned resting on the table against the contralateral leg. Place one hand on the lateral part of the tibial plateau, your thumb on the lateral part of the anterior joint space of the knee. This time, the patient glides his foot not against the other leg but parallel to his outstretched limb. Progressively draw the leg into adduction and medial rotation.

Be careful! Make sure this maneuver does not cause pain in the region of the medial meniscus. If the medial meniscus is injured, it will not appreciate this movement very much.

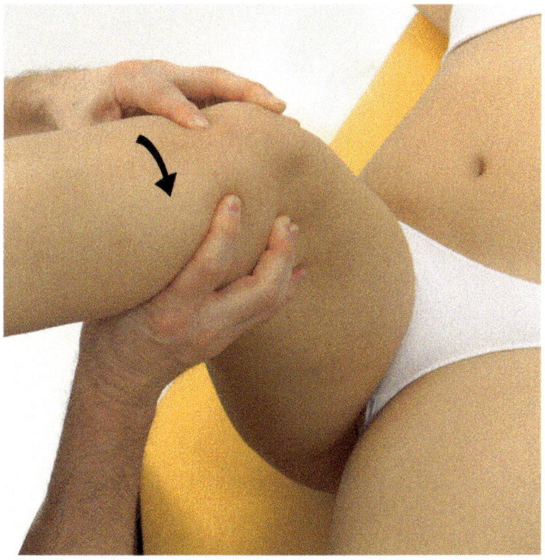

Fig. 16.23 Manipulation of the medial meniscus (second method).

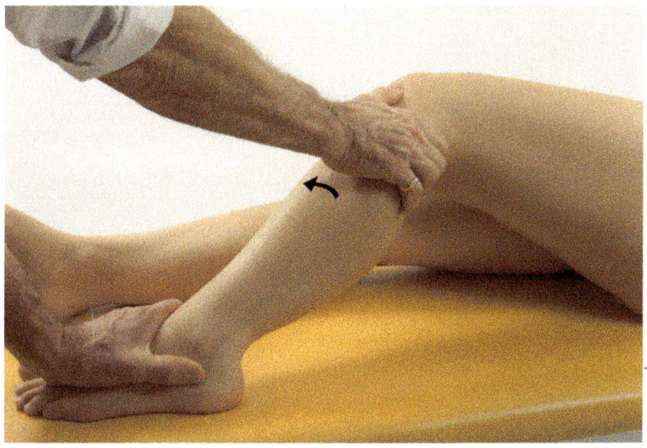

Fig. 16.24 Manipulation of the lateral meniscus.

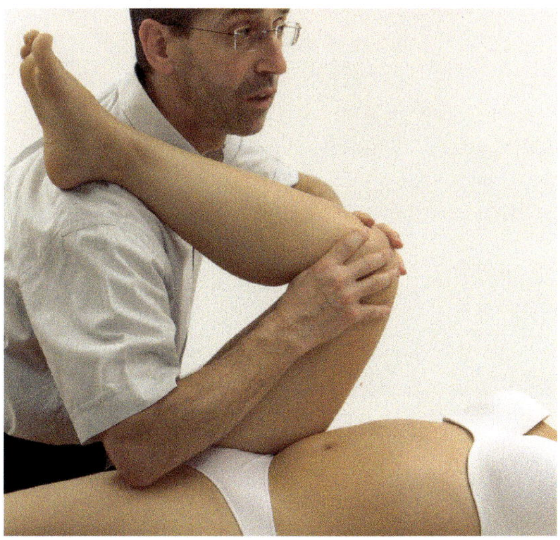

Fig. 16.25 Manipulation of the posterior horn of the medial meniscus.

Manipulation of the posterior horn of the medial meniscus (Fig. 16.25)

The patient is in decubitus. Sit on the table with the patient's foot on your shoulder. Position your fingers as for the meniscal rotation test. Your index fingers are on the anterior joint space facing the anterior horns of both menisci. Your thumbs are in the popliteal fossa on the posterior joint space, facing the posterior horns of the meniscus.

To manipulate the posterior horn of the medial meniscus, ask the patient to let his knee fall inward. This will cause hip adduction and inward angulation (valgus) of the knee, which opens the medial joint space. Ask the patient to laterally rotate the knee. During this movement, accompany the posterior meniscal horn toward the front with your thumb.

Next, maintaining the meniscal horn where it is, ask the patient to allow his knee to fall outward laterally. This will create abduction of the hip and inward angulation (varus) of the knee, which closes the medial joint space. Then ask the patient to rotate his leg medially and gently draw his foot toward the buttock. This will mobilize his knee in flexion and medial rotation.

Be careful! If this is done at all too vigorously, the flexion movement can very easily cause pain. Ask the patient not to move in a way that causes pain during the maneuver. The therapist should never force the movement. Follow the movement of flexion, performing induction with both of your thumbs on the posterior horn of the medial meniscus.

Before carrying out this technique, it is imperative to release the deep pes anserinus, particularly the meniscal attachments of the semimembranosus.

Manipulation of the posterior horn of the medial meniscus

For the very rare cases of dysfunction of the posterior horn of the lateral meniscus, it is appropriate to follow the opposite param-

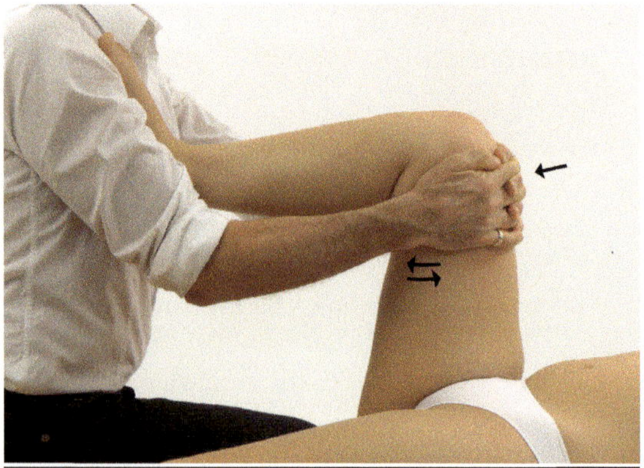

Fig. 16.26 Meniscocartilaginous smoothing in decubitus.

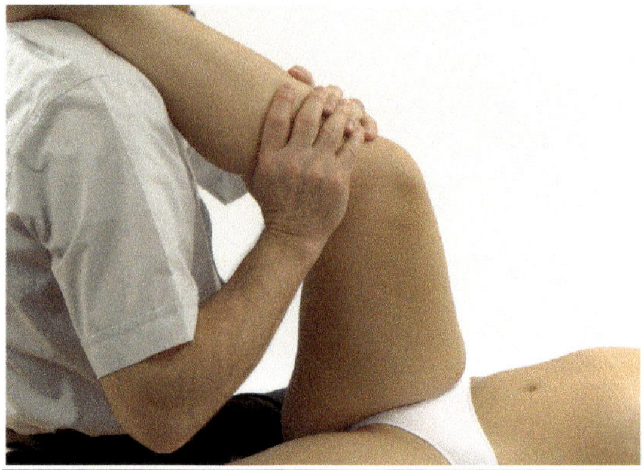

Fig. 16.27 Osteocartilaginous readjustment of the knee.

eters to those used in the maneuver of the medial meniscus maneuver. In such cases, tissular dysfunctions are mostly found posterolaterally. It is very important to check the popliteus muscle and release any tension you may find. While neither the lateral collateral ligament nor the arcuate popliteal ligament exchange fibers with the lateral meniscus, their fixations are nevertheless to be addressed.

16.3 ARTICULAR CARTILAGE

16.3.1 Techniques

Meniscocartilaginous smoothing in decubitus (Fig. 16.26)

The patient rests the foot of the knee concerned against your shoulder or belly; the knee is flexed. Place both your hands together above the patella, against the femur, and pull the knee up against you to compress the joint. Create small flexion-extension movements while maintaining the compression. This technique has the effect of relaxing both the meniscus and the cartilage. The main indications are meniscarthrosis and gonarthrosis.

Femoropatellar polishing

Time and again we have tried small flexion-extension movements at the knee while compressing the patella against the femur, with no apparent clinical results. What's more, in some people this maneuver resulted in synovitis.

Osteocartilaginous knee readjustment (Fig. 16.27)

An empirical observation

We often have been surprised at the end of our knee maneuvers to feel a very subtle gliding of the tibia on the femur. This small movement allows the tibia to readjust itself. Even while this motion is minimal, it is real. Small displacements of the tibia have grave repercussions for both proprioception and cartilage. This readjustment technique is best done at the end of the session, once the proprioceptive elements have been reinitialized.

Technique

The subject lies on the table, the foot or the Achilles tendon resting on your shoulder. Encircle the tibial plateau with both of your hands. The contact must be osseous and not muscular. Allow your hands to follow the listening. Most of the time they will follow the tibial plateau in rotation, which can be either medial or lateral. The maneuver consists of encouraging the amplitude of the listening, which is induction. It is important not to decide or choose the direction of the movement yourself.

Advice

To facilitate readjustment of the knee, it sometimes helps to exert a slight distal traction on the tibial plateau. Maintain the distal traction and allow the bone to go into induction. To be sure that the technique has been successful, always complete the maneuver with listening. Sometimes the listening pulls the tibia in the opposite direction of the one you felt at the start of the technique. Do not hesitate to begin again, following this new listening. The absence of listening proves that all is well.

Treatment of the osseous elements

17

17.1 REVIEW OF OSSEOUS TISSUE (FIG. 17.1)

The internal architecture of the bone is imbued with every constraint that the osteochondral system has ever been subject to. The layout of the trabecula and spongy bone, as well as any possible subchondral compressions, are all manifestations of the demands made on bones. Even stress created by a wrong step or a faulty stance leaves its mark on the bones of the knee.

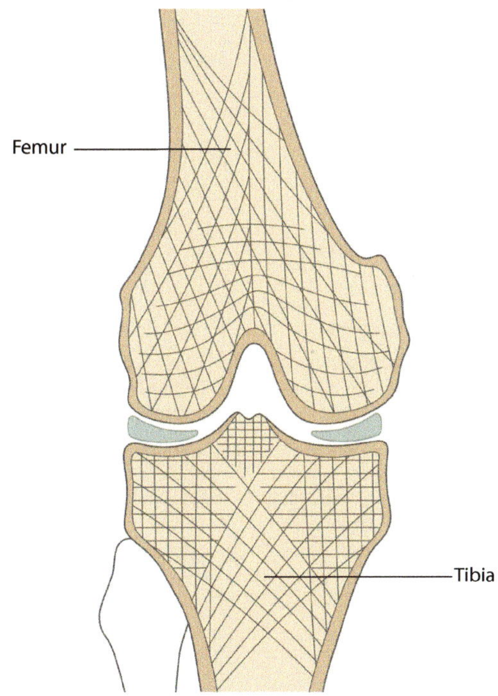

Fig. 17.1 Intraosseous structure of the femoral and tibial condyles (After Kapandji).

The osseous matrix also keeps in its memory all direct trauma it has ever experienced—cracks, fractures, inflammations, tensions generated by a malposition in utero, or the consequences of rickets and other systemic illnesses.

Osseous elasticity techniques are useful whenever the knee presents symptoms connected to arthritis. Osseous techniques restore and improve the cushioning capacity of subchondral bone, on which the health of cartilage depends. After treatment to restore bone elasticity, one can clearly feel a difference in terms of improved accommodation to compressive forces.

17.2 TECHNIQUES

17.2.1 In decubitus

Tibial bowing

The patient lies on the table, leg extended. You position yourself on the same side as the leg in question. Place your thumbs at either end of the lateral part of the leg while your fingers take hold of the medial aspect across from your thumbs. Evaluate and treat the elasticity of the bone by bending and releasing the tibia several times. Finish with induction.

Sagittal compression

Place your palms, one on top of the other, on the anterior part of the tibia, just off the tibial crest. If pressure on the tibia is at all uncomfortable, broaden and soften your contact. Progressively compress and release the tibia posteriorly, finishing with induction.

The tibia, like all bone, has lines of tension running through it. After trauma, these lines of force no longer transmit loads correctly, leading to destabilization of all the mechanoreceptors of the lower extremity. One is often astonished at the difference in bone density and elasticity that can be felt after the treatment.

Frontal compression of the condyles of the knee

The patient lies on the table, his leg nearly fully extended but not locked. Position yourself near the foot of the leg to be treated. Place your palms on the lateral and medial tibial condyles. Interlace your fingers behind the tibia in the popliteal fossa.

Stabilize yourself by placing your forearms on the table on either side of the leg. Exert compression on the tibial condyles in the frontal plane. Compress and release the bone several times. Next, perform induction, maintaining compression of moderate intensity, until you perceive a release deep in the tissues of the epiphysis.

Perform exactly the same technique on the femoral condyles.

Clinical application

Within bone there is a known synergism. Blood pressure and perfusion of the osseous epiphysis contribute to the mechanical capacity of bone, notably its powers of resistance and elasticity. These osseous elasticity techniques are effectively supplemented by treatment of the genicular arteries.

Neural manipulations

18

18.1 REVIEW OF NERVES OF THE KNEE (FIG. 18.1)

Many nerves provide sensitivity to the various parts of the knee. Medical literature is fairly limited on the subject of meniscal and ligamentous innervation.

18.1.1 Saphenous nerve

This branch of the femoral nerve passes through the adductor canal in company with the femoral artery. The saphenous nerve supplies:

- the medial part of the knee;
- the medial patella;

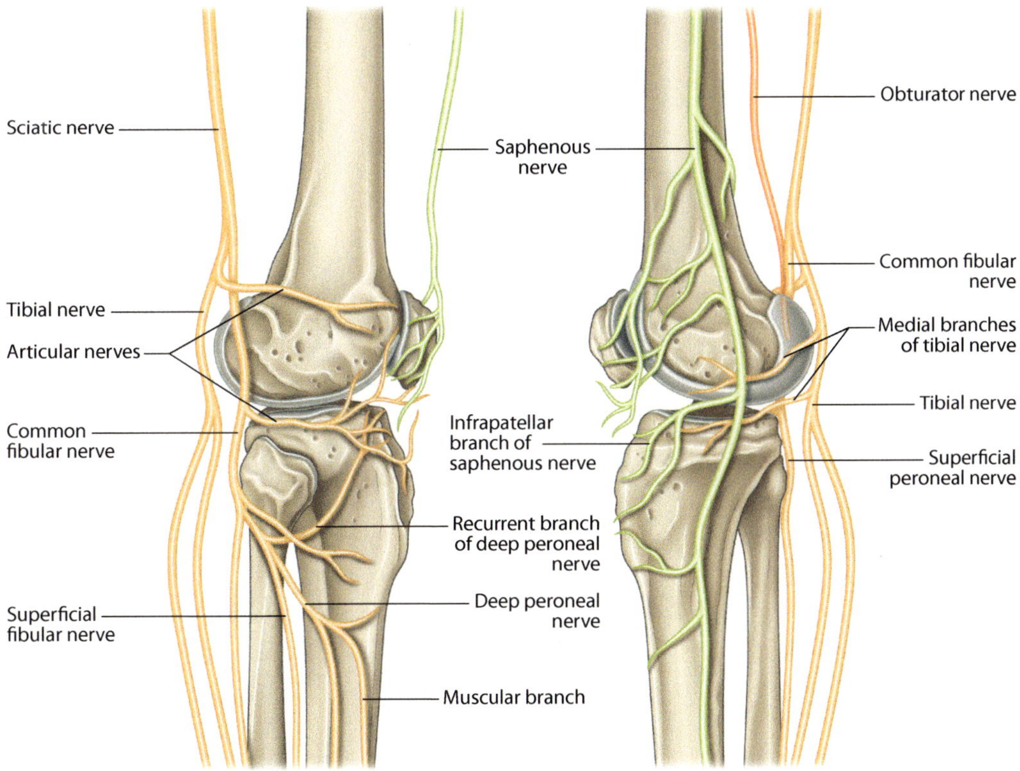

Fig. 18.1 Nerves of the knee.

- the infrapatellar region;
- the medial cutaneous surface of the leg.

It likely also sends a few branches to the medial meniscus.

18.1.2 Obturator nerve

This nerve supplies two branches to the knee. One is supplied by the nerve of the vastus medialis that runs to the medial knee. Another is provided by the nerve of the vastus lateralis that goes to the lateral part of the knee. It sends a few branches to the knee capsule and perhaps to the medial meniscus, as well.

18.1.3 Tibial nerve

This nerve is located laterally to the popliteal artery and medially in relation to the common fibular nerve. As a rule, it supplies three branches to the knee, innervating the posterior capsule and the two menisci.

18.1.4 Fibular nerve

This nerve supplies several branches to the knee and to the proximal tibiofibular joint.

18.1.5 Cutaneous innervation (Fig. 18.2)

It is important to be familiar with cutaneous innervation because you can affect deeper underlying structures through the skin. In this regard we find:

- the lateral femoral cutaneous nerve for the lateral part of the knee;
- the anterior cutaneous branches of the femoral nerve for the anterior knee;
- the saphenous nerve for the medial and posterior knee;
- the medial sural cutaneous nerve, a branch of the tibial nerve, which supplies the posterior part of the knee.

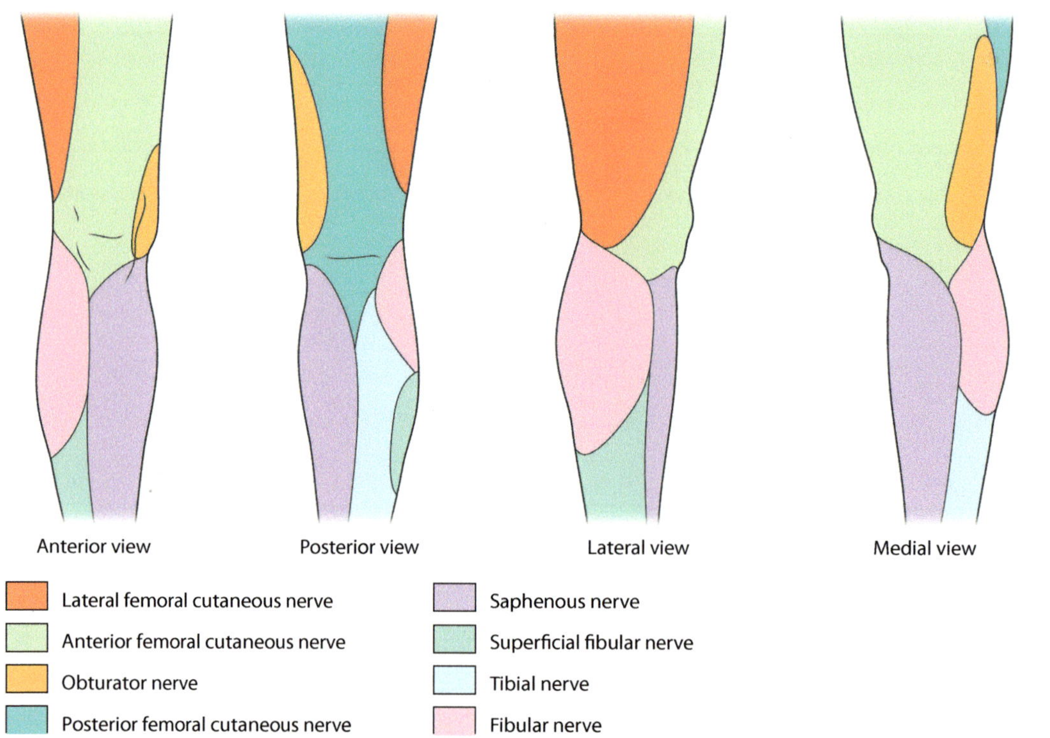

Fig. 18.2 Cutaneous innervation of the knee.

18.2 TECHNIQUES

All lower-extremity nerve branches supplying the knee are worthwhile to treat whenever they feel hardened and sensitive. Here we will describe specific techniques that give the best results.

18.2.1 Saphenous nerve

Adductor canal

Refer to chapter 19 concerning the adductors, specifically section 19.2.3, the technique at the junction of the adductor canal and the adductor hiatus. The saphenous nerve crosses the adductor canal in company with the descending genicular artery, a branch of the femoral artery. This canal is a key feature in neural manipulation at the knee.

18.2.2 Obturator nerve

The cutaneous branch of the obturator nerve runs as far as the medial aspect of the knee. It is located behind the saphenous nerve. The obturator nerve is also manipulated in the medial cranial quarter of the obturator canal, near the angle formed by the superior and inferior pubic rami. Refer to our book *Manual Therapy for the Peripheral Nerves* (Barral et al. 2004).

18.2.3 Tibial nerve

In lateral decubitus (Fig. 18.3)

The patient lies on the side of the knee to be treated, leg slightly flexed. Find the popliteal pulse located near the medial gastrocnemius muscle. The tibial nerve is situated laterally in relation to the popliteal artery. Stretch the tibial nerve distally five to six times. This technique should never cause numbness of the leg. Tingling indicates that you are applying too much compression. Lighten up.

Note: Stretching a nerve naturally involves neighboring tissues. Stay lateral of the artery to be sure to have an effect on the nerve.

18.2.4 Fibular nerve

In lateral decubitus (Fig. 18.4)

The patient lies on the side opposite the knee concerned. Place one of your thumbs on the lateral part of the lateral gastrocnemius muscle, and direct it progressively toward the femoral head. Here the fibular nerve is rather superficial, running lateral to the biceps and medial to the lateral gastrocnemius.

Carry out small stretches in a distal and slightly caudal direction, using very light compression.

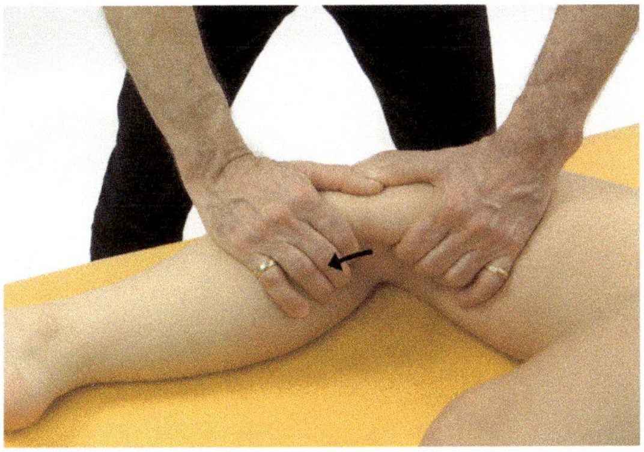

Fig. 18.3 Tibial nerve in lateral decubitus.

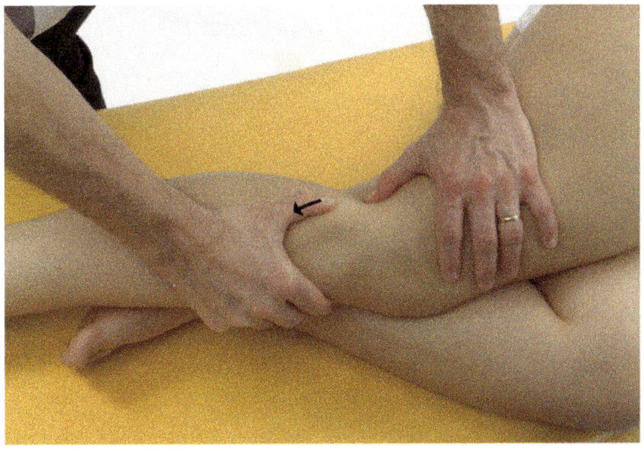

Fig. 18.4 Fibular nerve in lateral decubitus.

18.2.5 Cutaneous treatment

Treating the skin over the knee produces excellent results. We have made a study of the most effective zones. There are fundamental differences in cutaneous sensitivity between the medial and lateral parts of the knee. The medial knee is considerably more sensitive, which certainly factors in the framework of proprioceptive knee protection. This also happens to be an erogenous zone, a topic beyond the scope of this book.

18.2.6 Obturator nerve

In decubitus or lateral decubitus

The cutaneous zone that yields the best results is located on the medioposterior region of the knee, very near the adductor hiatus (Fig. 18.5). We locate the hiatus somewhat distally compared to classic topographical descriptions.

Be aware that the medial part of the thigh is very sensitive. Proceed gradually in progressively stretching the skin in induction. It is amazing to witness the difference in sensitivity after each skin treatment.

18.2.7 Lateral femoral cutaneous nerve

We have described treatment for this nerve as it perforates the iliotibial tract (see chapter 14).

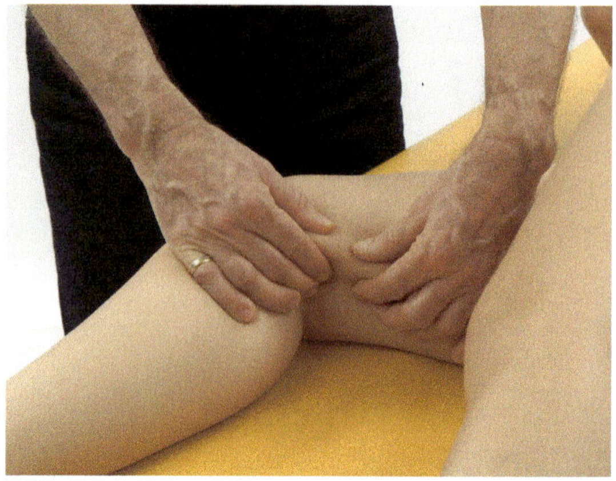

Fig. 18.5 Obturator cutaneous zone.

In decubitus

The patient lies on his back with his knee flexed. Glide your thumb along the lateral surface of the thigh, following along the fascia lata. The restricted nerve is at the place where your thumb cannot glide. You will have the impression that the thumb sinks into a sort of pit in the fascia lata. This usually indicates a small perforating branch of the nerve that is surrounded by a fascial ring. It will be sensitive.

Place your thumbs on either side of the sensitive spot. One thumb stretches the fascia lata distally while the other stretches it proximally as the leg is slowly extended. The goal is to open the ring.

Once the nerve is less sensitive, carry out a slight compression-stretch induction directly on the sensitive nerve.

Vascular manipulations

19

A good joint requires quality arterial and venous circulation and a nervous system that is perfectly able to fulfill its sensory, proprioceptive, and motor functions.

Arteries and nerves are vulnerable to constraint due to the various tissues that surround them. We begin with the adductor canal, a key passageway that transmits the saphenous nerve together with the descendent genicular artery, whose branches supply the joint. Next we look at the adductor hiatus, through which the femoral artery passes to become the popliteal artery.

19.1 ADDUCTOR CANAL (FIG. 19.1)

The adductor canal is an aponeurotic tunnel constituted by the vastoadductor septum, also known as the vastoadductor membrane, which incorporates the adductor magnus, vastus medialis, and adductor longus muscles.

19.1.1 Features

The adductor canal extends to an aperture called the adductor hiatus.

19.1.2 Contents

- The saphenous nerve, a branch of the femoral nerve that is unusually sensitive
- The femoral artery, which courses medially, and the descending artery, which passes in the front of the canal
- The femoral vein

19.2 ADDUCTOR HIATUS (FIG. 19.2)

The hiatus is a gap in the distal adductor magnus tendon. This opening communicates with the adductor canal.

19.2.1 Adductor magnus

This muscle arises from the inferior ramus of the pubis and from the inferior ramus of the ischium. Portions of the muscle insert into the linea aspera, while other fibers reach the adductor tubercle. Between these two insertions lies a slit-like opening called the adductor hiatus.

19.2.2 Contents

- Once through the hiatus, the femoral artery continues as the popliteal artery. Branches of the popliteal artery include articular branches to the knee: the superior medial genicular artery and the lateral genicular artery.
- The femoral vein also passed through the hiatus.

19.2.3 Techniques

Palpation of the hiatus

The hiatus is deeply situated behind the semimembranosus and semitendinosus muscles. Position yourself posteriorly and medially to the vastus medialis. Landmark the adductor tubercle on the medial epicon-

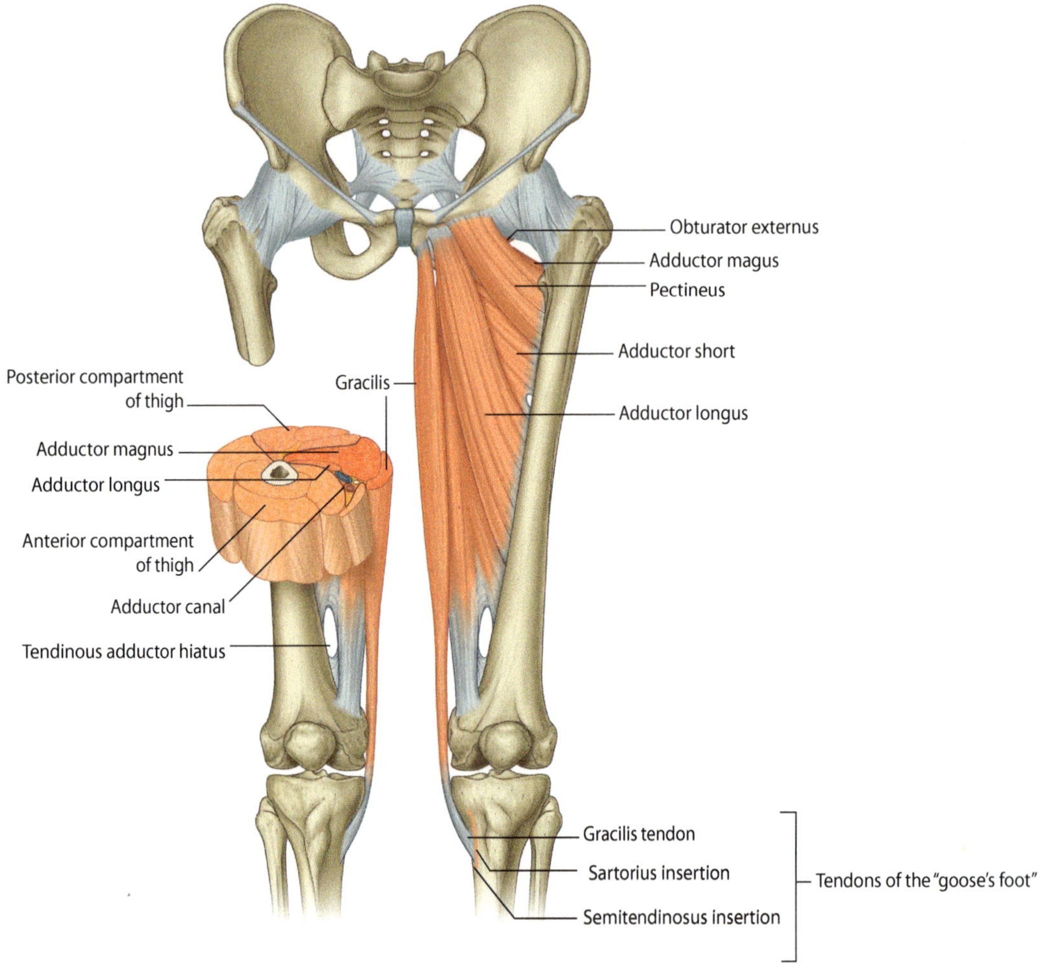

Fig. 19.1 Adductor canal.

dyle where the adductor magnus inserts. Move your fingers cranially and move the semimembranosus aside. Separate the adductor magnus fibers that insert onto the femur from the fibers that attach to the adductor tubercle. Your fingers will find themselves on the femorotibial intermuscular septum.

The part of the adductor magnus that is attached to the linea aspera acts as a lateral rotator. The part that reaches the medial epicondyle acts as a medial rotator when the knee is flexed.

Hiatus technique in lateral decubitus (Fig. 19.3)

The patient lies on the side of the leg to be treated. Position yourself in front of the patient. Grasp the semitendinosus and semimembranosus with your fingers; draw both muscles medially. Glide your thumbs along and behind the vastus medialis until you encounter fibers of adductor magnus. Stretch the adductor magnus and move off the semimembranosus medially.

Hiatus technique in decubitus (Fig. 19.4)

The patient lies on the table with his foot on your shoulder. Glide one thumb under the adductor magnus fibers where they insert on the adductor tubercle. Spread these fibers medially while your other thumb laterally stretches the semimembranosus and semitendinosus.

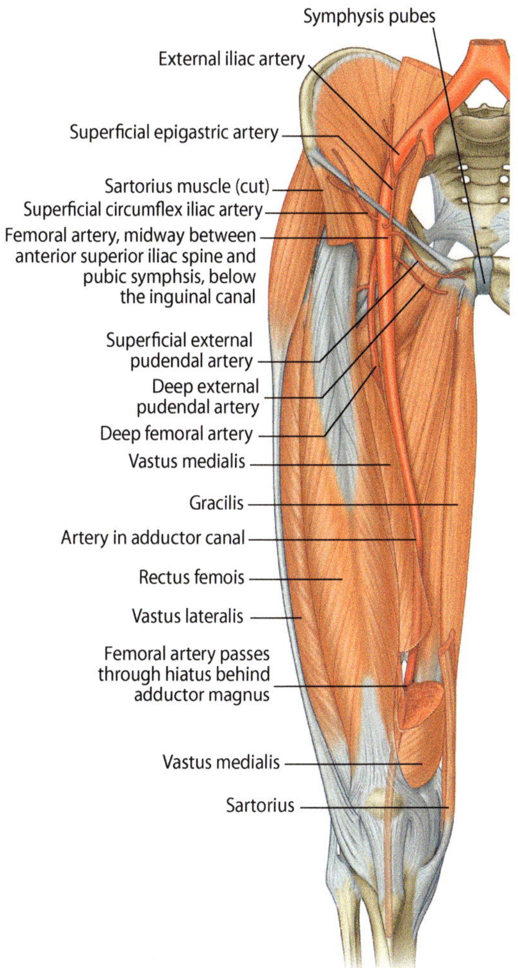

Fig. 19.2 Adductor hiatus.

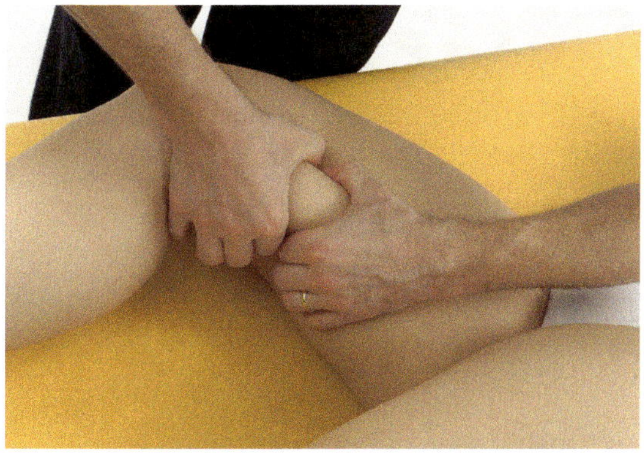

Fig. 19.3 Adductor hiatus in lateral decubitus.

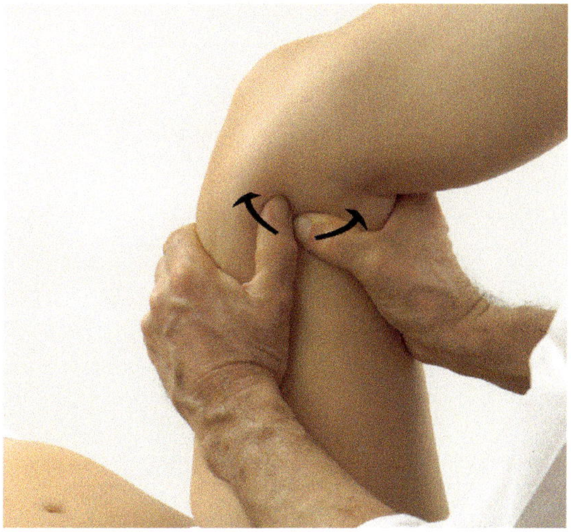

Fig. 19.4 Adductor hiatus in decubitus.

Clinical note

The saphenous nerve innervates the medial surface of the knee and leg. It provides an infrapatellar branch, as well. This nerve is important for knee proprioception.

To locate it, find the adductor tubercle. Use your index finger to gently press the inner thigh, making your way in a lateral and cranial direction. At first, you will feel the relatively soft muscle fibers of the vastus medialis and adductor magnus. All of a sudden you will come across something much firmer at the level of the adductor canal. This is the saphenous nerve.

Vastoadductor membrane technique in lateral decubitus (Figs. 19.5 and 19.6)

Unlike the technique for the adductor hiatus, treat the membrane with your thumbs parallel. Using induction, separate the fibers of the vastus medialis from those of the adductor magnus and adductor longus. There is almost always a point that is sensitive to your compression. This is the saphenous nerve where it emerges across the surrounding fascia. To release it, stretch the vastoadductor septum fibers on either side of the sensitive point. When the sensitive point releases, treat the nerve directly with a compression-induction technique.

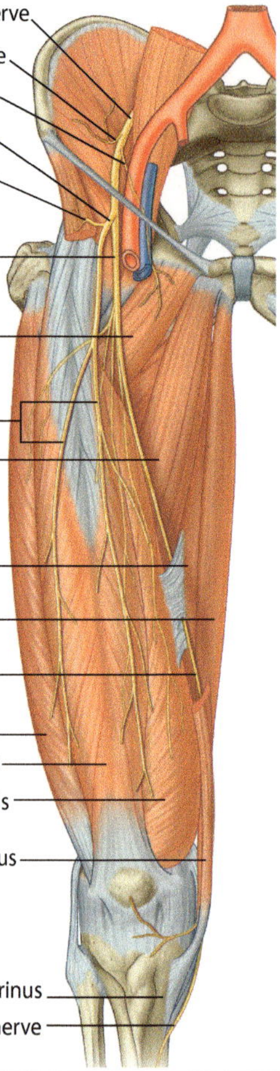

Fig. 19.5 Vastoadductor membrane

Technique for the junction of the adductor canal and the adductor hiatus (Figs. 19.7 and 19.8)

A valuable technique

This is a key zone for treatment of the knee and leg. As described above, the saphenous nerve passes through the adductor canal to innervate a good part of the knee and leg. The descending genicular artery also runs in the canal. The adductor hiatus transmits the femoral artery, which becomes the popliteal artery once it passes through the hiatus. The canal and hiatus communicate. We describe a maneuver that includes these three structures as having a simultaneous neural and vascular effect.

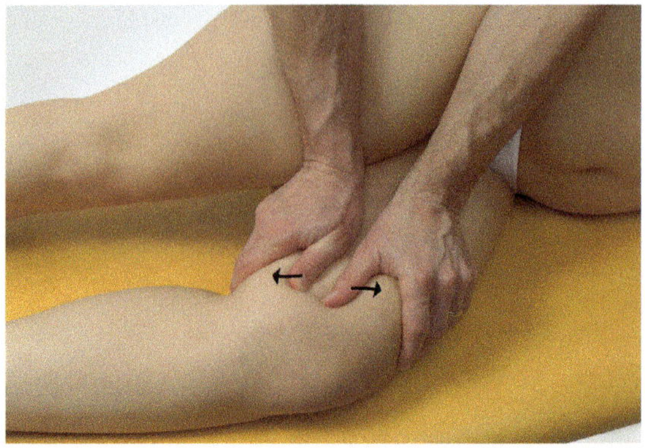

Fig. 19.6 Releasing vastadductor membrane.

In lateral decubitus

The patient lies on the side of the lower limb to be treated, knee slightly flexed. Stand behind the patient and place your thumbs side by side on the adductor canal that is formed mainly by the vastus medialis and adductor magnus. Your thumbs progressively open the walls of the canal with a spreading-induction technique.

Your middle and index fingers pass behind the adductor canal, fingers pointing in a distal direction. Use your fingers to separate the adductor magnus from the femur as it inserts on the linea aspera and at the adductor tubercle.

Your thumbs and fingers penetrate the canal and the hiatus at the same time, progressively and deeply, as if wanting to join each other. Finally, carry out a double separation-induction of the canal and hiatus together, and maintain the lift for several seconds.

19.3 ARTERIES OF THE KNEE (FIG. 19.9)

The femoral and popliteal arteries are released by the adductor canal/hiatus maneuver above. Below are techniques and applications for the main arteries of the knee.

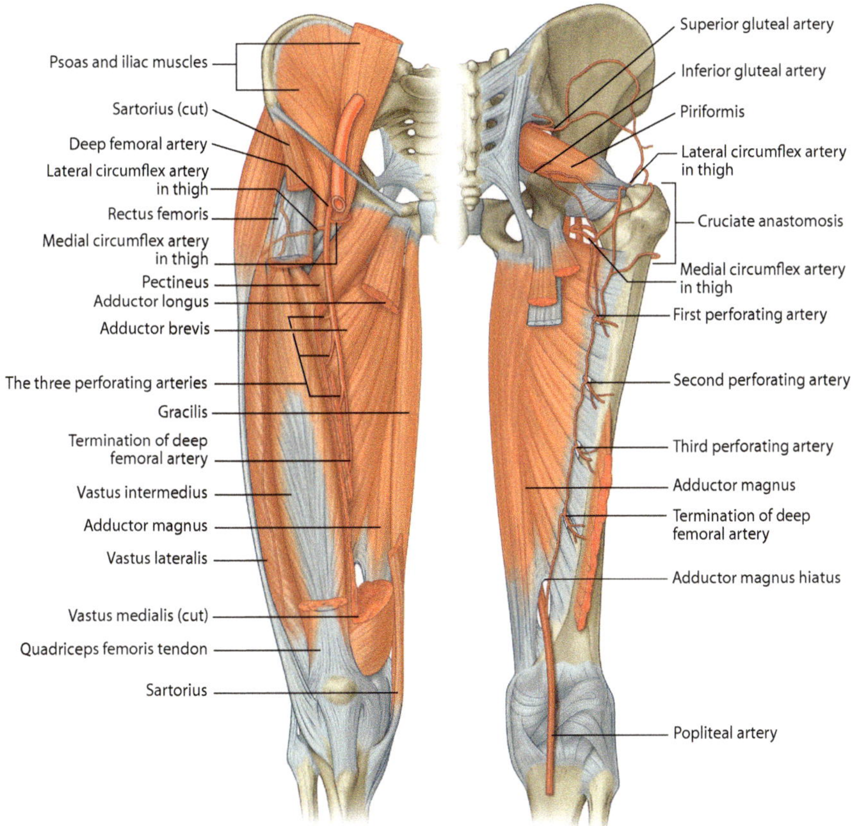

Fig. 19.7 Contents of adductor canal and hiatus.

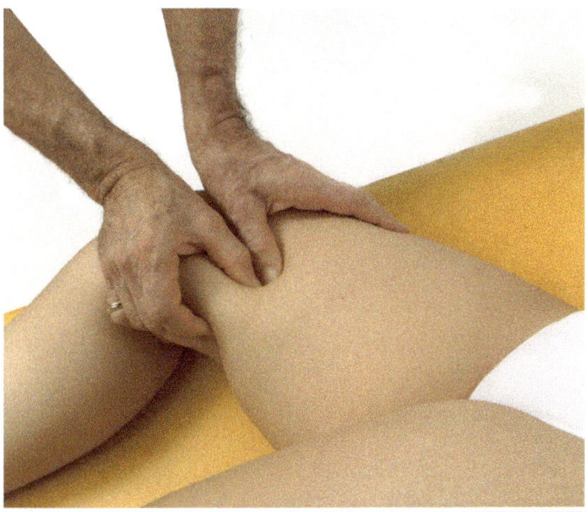

Fig. 19.8 Manipulation of adductor canal and hiatus.

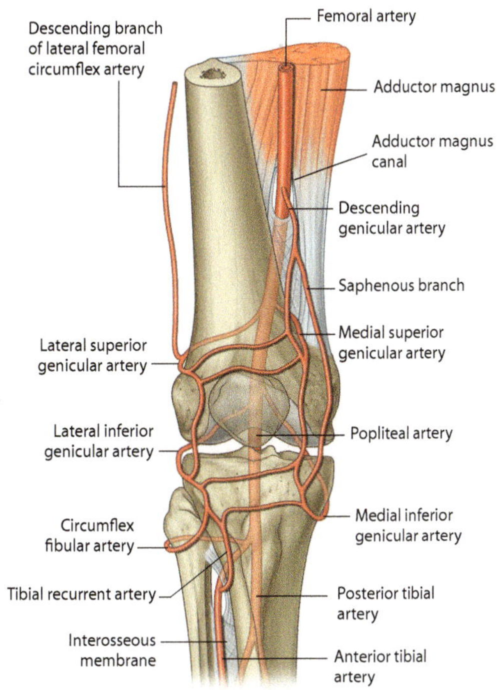

Fig. 19.9 Arteries of knee.

19.3.1 Review

Descending artery of the knee

This branch of the femoral vessel crosses the adductor canal in company with the saphenous nerve to which it runs laterally. The descending genicular artery irrigates the medial part of the knee joint; after this, it descends in the leg together with the saphenous nerve. The adductor canal and hiatus techniques apply to this artery.

Popliteal artery

The popliteal artery is deeply situated in the popliteal fossa. The superior medial and superior lateral genicular arteries arise from it to supply the knee. Distally, blood is carried to the foot directly from the popliteus by the anterior and posterior tibial arteries.

Clinical note

Popliteal artery entrapment syndrome
The popliteal artery can become compressed behind the knee due to unresolved muscle strain at the gastrocnemius muscle junction. This muscle strain compresses the popliteal fascia and the fascia surrounding the popliteal vessels. The patient experiences "restless leg," which can sometimes present as pseudoclaudication.

Popliteal vein syndrome
This condition is caused by the same myofascial compression, this time affecting the popliteal veins.

Identifying the syndrome
Take the pulse of the anterior and posterior tibial arteries with the leg flexed. We chose the posterior tibial artery because its pulse is generous and easier to find. Next, extend the leg and take the pulses again to see if there is any variation or abolition of the pulses.

It is easier to confirm an arterial problem than a venous problem because of the pulse. Veins can be visually noted, whereas a disturbed venous return is identifiable by the blush coloration of the integument.

Special note

The medial gastrocnemius muscle has a more important vascular role than the lateral counterpart. It drains as much as seven times more venous blood!

19.3.2 Techniques

Evaluation of the posterior tibial artery

As aforementioned in terms of the hip, the posterior tibial pulse is an excellent witness to the arterial condition of the lower extremity, and it doubles as a good indicator of the effectiveness of your maneuvers. Refer to chapter 10, where you will find a paragraph titled, "The posterior tibial arteries as witness pulses" (also reference Fig. 10.3).

Palpation of the popliteal fossa

Palpate the popliteal fossa with the knee somewhat flexed in decubitus, procubitus, or lateral decubitus.

Popliteal fossa, a diamond-shaped space (Fig. 19.10)

Cranial boundaries from superficial to deep

At the skin level are the small saphenous vein and the medial sural cutaneous nerve.

The muscle borders of the popliteal fossa are:

- the superiorlateral—the biceps femoris;
- the superiormedial—the semimembranosus (medial and posterior to which is the semitendinosus tendon);
- the more inferior—the lateral and medial heads of the gastrocnemius.

More anteriorly

Staying cephalad, separating the gastrocnemius, biceps, and semimembranosus muscles from lateral to medial reveals the contents of the fossa.

From lateral to medial are:

- the common fibular nerve;
- the tibial nerve;
- the medial sural cutaneous nerve,

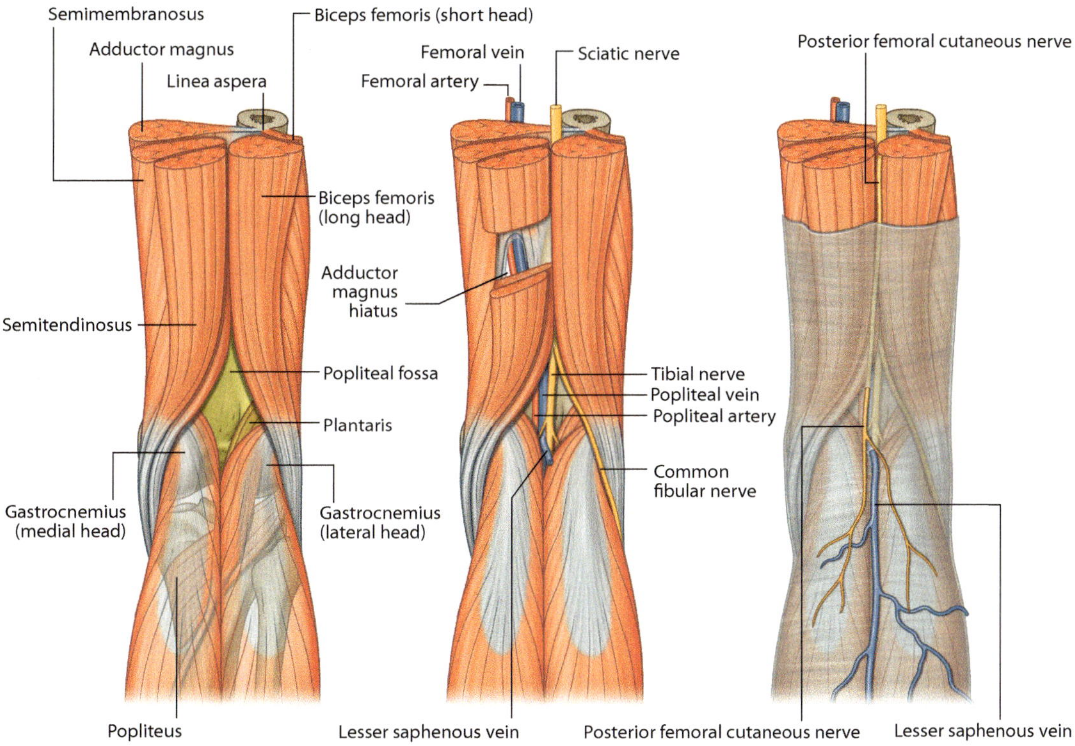

Fig. 19.10 Popliteal diamond-shaped fossa.

situated more posteriorly, thus more superficial than the others;

- the popliteal artery;
- the medial sural cutaneous vein, which covers part of the artery.

Deepest structures

Behind the boney knee, from lateral to medial are:

- the joint capsule;
- the collateral fibular ligament;
- the arcuate popliteal ligament;
- the popliteal muscle, beneath the arcuate popliteal ligament;
- the oblique popliteal ligament;
- the direct tendon of the semimembranosus.

Popliteal artery in procubitus (Fig. 19.11)

The patient lies prone with the knee slightly flexed, foot resting on a pillow or on your knee. The more flexed the knee, the more difficult it is to find the popliteal pulse, as it moves anteriorly and tissues are tighter.

Once you locate the popliteal pulse, stretch the artery distally several times, maintaining the elongation for 15 seconds. The goal is to have an effect on the mechanoreceptors of the arterial walls.

Caution

Avoid compressing the tibial and fibular nerves that run laterally to the artery. The technique should not be painful. Any pain signifies that your pressure is too firm or you are on the sciatic nerve.

Popliteal artery in lateral decubitus

The patient lies on the side of the knee to be treated. You position yourself facing him. Begin by searching for the popliteal pulse toward the medial part of gastrocnemius. After finding the pulse, fix the proximal part of the artery with one thumb; maintain distal axial stretch of the artery with the other thumb.

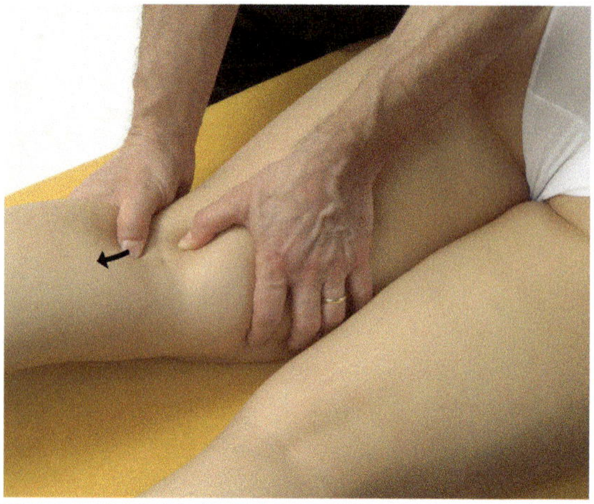

Fig. 19.11 Popliteal artery in procubitus.

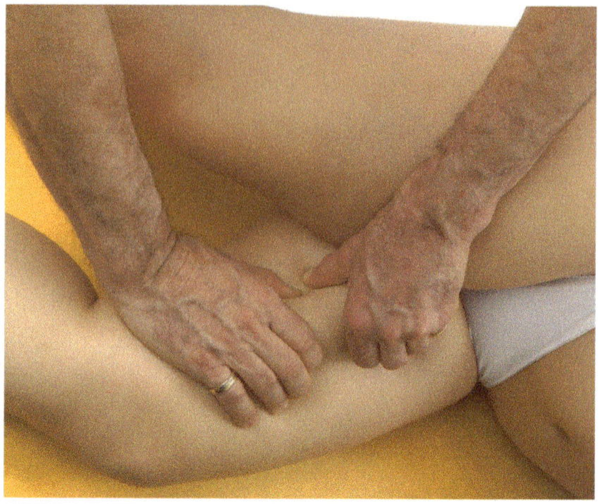

Fig. 19.12 Technique for perforating arteries in lateral decubitus.

Popliteal veins

Perform the same technique, stretching the vein proximally. Maintain vessel traction with a minimum of compression.

Exercise

Ask the patient to lie on his back near a wall or a door. Bend the knees and place the feet up against the wall. Place two tennis balls under the feet on the wall. For one to two minutes, roll the feet around the balls, trying to touch each section of the bottom of the feet. This is an excellent way to facilitate venous and lymphatic return from Lejars' famous plantar venous insole and, at the same time, stimulate the foot's proprioceptive innervation.

Perforating arteries

Three perforating branches arise from the deep femoral artery, which is a branch of the femoral artery.

Anatomy review

Cranially, the perforating arteries cross the adductor brevis. The first travels cranially to the adductor brevis; the second passes in front of that muscle, and the third passes immediately caudally to it. The three arteries pierce the adductor magnus through its tendinous insertions on the linea aspera. They give branches that anastomose with each other to irrigate the hip and the posterior knee.

Technique in lateral decubitus (Fig. 19.12)

This maneuver is the same as the one described above for the adductor hiatus, except the fingers work more cranially. Place yourself behind the patient, who lies on the side of the knee to be treated. With your thumbs, go deeper than the adductor magnus and brevis muscles to be as close as possible to their femoral insertions on the linea aspera. Spread the myofascial insertions with your thumbs, while your fingers stretch the muscle bodies back and medially. Proceed by sections, from caudal to cranial, maintaining the stretch for 12 seconds.

Genicular arteries (Figs. 19.13 and 19.14)

To locate these arteries, proceed in three steps so that you do not miss anything:

1. Two finger widths above the knee crease
2. At the knee crease
3. Two finger widths below the knee crease

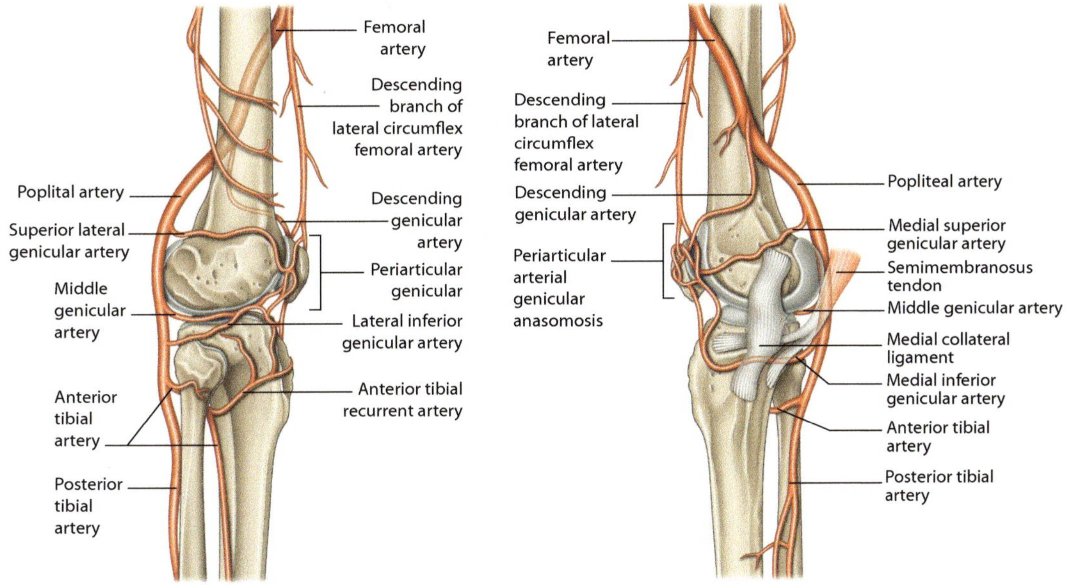

Fig. 19.13 Geniculate arteries.

Technique in decubitus

Descending genicular artery

Locate the descending genicular artery, just above the adductor hiatus. This technique is performed in the same position as for the adductor hiatus. Place one thumb just inferiorly to the hiatus and stretch the artery several times in a distal direction.

Lateral and medial superior genicular arteries

Feel for the pulse of these arteries on either side of the proximal part of the patella. They are not always easy to landmark. Even if you do not perceive the pulse, apply a transverse stretch of the soft tissue on either side of the quadriceps tendon. Next, keeping to either side of the patella, distally stretch each artery, in turn. Remember to maintain these stretches for 12 seconds, as we do with all vascular techniques.

Technique in lateral decubitus

The patient lies first on the side of the artery to be treated and then on the opposite side. The medial side is the most interesting to manipulate. Place one thumb against the cranial border of the patella and the other more laterally, where you feel the pulse. Stretch in a posterior direction. In this position it is possible to feel the medial genicular artery that passes over the knee joint. Maintain the stretch without compressing the artery for 12 seconds.

19.4 VEINS OF THE KNEE

19.4.1 Popliteal vein

This vein is located laterally to the popliteal artery. Find it between the femoral condyle and the tibial nerve. When the knee is extended, it is pressed against the bone.

Vascular entrapment

After a trauma, it is best not to immobilize the knee in hyperextension. Always allow a few degrees of flexion. Prolonged hyperextension can cause soft tissues to compromise venous and lymphatic circulation. In people with fragile vessels, such compression can even lead to phlebitis or veinitis.

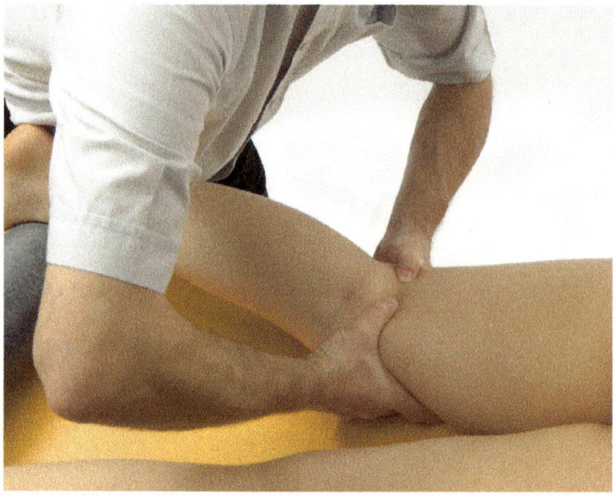

Fig. 19.14 Bilateral stretch of the superior geniculate arteries.

19.4.2 Popliteal vein enfolding

The popliteal vein folds during knee flexion. The most significant pleating occurs just below the adductor hiatus due to a fibromuscular ring in the adductor magnus that surrounds it. We have seen major vascular lesions in tilers following prolonged kneeling. It shows up as synovitis, venolymphatic circulatory retention, and sometimes even aneurism of the popliteal artery, all due to working on their knees.

19.4.3 Arteriovenous entrapment

Such entrapments contribute the same canal syndromes that impinge on peripheral nerves. At the knee, fibrosis of the aponeurotic fibers, between the medial gastrocnemius muscle and the lateral femoral condyle, can compromise the great saphenous vein. Recall that the medial gastrocnemius vein drains seven times more blood than its lateral counterpart, and most compressions are found medially.

The emotional knee

20

20.1 POSTURO-EMOTIONAL REPRESENTATIONS

How we hold our knees reveals a particular psychological attitude. Whether one stands with the knees straight or somewhat flexed is a function of what one is and what one wishes to express. Some of these attitudes are transient; others can become set and more telling with the trials of life.

Below are posturoemotional attitudes we have observed in hundreds of patients. As usual, exceptions exist. Needless to say it is difficult and rather pointless to characterize a person with a single word or phrase. In any event, it is clear that our bodies are very expressive, and it is next to impossible to prevent them from showing our true natures. It is easier to fool people with our words.

20.2 POSTURES

20.2.1 In extension

A standing position of knees straight, legs a little apart, and the lower extremity in lateral rotation may express these characteristics:

- confidence;
- ambition;
- seduction;
- need for action;
- challenge;
- appearance;
- conviction;
- determination;
- need to succeed;
- territorial;
- willpower;
- combativeness;
- responsiveness;
- domination;
- confrontation;
- arrogance;
- vanity.

20.2.2 In flexion

A standing position of knees slightly bent and lower extremities held in medial rotation may express these characteristics:

- lack of confidence;
- uncertainty;
- insecurity;
- need for protection;
- fear of confrontation;
- vulnerability;
- fragility;
- instability;
- withdrawal;
- docile nature;
- timidity;
- modesty;
- passivity;
- servitude;
- self-effacement;
- lack of fighting spirit ;
- victimization;
- doubt;

- lack of energy;
- fear of others (of being judged);
- submission.

20.2.3 Discussion

We are speaking here of attitudes and posture. Post-traumatic flexion contracture is not in the same category, at least when it first appears. There is also the question of degree. Nothing is categorical, but as Labruyère wrote a long time ago, "Leopards cannot change their spots."

What is interesting is that the person who stands with flexed knees has a tendency to develop patellar problems in the form of irritation of the patellar retinacula and muscles of the superficial pes anserinus, as well strain on the anterior cruciate ligament.

The person who stands with knees in extension is more likely to experience problems of the anterior meniscal horns, anterior cruciate ligament, and tibial collateral ligament.

Can a natural tendency be changed?

Each of us has a unique personality and way of being. What is innate joins with the events of our lives and marks us profoundly. On the other hand, we can always evolve in the way we adapt and compensate around life's difficulties.

Teaching people to hold themselves differently will alter their self-image and allow them to better confront life's challenges. We advise timid people to stand up straight, head held high, shoulders back, legs straight and slightly apart, with feet firmly planted on the ground. The transformation can be remarkable. It can even include voice alterations, in which expression becomes more clear and audible.

Old habits naturally return, but, through work and awareness, attitudes can transform. Even if such change is not as long-lasting as we might hope, the experience can be drawn upon to help us behave in a new way at difficult moments or in facing anxious situations.

The knee and the genital organs

The knees have a well-known relationship to the genital system. Knee pain can develop in girls during puberty. The obturator and saphenous nerves sometimes become irritated by the awakening ovary, which lies adjacent to them in the pelvis.

It is useless to try to manipulate the symptomatic knee. Better to explain to the adolescent that the pain will go away by itself and there is nothing to be concerned about.

As a rule, knee pain in pubescent girls is anterior, involving the patellar and medial ligaments, making you think of a meniscal problem. The same phenomenon does not occur in boys.

In women at perimenopause or menopause, knee pain is commonly medial and posterior, often brought on by uterine disorders or fibroids.

The knee and sexuality

Everyone can experiment with medial knee caresses to discover that the medial surface of the knee is more sensitive than the lateral aspect. The medial parts of the knee and thigh are natural erogenous zones due to their great sensitivity and their proximity to the genital organs.

4

Ankle and foot

Functional anatomy

21

The ankle and foot are a mosaic of bones that amount to a complex anatomical whole. This flexible structure must provide functions that are sometimes contradictory. It lets us stand upright, bear great loads, and adapt to changing surfaces when we walk or run. All the while it provides proprioceptive and exteroceptive information to the brain for the regulation of posture. The foot is an anatomical and architectural triumph! This mechanical marvel is able to withstand forces many times greater than the weight of the body.

The foot consists of 26 bones (28 if we count the tibia and fibula), 114 ligaments, 28 joint units formed by at least 49 different boney contacts, and an elaborate network of blood vessels and nerves. All of these are subject to frequent trauma. It is a lifelong challenge for bipeds to stand upright in defiance of the law of gravity. Numerous adaptations and compensations are required.

The feet are a goldmine of somatic dysfunctions. We routinely make a careful examination of patients' feet. It is rare that any escape without some problem unearthed. In addition, mechanical problems of the foot can generate major general structural imbalances that affect the entire body.

In view of the disastrous proprioceptive consequences caused by even a mild foot fixation, it is our job to understand as much as possible about the inner workings of the foot.

21.1 ANATOMICAL REVIEW (FIG. 21.1)

21.1.1 Terminology

Those of you who have made a long-time study of anatomy surely know that certain anatomical terms have fallen out of current usage. Descriptions of the foot and ankle have collected into an avalanche of new terms devised to be easier to remember. For those of us stumbling about with this new terminology, we have provided a nomenclature equivalency chart (Table 21.1).

Table 21.1
Anatomical nomenclature of the foot

Old nomenclature	New nomenclature
Bone	
Peroneus	Fibula
Astragale	Talus
Scaphoid	Navicular
Calcaneum	Calcaneus
Joints	
Ankle	Talocrural
Superior peroneotibial	Proximal tibiofibular
Inferior peroneotibial	Distal tibiofibular
Tibiotarsal	Talocrural
Subastragalar	Subtalar
Mediotarsal (Chopart)	Transverse tarsal
Lisfranc joint	Tarsometatarsal
Muscles	
Lateral peroneus brevis	Fibularis brevis
Lateral peroneus longus	Fibularis longus
Quadrate muscle of Sylvius	Quadratus plantae

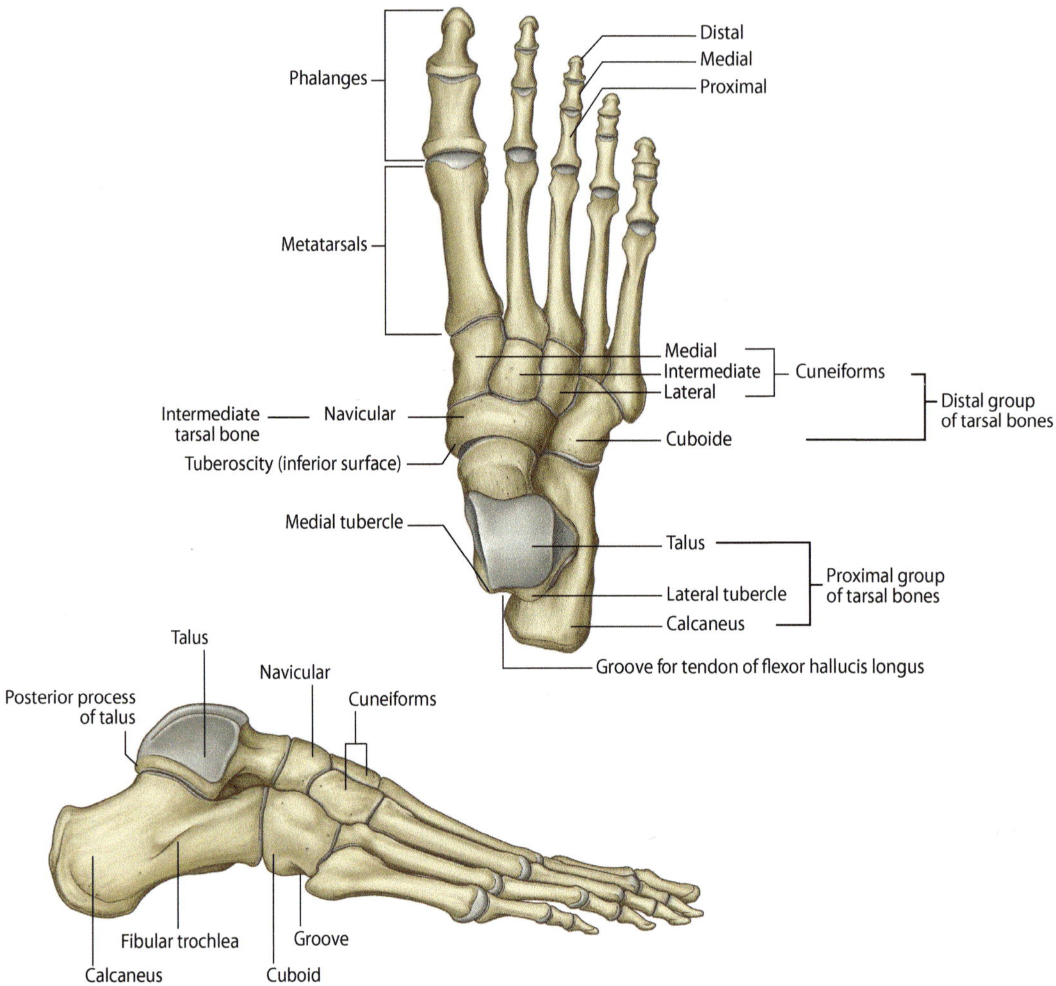

Fig. 21.1 The foot, general view.

21.1.2 Bone

Of the 206 skeletal bones, a full 52—slightly more than a quarter—are in the feet. The skeleton of the foot divides into three parts: tarsus, metatarsus, and phalanges.

Posterior tarsus

The proximal tarsus has two levels:

- The superior level, the talus (old nomenclature astragale), is a polyarticular bone. The long axis of the talus is inclined anteromedially and inferiorly. No muscles attach to the talus, which explains its tenuous vascularization. It is essentially stabilized by many ligaments that attach to it and by tendons that cross it medially.
- The inferior or plantar level, the calcaneus (formerly calcaneum), constitutes the heel. The calcaneus is oriented upwardly and laterally, meaning that the two bones of the posterior tarsus are divergent.

Anterior tarsus

The anterior tarsal comprises the bones that extend from the posterior tarsus. The navicular (formerly scaphoid) is the interme-

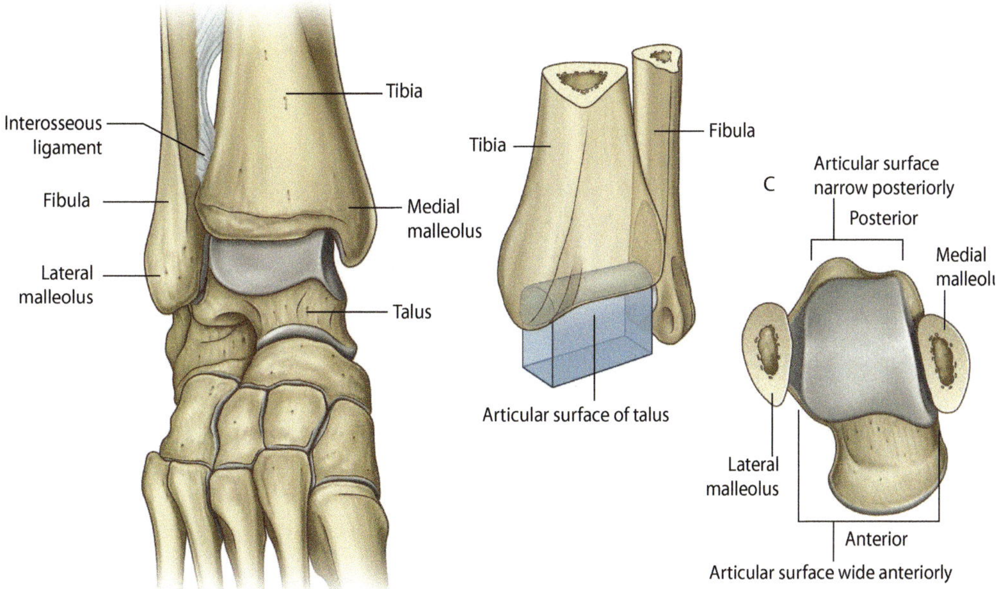

Fig. 21.2 Ankle joint (talocrural joint).

diate tarsal element, situated fairly high on the medial foot. The cuboid lies in front of calcaneus and is the most lateral bone in the tarsal arrangement.

Three cuneiform bones articulate proximally with the navicular and distally with the first to third metatarsals. The three cuneiform bones are the medial, intermediate, and lateral.

Metatarsus and phalanges

The metatarsus consists of five long bones that connect the tarsus and phalanges. The first four have three phalanges, while the hallux possesses only two. A pair of sesamoid bones is located on the plantar surface of the first metatarsophalangeal joint.

21.1.3 Articulations

Talocrural joint (Fig. 21.2)

This joint is located where the vertical axis of the leg meets the horizontal line of the foot. It supports the entire weight of the body and must control the hindfoot regardless of what position the foot lands. It is formed by the flexible union of the tibia and fibula into which the upper part of the talus fits.

A fibrous capsule attaches to all three bones. The anterior and posterior parts of the joint capsule are thin. Laterally the capsule is somewhat thickened by powerful collateral ligaments. The lateral ankle ligament (Fig. 21.3), or fibular collateral ligament, is composed of three separate bands:

- the anterior talofibular ligament;
- the posterior talofibular ligament;
- the calcaneofibular ligament.

The medial ankle ligament (Fig. 21.4), also known as the deltoid ligament, radiates out to insert distally on the talus, calcaneus, and navicular bones. It is composed of four adjacent but continuous fiber bands that insert onto the inferior tarsal bones. The arrangement from front to back is the:

- anterior tibiotalar ligament;
- tibionavicular ligament;
- tibiocalcaneal ligament;
- posterior tibiotalar ligament.

The talocrural ligaments do not insert exclusively on the talus. They extend to the calcaneus and navicular. Because of this, the talocrural joint is mechanically linked to

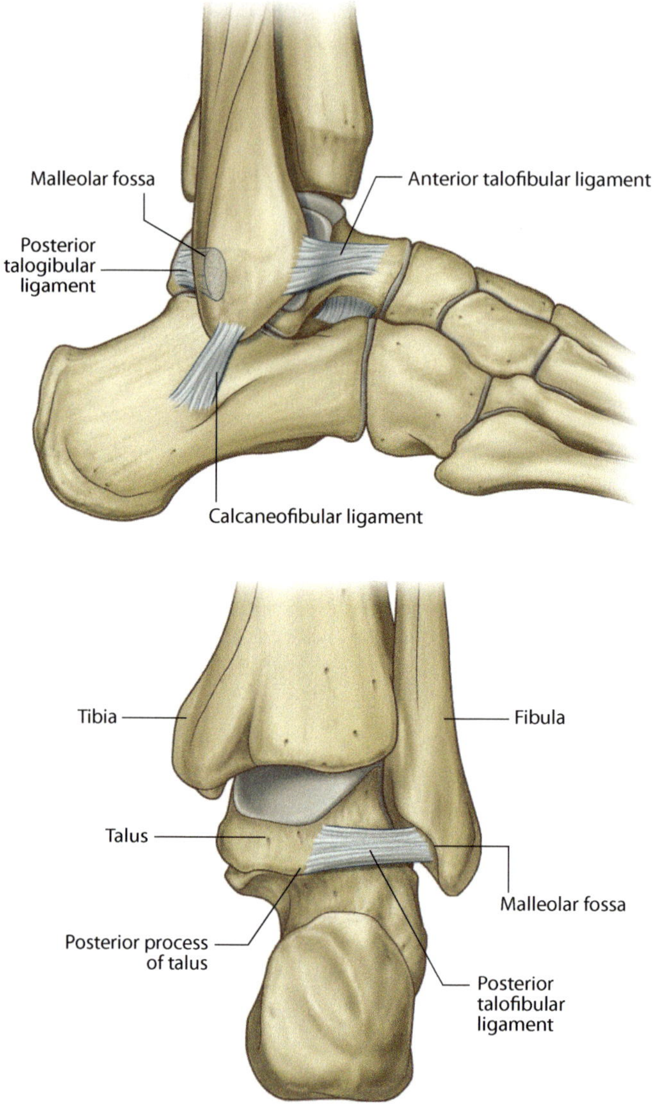

Fig. 21.3 Lateral (fibular) collateral ligament.

both the subtalar joint and the transverse tarsal joint (formerly mediotarsal). No muscles attach to the talus. Mobilization of the tibiotalar joint can only happen through the subtalar and mediotarsal joints. Tarsal mobilization is achieved though muscles that bridge around the tibiotarsal joint.

The ankle's greatest challenge is in stabilizing varus and valgus rocking motions in the tibiofibular mortice.

Subtalar joint (Fig. 21.5)

This joint is the meeting point of two bones that are juxtaposed and superimposed. The body of the talus articulates with the cranial surface of calcaneus. The capsule attaches to the borders of the joint surfaces. It is reinforced by the lateral talocalcaneal, medial talocalcaneal, and posterior talocalcaneal ligaments. The interosseous talocalcaneal ligament is the chief bond between the two bones.

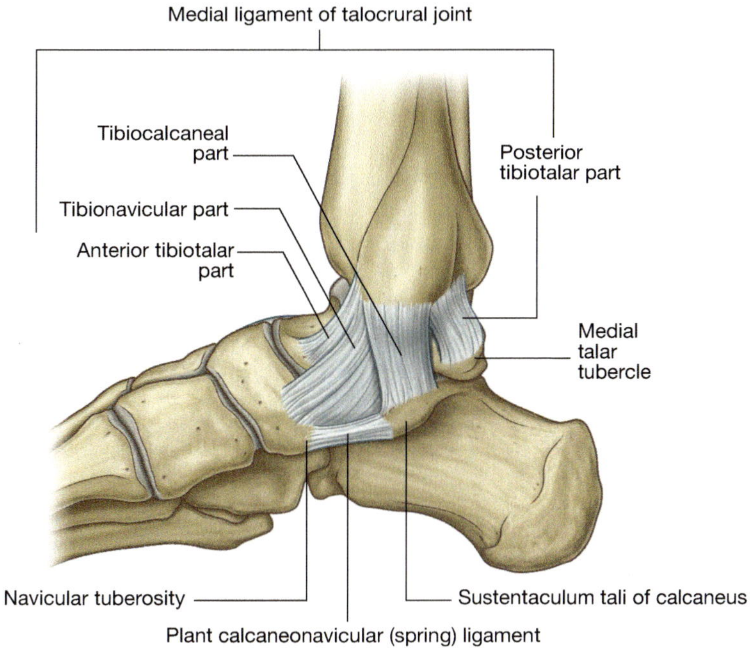

Fig. 21.4 Medial (tibial) collateral ligament.

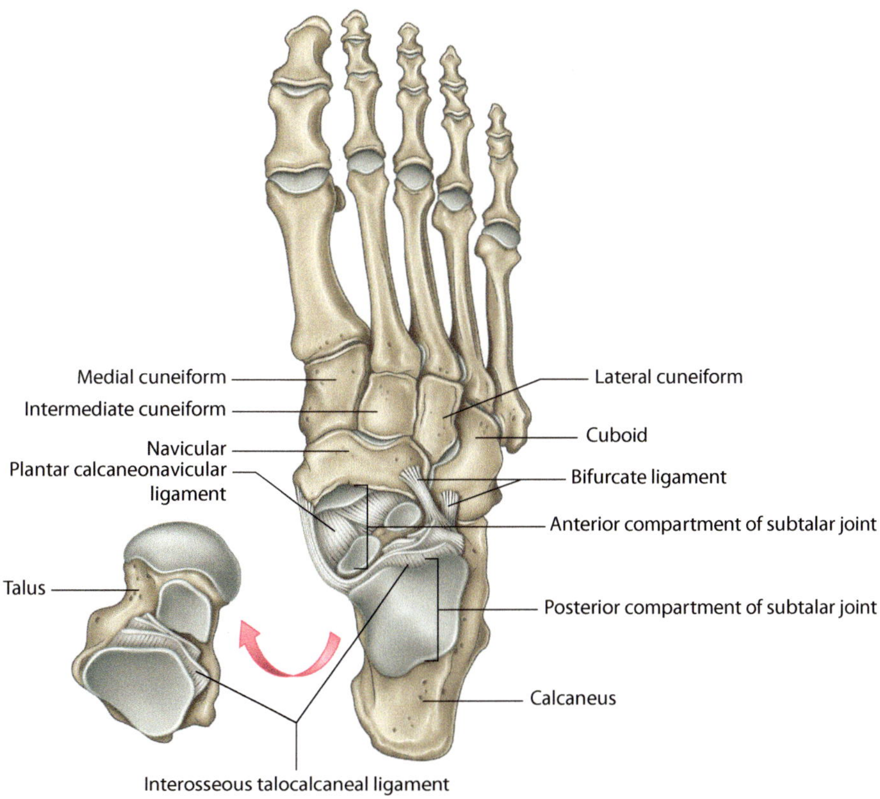

Fig. 21.5 Subtalar joint.

More and more authors consider this joint to be part of the talocalcaneonavicular complex in view of their common function. This ensemble is often identified as the subtalar joint complex or even the calcaneal pedal block.

The subtalar joint is important in allowing inversion and eversion of the foot. It plays a vital role in adapting the mobile foot to ground surfaces it walks over, as we shall see in upcoming sections devoted to function.

Transverse tarsal Joint (Chopart's joint)

Viewed from above, the midtarsal joint line appears like an S or a wave. This functional unit is composed:

- medially by the spherical talocalcaneonavicular joint;
- laterally by the calcaneocuboid joint, a reciprocal interlocking or saddle union.

Talocalcaneonavicular articulation (Fig. 21.6)

In this joint the rounded surface of the talus meets the calcaneus and the navicular bones. The plantar calcaneonavicular ligament ("spring" ligament) supports the head of the talus.

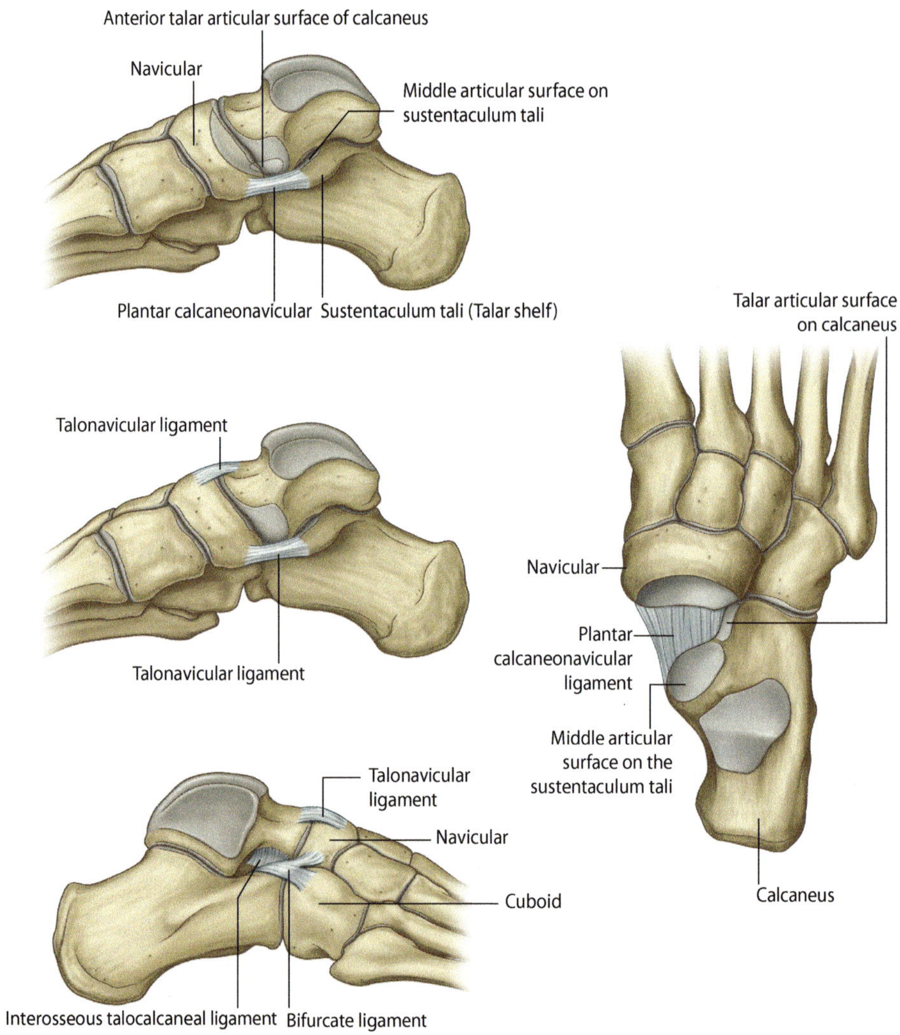

Fig. 21.6 Talocalcaneonavicular articulation.

Calcaneocuboid articulation

The anterior end of the calcaneus articulates with the posterior surface of the cuboid. A fibrous capsule encloses the joint completely. The ligaments that serve to support and strengthen the joint are the dorsal calcaneocuboid and the plantar calcaneocuboid.

The long plantar ligament on the underside of the foot supports the calcaneocuboid joint. On the dorsal surface these two joints are connected by the bifurcate ligament. As much as these two joints are morphologically distinct, they participate functionally in the same movements and associate with the subtalar joint.

Distal tarsal joints

There are five classified joints:
- cuneonavicular joint—a synovial articulation of the condylar variety;
- cuboidnavicular joint—a syndesmosis;
- medial intercuneiform joint—synovial articulation of the planar type;
- lateral intercuneiform joint—synovial articulation of the planar type;
- cuneocuboid joint—synovial articulation of the planar type.

A single fibrous capsule envelops these joints. Dorsal and plantar cuneonavicular ligaments reinforce the capsule.

Tarsometatarsal joint (Lisfranc joint) (Fig. 21.7)

This is the area where the cuneiform and cuboid bones unite to articulate with the bases of the metatarsals. Each articulation has its own joint capsule. The bones are connected by these ligaments:
- dorsal tarsometatarsals;
- plantar tarsometatarsals;
- interosseous tarsometatarsals.

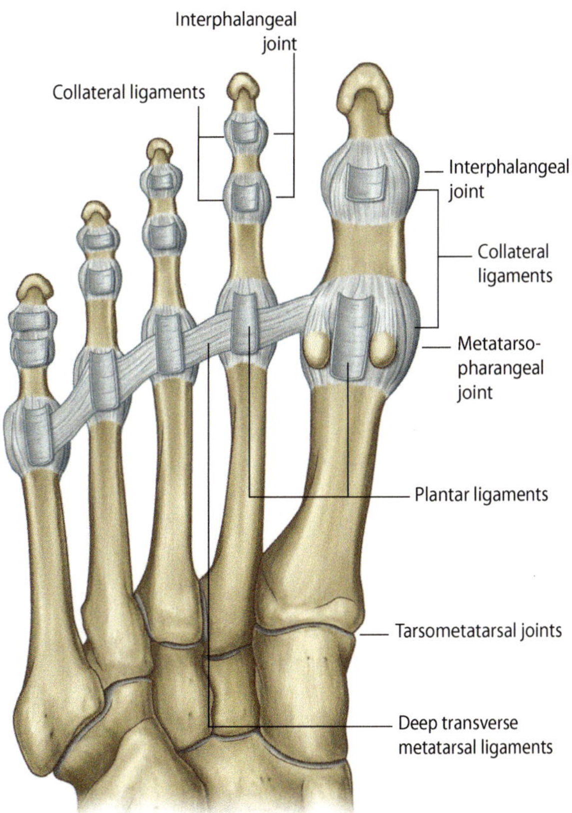

Fig. 21.7 Articulations of the forefoot.

This joint formation permits flexion, extension, and some lateral glide of the forefoot in relation to the rear foot. There is more mobility between the metatarsal of the big toe and the medial cuneiform than there is between the other tarsometatarsal joints.

Metatarsophalangeal joints

The rounded surfaces of the metatarsal heads are linked with the shallow cavities of the proximal toe phalanges. Movements permitted at this articulation are toe flexion, extension, and some adduction, abduction, and circumduction.

Fibrous joint capsules enclosing each joint are reinforced by:

- the medial collateral ligament;
- the lateral collateral ligament;
- the plantar ligaments that are concave inferiorly to allow for passage of the flexor digitorum longus tendons.

Four deep transverse metatarsal ligaments band the metatarsal heads together, allowing them to be interconnected as a single functional unit.

21.1.4 Main plantar ligaments (Fig. 21.8)

Certain plantar ligaments play a great role in supporting the architecture of the foot. Following are the principal ligaments of the plantar surface of the foot that assist in that function.

Plantar calcaneonavicular ligament

The plantar calcaneonavicular ligament or spring ligament (formerly known as the inferior calcaneoscaphoid ligament) extends from the talar shelf (sustentaculum tali) to the plantar surface of the navicular bone. It fills the wedge-shaped gap between these two bones. This ligament plays an important role in maintaining the longitudinal arch of the foot. It does this by supporting the head of the talus, which acts as a keystone of the arch and therefore enables us to bear the majority of our body weight on it.

Long plantar ligament

The plantar ligament (formerly known as the great plantar ligament) links the plantar surface of the calcaneus to the cuboid tuber-

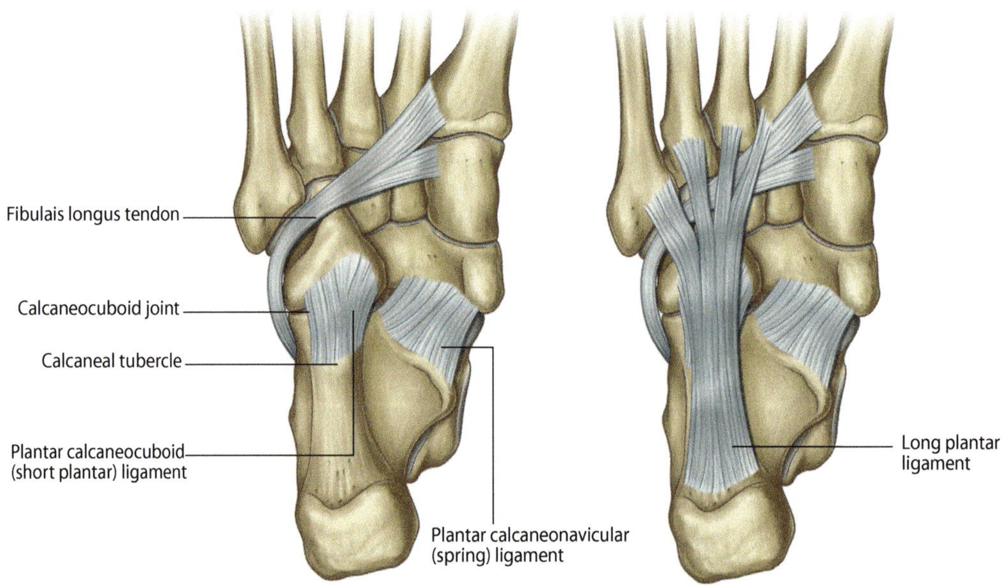

Fig. 21.8 Plantar ligaments of the foot.

osity and groove. Some fibers extend to the bases of the metatarsals, converting the plantar surface of the cuboid into a tunnel for passage of the fibularis longus tendon. The long plantar ligament plays an important role in maintaining the longitudinal arch of the foot.

Plantar calcaneocuboid ligament

The plantar calcaneocuboid (previously designated the short plantar ligament) runs deep to the long plantar ligament and is adjacent to the plantar calcaneonavicular band. It connects the anterior part of the inferior surface of the calcaneus to the inferior surface of the cuboid. It is an integral component of longitudinal arch support.

21.1.5 Muscles and tendons

The 28 muscles of the foot divide schematically into two groups:

- Extrinsic muscles have a proximal insertion on the leg and a distal insertion on the foot. They control movements of the tarsus and the foot arches.
- Intrinsic muscles relate to the foot only and have to do primarily with the toes.

Detailed anatomical reviews are provided for each muscle in the manipulation chapters.

21.2 FOOT FUNCTIONS

Effective treatment of the foot must be founded on some theoretical basis as to its function. It is worthwhile to study foot kinesiology to gain a detailed understanding of how each joint operates. But this knowledge must not eclipse your understanding of the complexity of the structure as a whole.

While this book is not intended as an exhaustive guide to the biological and functional mechanics of the foot, some considerations stand out in their importance to the overall scheme of things. Set out below are a few concepts we consider indispensable to understanding how our actions affect the foot.

21.2.1 A versatile design

For the foot to function correctly it must marry several demands that seem to be in opposition:

- on the structural plane—lightness and power;
- on the mechanical plane—rigidity and flexibility;
- on the cutaneous plane—sensitivity and resistance.

Rigidity

Resistance

The foot has the strength to withstand all loads that land on it. It must support and balance the weight of the body. We humans must be able to stand securely on two feet without undue effort. The foot receives enormous stress, equivalent to or greater than several times our body weight, but only for a short duration.

Power and propulsion

Strength and rigidity allow the foot to make powerful movements, often for just brief intervals, such as when the body is propelled forward in walking or running.

Flexibility

Adaptation

Flexibility gives the foot the mobility to adapt to different surfaces while walking or running.

Shock absorption, reception

Deformability permits the foot to cushion vibrations created by displacement as well as shock waves generated when the foot hits on the ground.

21.2.2 Mechanical duality

Changes of state

Thanks to the complexity of its anatomical

structure, the foot is capable of a large range of movements that allow it to virtually "change state" (Maestro et al. 2011). The foot can go from being flexible, adaptive, cushioning, or supportive to something solid, rigid, and powerful enough to digitigrade, such as when ballerinas dance on their toes. The foot possesses systems that play the role of tissular stiffeners. Many studies provide an understanding of just how the foot conjugates stability and mobility.

Pierre Rabischong (2011) describes the foot as acting mechanically like a viscoelastic structure of variable compliance. He conceives of the foot as having properties that make it "highly adaptive to mechanical conditions in both static and kinematic motion."

The double foot

Dolto (1976) emphasized the duality of the human foot, especially in terms of its dynamic aspects. He characterized the human foot as a "forked" structure (Fig. 21.9) divided into:

- the talar or superomedial foot, made up of the talus and the navicular and cuneiform bones together with the skeleton of the three first rays;
- the calcaneal or inferior lateral foot, comprising the calcaneus, cuboid, and the skeleton of the last two rays.

This perception of the foot as two subunits, each governed by one of the two bones of the rear foot, is interesting to us. It serves as a basis for understanding certain dysfunctions, and it guides our diagnostic approach to the foot.

The three palettes of the foot (Fig. 21.10)

E. De Doncker and C. Kowalski (1976) analyzed the functioning of the forefoot. In comparing mobility of the five rays of the foot, they subdivided the foot into three distinct units called palettes (Fig. 21.10a).

The axial palette corresponds to the middle zone of the foot. It is comprised of the second and third rays, which are the least mobile because they are recessed in the tarsometatarsal joint space. On the other hand, the axial palette offers remarkable stability as soon as the foot is on the ground.

The medial palette corresponds to the first ray, which is much larger than the others. It is also the most mobile metatarsal.

The lateral palette corresponds to the fourth and fifth rays together with the lateral cuboid tarsometatarsal junction. These two metatarsals are much more mobile than the other long bones of the axial palette; they are a little less mobile than the first metatarsal.

This longitudinal division of the foot reflects anatomical and physiological reality. The foot possesses one component of stability in the axial palette. It has two components of dynamic stability in the lateral and medial palettes, which sit on either side of the central element. De Doncker and Kowalski liken this arrangement to a sailboat or a child's tricycle (Fig. 21.10b).

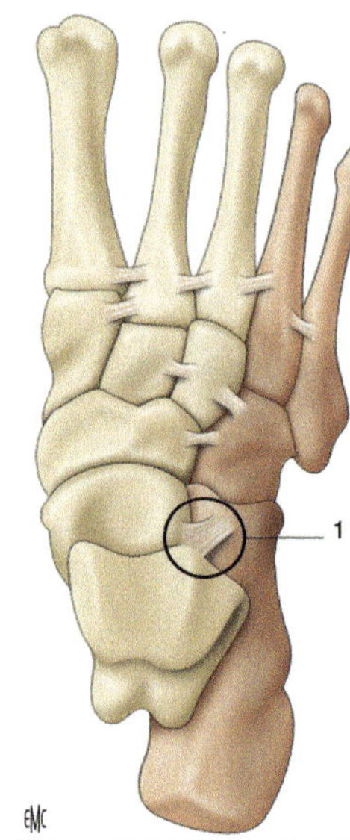

Fig. 21.9 The talar and calcaneal foot. In red, the calcaneal foot of reception and stabilization; in beige, the talar foot of propulsion. (1) Pivot. (A. A. Lopez and A. Goldcher. 2010. "Historical understanding of the biomechanics of bare feet." EMC Podiatry 27-010-A-10: 1–15. Paris: Elsevier Masson. All rights reserved.)

21.2.3 Solidity

Numerous conceptual schemes have been proposed to represent the mechanical structure of the foot. Architectural foot models have evolved considerably over the past 100 years. In the early days, rather static aspects related to form were emphasized. Functional representations developed through the years. While some conceptual frameworks have fared poorly over the years, others have stood the test of time, and we have made advances of our own.

Arches of the foot (Fig. 21.11)

The bones of the foot do not lie on the horizontal plane. They are arranged in longitudinal and transverse arches, passively supported by ligaments and actively strengthened by flexible tendons. These arches contribute to the weight-bearing capabilities and resiliency of the foot.

Longitudinal arch

The longitudinal arch of the foot runs from the plantar surface of the calcaneus posteriorly to the heads of the metatarsals anteriorly. It is composed of a medial and a lateral part.

The medial longitudinal arch is higher and more important than its lateral counterpart. It is made up of the calcaneus, talus, navicular, three cuneiforms, and three metatarsals. The talar head is the keystone of the medial longitudinal arch.

The lateral longitudinal arch is much flatter than the medial one and rests on the ground during standing. It is formed by the calcaneus, cuboid, and lateral two metatarsals.

The ligaments that maintain the longitudinal arch are the calcaneonavicular, plantar calcaneocuboid, and long plantar together with the plantar aponeurosis. The tibialis anterior inserts on the base of the first metatarsal and the medial cuneiform to help

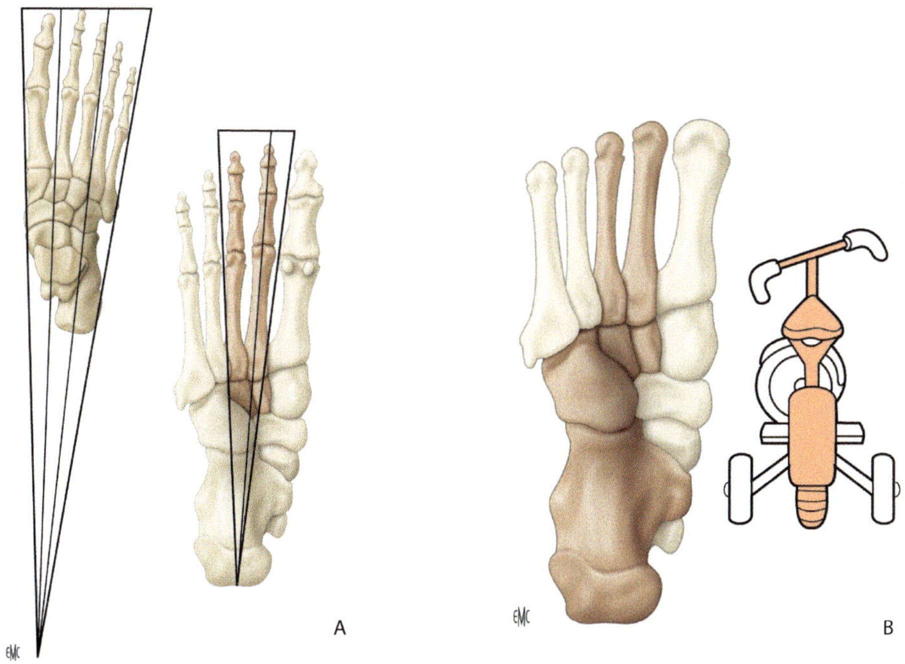

Fig. 21.10A and B The three pallets of the foot. (A) In red, 2nd and 3rd rays represent the median pallet; (B) The lateral and medial pallets provide stabilization like the small wheels of a child's tricycle. (A. A. Lopez and A. Goldcher. 2010. "Historical understanding of the biomechanics of bare feet." EMC Podiatry 27-010-A-10: 1–15. Paris: Elsevier Masson. All rights reserved.)

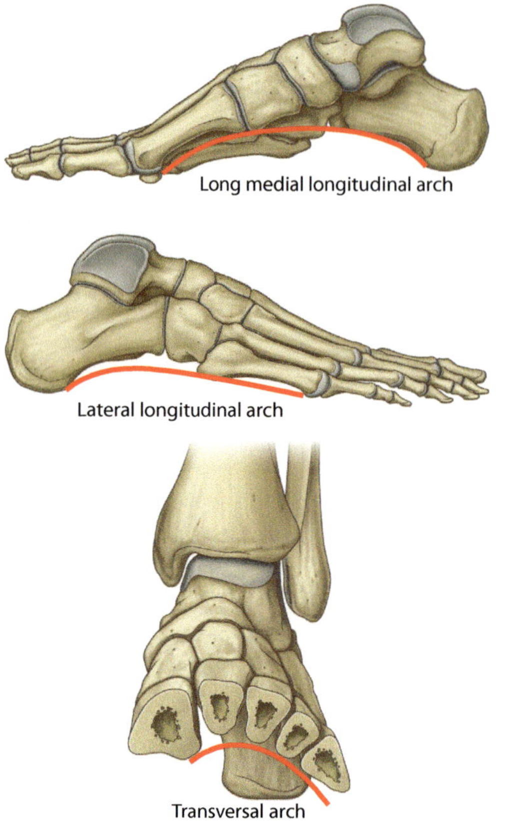

Fig. 21.11 Arches of the foot.

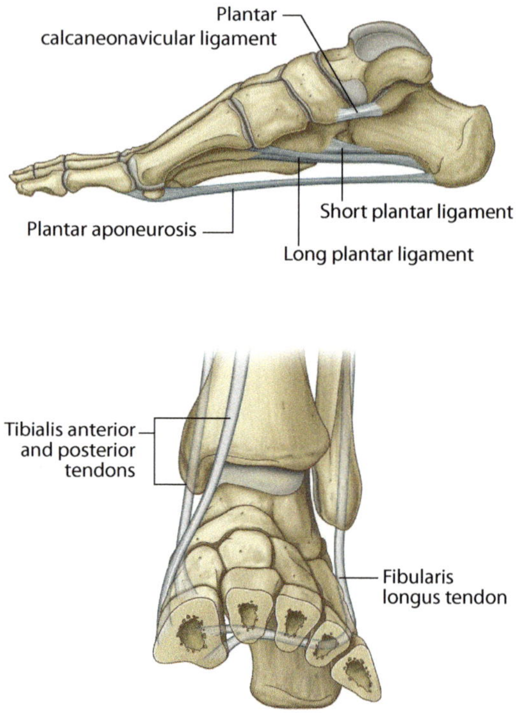

Fig. 21.12 Foot arch support.

strengthen the medial longitudinal arch. It is aided in this action by the fibularis longus tendon that crosses the sole of the foot from lateral to medial (Fig. 21.12).

Transverse arch

This arch extends from side to side, formed by the cuboid, cuneiforms, and bases of the metatarsal bones. The medial and lateral parts of the longitudinal arch serve as pillars for the transverse arch. The tendons of the fibularis longus and tibialis posterior extend across the sole of the foot like stretchers helping to maintain the curvature.

Podal architecture

De Doncker and Kowalski (1976) described an architectural arch or vault as an arrangement designed to maintain itself under the weight of its constituent parts alone. This model supposes permanent contact with the ground (Fig. 21.13). As such, the term vault cannot really be applied to the foot, which sometimes bears weight and sometimes does not.

The more appropriate architectural term is the dual-pitched farmhouse roof, which is formed by two oblique rafters, called top cords, linked at their bases by a bottom cord or tie beam. This ensemble presents an internal coherence, making it possible to manipulate it.

The foot has two pitched sides, an anterior top cord and a posterior top cord (Fig. 21.14). The anterior top cord is made up of bones that run from the talus to the heads of the metatarsals. The posterior top cord is formed by the talus superimposed on the calcaneus.

The tie beam maintaining the boney arch of the foot is composed of multiplanar liga-

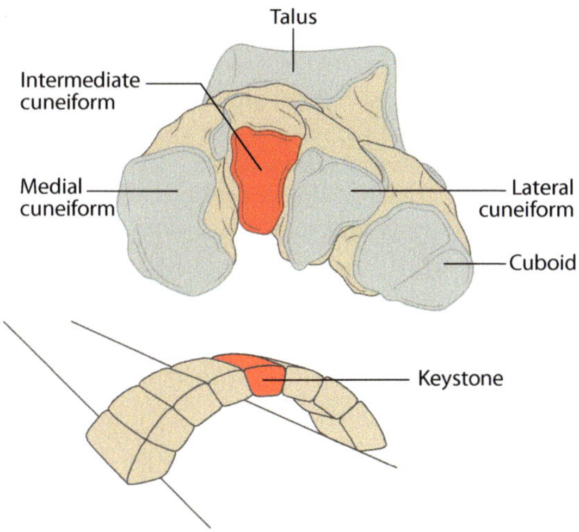

Fig. 21.13 Vault concept. (After Klein and Sommerfeld. 2008. Biomechanics of the lower extremities 60: 395. Paris: Elsevier Masson.)

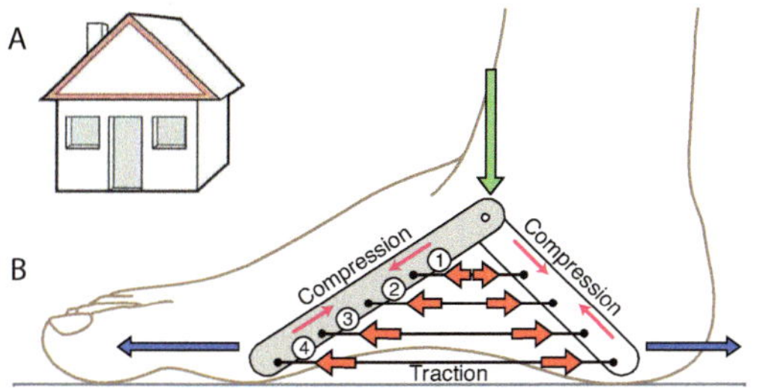

Fig. 21.14 Concept of farm roof. (A) Doncker and Kowalski's podal roof model. The structure of a foot is comparable architecturally to a pitched roof rather than a vaulted construction. (A. A. Lopez and A. Goldcher. 2010. "Historical understanding of the mechanics of bare feet." EMC Podiatry 27-010-A-10: 1–15. Paris: Elsevier Masson. All rights reserved.) (B1) Deep plantar ligaments; (B2) Intrinsic muscles; (B3) Extrinsic muscles; (B4) Middle plantar aponeurosis. (After Klein and Sommerfeld. 2008. Biomechanics of the lower extremities 60: 395. Paris: Elsevier Masson.)

ments. Among these deep ligaments are the plantar calcaneonavicular (spring ligament), the long plantar ligament, and the plantar calcaneocuboid ligaments.

These bands are reinforced by the short plantar muscles and superficial plantar ligamentous elements (plantar fascia). In static conditions, only ligamentous elements play the role of tie beam. In dynamic conditions such as walking, plantar muscles help to maintain the arches under the stress of increased load.

If you cut the ligamentous tie beam, the pitched roof collapses!

Fragmentation

The foot supports weight loads of up to seven to eight times the weight of the body, depending on position. According to Rabischong (2011), the foot is strong because it is a prefragmented mosaic structure. A good way to increase the resistance of any rigid structure is to break it up and then reconnect the resulting pieces in a way that allows small movements. This is a good description of the foot, whose numerous bones are linked by a great many ligaments capable of flattening under strain and then resuming their curvature when load is removed.

Locking

The foot is integral to the articular chain of the lower limb. When the foot is on the ground, its range of motion is reduced by tension in the weight-bearing soft tissues. When the weight of the body is transmitted from the tibia to the talus, the foot naturally pronates. In this position, joints of the foot are compressed together to increase stability. This is McConnail's close-packed position.

All joints but one are fully locked together. The exception is the transverse tarsal, or Chopart joint, whose bones are interlocked less firmly. This flexibility makes the foot adaptable to uneven terrain by allowing balancing movements (Maestro et al. 2011).

Eversion position of the foot

Maestro et al. (2011) noted that force is required to put the foot into eversion—either the force of gravity in weight bearing or muscle action when the foot is unloaded. Eversion only happens when enough force is exerted to overcome inherent pretension.

The spontaneous tendency of the foot is always toward inversion due to the influence of the soft tissues. Moreover, following ankle sprain, burn, or paralysis, the foot has a tendency to heal in the position of inversion, creating a vicious cycle where the arch of the foot supinates, predisposing it to reinjury.

21.2.4 Flexibility

The foot is also well-adapted to dynamic function. Following are ways that flexibility factors in:

- Propulsion: During the swing phase of gait, flexibility allows the foot to "spring" by retaining some of the energy and mechanical forces that it receives in the stance phase.
- Adaptation: On uneven surfaces, resiliency gives the foot tremendous plasticity whereby it can adapt to variable terrain.
- Shock absorption: Controlled flexibility allows the foot to absorb changes in load, vibrations, or shock waves when it hits the ground.

Triangles of the foot (Fig. 21.15)

According to Rabischong and Bonnel, the static foot is not a tripod as it is so often depicted. These authors liken the sole of the foot to a pair of triangles joined by a common base.

The anterior triangle is formed by the toes and their metatarsophalangeal joints. This is called the propulsion triangle, in which the plantar surface of the hallux appears prominent.

The posterior triangle is formed by the cutaneous plantar sole of the foot, running from the calcaneus to the distal metatarsophalangeal balls of the foot. This statodynamic triangle balances an apparently static body through numerous dynamic adjustments in relation to the center of gravity.

Foot unlocking

When the foot is in inversion, when body weight is removed, or when the heel is actively lifted in walking, all the joints are in McConnail's unlocked, loose-pack position. The foot is at its greatest flexibility and maximum mobility when unloaded.

All the joints unlock except for the transverse tarsal joint (Chopart), which locks down in this phase. The foot becomes dependent on movement through the subtalar joint to place the foot in inversion dynamically.

This mechanism of inverse locking changes the angle of the joint axis. It allows the foot to adapt almost instantaneously to functional dynamic conditions. Active joint muscle locking entails no loss of foot rigidity (Blackwood et al. 2005).

Shock absorption

According to De Doncker and Kowalski (1976), whose work we draw on here, several boney and musculoligamentous arrangements function as shock-absorbing systems. Certain plantar features are key contributors to this function.

The authors identified several cushioning levels in the foot and lower limb:

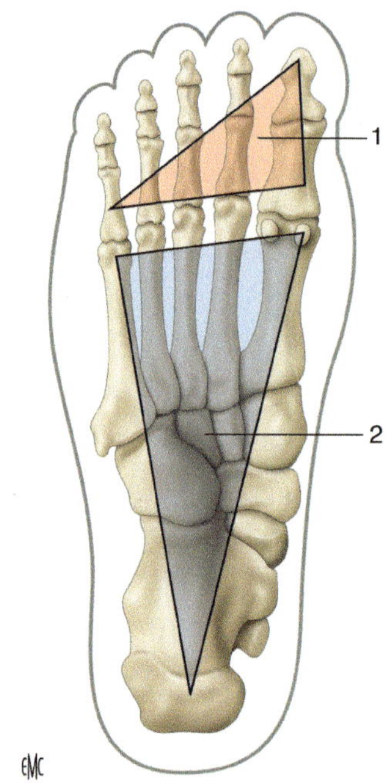

Fig. 21.15 Triangle of the foot. (1) Anterior triangle of propulsion; (2) Posterior triangle of reception (A. A. Lopez and A. Goldcher. 2010. "Historical understanding of the biomechanics of bare feet." EMC Podiatry 27-010-A-10: 1–15. Paris: Elsevier Masson. All rights reserved.)

- shock absorption of the sole of the foot;
- shock absorption of the hindfoot;
- shock absorption of the forefoot;
- shock absorption of the top of the foot triangle (elastic arches);
- adjacent articulations.

Shock absorbers of the plantar aspect of the foot (Fig. 21.16)

This is the first part of the foot to touch the ground. The subcutaneous tissues on the underside of the foot are very thick, and their elastic function can be compared to car tires. It is made up of a particular fatty tissue distributed through small, quite separate microchambers of connective tissue arranged like a honeycomb. This feature is covered in greater detail in the section on foot viscoelasticity (21.2.5).

The plantar fibroaponeurotic system is organized in a complex scheme, in which fat pads cushion the foot as soon as the fibrous network is tensed by the metatarsals during weight bearing. It behaves like a three-dimensional spider web that allocates pressures to protect the foot from forces transmitted to it from some distance away.

Shock absorption of the hindfoot (Fig. 21.17)

At the subtalar joint, the calcaneal axis runs laterally in relationship to the leg and the talus. This cantilevering is supported by the medial ankle ligament and maintained by the posterior tibial muscle. This arrangement constitutes a cushioning mechanism.

Shock absorption of the forefoot (Fig. 21.18)

At the forefoot, the transverse arch operates like a spring composed of the intermetatarsal ligament and transverse fascicles of the abductor hallucis muscle. These structures stretch under load, allowing the metatarsal heads to make contact with the ground. Once body weight is removed in the stepping phase of gait, elasticity and tone bring the metatarsal heads up to form the arc of a circle.

Shock absorption of the top of the foot triangle

Weight is also distributed along the axis of the foot by an arrangement comparable to a Hendrix torsion bar (Fig. 21.19) involving the calcaneus, cuboid, and lateral and intermediate cuneiforms together with the second and third metatarsals.

Traditional mechanics describes a type of shock absorption created by a relatively elastic bar, called a torsion bar, that extends between two solid lever arms. A pad is placed on the bar and load is applied. When laden, the angle between the lever arms and the ground is proportional to the weight of the charge and the elasticity of the bar.

In the anatomical analogy, the torsion bar is formed by the cuboid together with the lateral and intermediate cuneiform bones. The lever arms are made up of the calcaneus and the second and third metatarsals, respec-

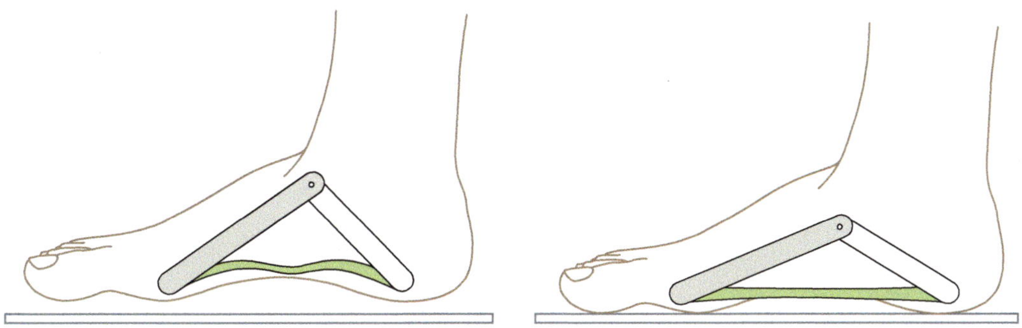

Fig. 21.16 Plantar shock absorption. (After Klein and Sommerfeld. 2008. Biomechanics of the lower extremities 74: 411. Paris: Elsevier Masson.)

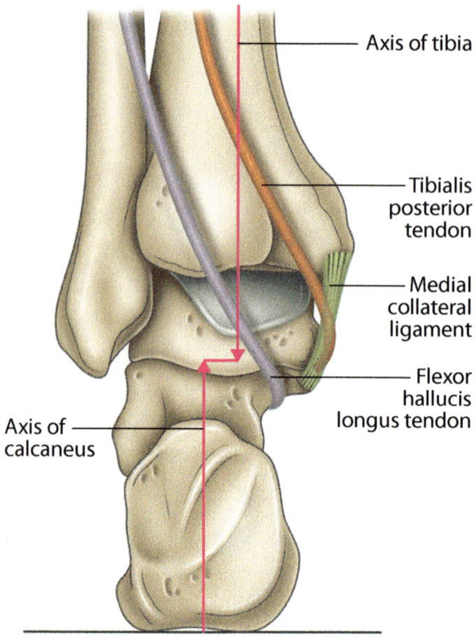

Fig. 21.17 Shock absorption of the hindfoot.

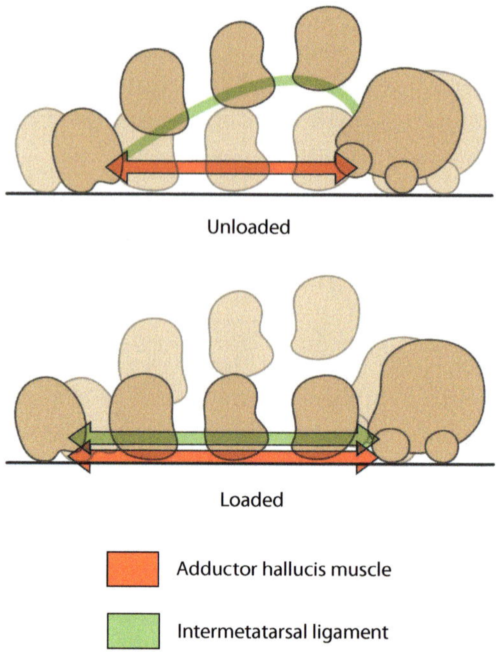

Fig. 21.18 Shock absorption of the forefoot.

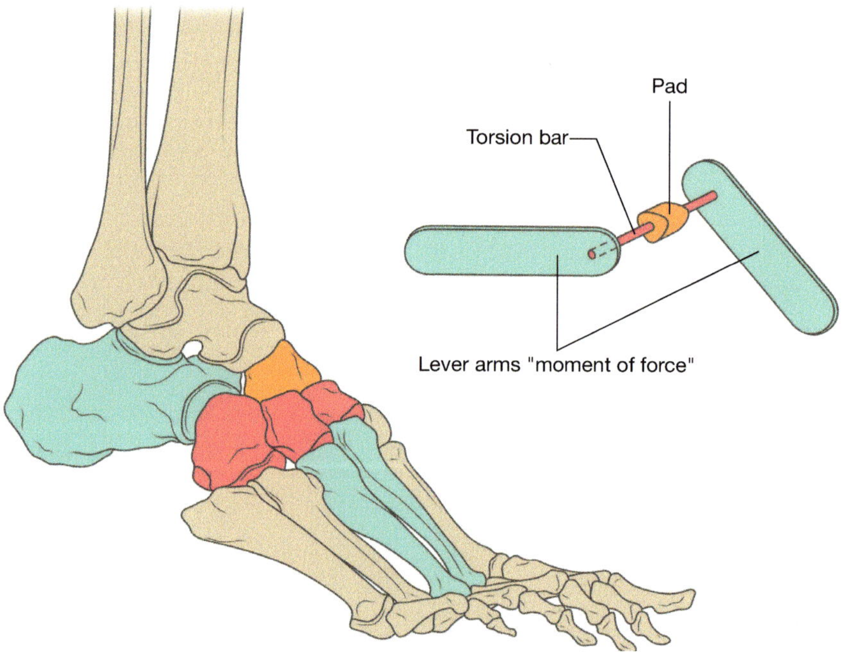

Fig. 21.19 Hendrix torsion bar—the distribution of weight along the axis of the foot.

tively. The navicular acts as the cushion onto which the weight of the body is transmitted through the talus.

Adjacent articulations

The joints of the foot are not alone in protecting the foot from shocks and vibrations. All the joints of the lower extremity contribute to this endeavor. The hip and the vertebral column do their part, as well.

Most of the joints have some slight overhang that plays a role in cushioning shock. At the hip, the angulation of the femoral head acts as a lever arm that is strongly counterbalanced by the gluteus medius. The knees angle slightly inward under constant tension of the medial collateral ligament and the pes anserinus muscle group. Most of the time, this cantilevered effect in the frontal plane is doubled by slight flexion of the knee, allowing the quadriceps to provide a degree of cushioning in the sagittal plane.

Clinical importance of lower-extremity shock absorption properties

Functional unity

The structures and force-dampening devices of the lower extremity cushion the shock waves and vibrations caused by walking or jumping. Their complementary actions constitute a true function. When well done, this action happens transparently and silently.

Shock absorption is an invisible mechanical function. We do not suspect it at first glance. While it is of the utmost importance to the economy of the body, it has been little studied and barely touched upon in osteopathy.

Similarities

While a great diversity of cushioning devices exist in the foot, the overhang arrangement predominates, just as it does in many areas of the body. A joint connects two bones whose axes are not quite aligned. This noncoincidence is passively supported by one or more ligaments and actively maintained by one or more muscles.

When the lower extremity is carried in static situations, practically all the effort linked to weight bearing is buttressed by ligaments and passively reinforced by muscles and their tendons. In dynamic situations, such as standing and walking, muscles actively assist ligaments.

Complementary considerations

None of the cushioning elements of the lower extremity are sufficient in themselves. If even one of them becomes dysfunctional, all other components must immediately absorb the additional work that befalls them. Their only option in distributing this overload is to deform a little more to compensate for the deficient element.

In this mechanical compensation scenario it is not unusual that certain components find themselves strained, even overwhelmed and incapable of doing more than they ordinarily do.

The plantar skin can form calluses, corns, and ulcers as a testament to faulty load distribution of the cushioning function. Joints can lose some of their initial elasticity and become too stiff to assume the increased deformation required to offset loads. This tends to occur with aging or in the aftermath of trauma or surgery. It is not uncommon for an old pain to reappear after a seemingly minor traumatic event or for a familiar discomfort to return by wearing a new pair of shoes.

Interdependence

Foot shock absorption extends beyond mere localized mechanics. It is part of an overall joint surface management and protective mechanism plan, both local and distant.

In any cushioning insufficiency, the last recourse is the cartilage. Locomotor strain can become a constant cartilage irritant, inevitably wearing down joint surfaces. This is very likely how a long-standing foot fixation eventually harms joint surfaces of the knee, hip, or lumbosacral junction, leading to arthritis.

Imagining shock absorption as a noble function causes us to reconsider our manual actions. The fair allocation of pressures depends on the harmonious deformability of an entire mechanical system. The slightest soft tissue or joint restriction within any of these units assumes great importance. Any correction must be planned out, as it concerns the heart of an inventory of cushioning mechanisms.

21.2.5 Viscoelasticity

Bones and musculoligamentous structures provide part of the foot's shock-absorption qualities. Viscoelastic capacities are the other component.

Viscoelasticity involves:

- plantar cutaneous resistance;
- plantar fat;
- the special venous system of the foot, whose vascular pad functions as a "waterbed," to use Dufour et Pillu's comparison (2006).

Cutaneous sensitivity and resistance

The skin of the foot, like skin everywhere, assumes the classic role of protection. It has additional, sometimes paradoxical, features, as well. In places such as the back of the foot or outside the sole of the foot, the skin is delicate and ultrasensitive, contributing to its sensory function.

At other locations, such as the plantar surface, it is sufficiently resistant to support considerable loads. No other cutaneous part of the body can resist the same level of stress.

The skin is especially sensitive where it is the thinnest:

- the plantar surface of the hallux;
- the plantar surface of the third toe;
- the base of the first and fifth metatarsals.

Fat: a resistance factor

Apart from functioning as a metabolic reserve, fat offers mechanical protection. The body requires adipose for tissue protection, cushioning, load distribution, and proprioception, especially at the feet.

The foot is made to resist loads that few other parts of the body could withstand. The stress to which the skin is submitted would scar the skin of any other area of the body. These seemingly excessive loads are well tolerated through the agency of adipose tissue, venolymphatic circulation, and a myofascial system that is a model of bipedal adaptation.

For example, when the heel strikes the ground in walking, structures resist and absorb a portion of the energy produced when the weight of the body is exerted on an area that is just a few centimeters in size. Jumps generally land on the forefoot, where cutaneous padding under the metatarsal heads makes it more resilient. The importance of these soft tissues that "quilt" the sole of the foot can be seen in Fig. 21.20.

Subcutaneous plantar fat lobules are organized in a honeycomb structure. The padded foot is able to dampen and distribute pressures over and above what bones could ever support.

A special hydraulic system

The plantar venous mass forms a cushioning "hydraulic chamber" that empties on contact and refills on discharge to help spread forces landing on the foot. (Dufour and Pillu 2006) (Fig. 21.21).

The foot is the part of the body farthest from the heart and situated the lowest. Its venous circulation, together with that of the entire lower extremity, must constantly fight against gravity.

Alternating weight-bearing and non-weight-bearing action helps the foot to pump venous blood upward against gravity, operating as a "peripheral heart." Be aware that the foot's venous circulation is activated by walking and not just by standing about. Some authors are so specific as to describe the venous return engine as "starting up from the seventh step" (Gillot 1995).

Deep plantar veins drive the blood into the posterior tibial vein toward the medial and lateral marginal veins that become the saphenous vein. Normally the superficial veins drain into the deep veins and not the reverse. This is particularly apparent at the feet. Clini-

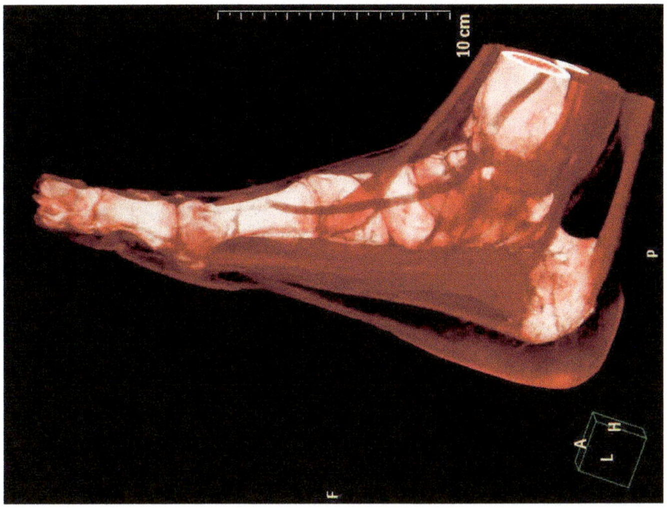

Fig. 21.20 The structures of the footpad. TDM with volume rendering. (TDM with volume rendering. Photo credit: Dr. M. Behr.)

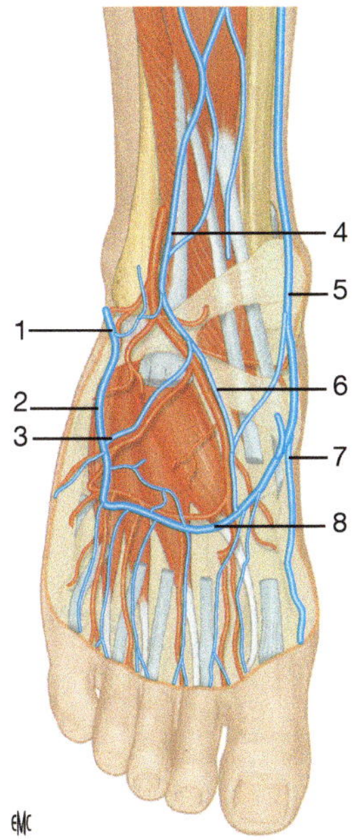

Fig. 21.21 Venous organization of the foot. Dorsal view of the veins of the foot showing their organization and relationship of tendinous and arterial structures. Note their plexiform pattern. (1) Small saphenous vein; (2) Lateral marginal vein; (3) Anterior dorsolateral satellite vein; (4) Anterior satellite vein; (5) Anterior dorsomedial satellite vein; (6) Superficial dorsal arcuate vein; (7) Medial marginal vein; (8) Dorsal venous arch. (F. Bonnel, P. Teissier, and C. Bonnel. 2010. "Arterial and venous vascularization of the foot." EMC Podiatry 27-000-A-15: 1–8. Paris: Elsevier Masson.)

cally we often find that if the superficial veins of the leg are distended and varicosed, the dorsal veins of the foot are as well.

In summary

The skin and the hydraulic system of the foot are key players in:

- cushioning forces exerted on the foot;
- load distribution;
- proprioception and postural balance;
- providing instantaneous information as to pressure changes.

21.2.6 Sensitivity

The foot as a sense organ

The foot is not just an organ of action but an important sensory organ for the nervous system. Many receptors send a stream of information to the brain, allowing it to create movement patterns for the body. This makes the foot a critical sensory organ, no different than the eye and inner ear.

The foot is extraordinarily good at analyzing the exact terrain underfoot, as well as any movement of its own. This data is transmitted to the cerebellum and medulla oblongata to permit instantaneous muscular feedback.

Nerve impulse travels at about 300 km/h to trigger optimal muscle response at the correct location and moment. It is worth noting that practically all nerve branches of the proprioceptive system derive from the sciatic nerve.

Rabischong (2011) describes a sensory foot that is actively involved in the dynamic stabilization of upright posture, a distinguishing characteristic of the human species. The following sections on plantar force platform and postural servomechanism summarize his views.

Plantar force platform

Baroreceptors are located in the dermal layer of the plantar skin. They differ from cutaneous sensory receptors. Pressure sensors are distributed along the sole of the foot, at the contact surface of the heel and the metatarsophalangeal bar. They make up what Rabischong called a plantar force platform capable of detecting local pressure excesses.

In view of the precise nature of information relayed, plantar receptors have been compared to tactile retina (Misery 2000). Plantar receptors can identify minute topographical surface imbalances and initiate postural reflexes that support a more stable position.

Stimulation originating outside the body is picked up in the thickness of the skin and is integrated very similarly to proprioceptive input. It is interesting to note that the usual boundary between proprioception and exteroception is blurred at the foot.

Postural servomechanism

According to Rabischong, a biological servomechanism links two mechanical systems in a relationship of functional servitude (servus, slave) with one abiding rule—anticipation.

Standing on one or both feet is a highly automated function. Incessant postural adjustments and involuntary movements that counter multidimensional disturbances to standing posture are regulated unconsciously by four complementary and abundant sources of data: visual input, cutaneous input, vestibular input, and tendinomuscular input.

Elements of diagnosis

22

22.1 FOOT EXAMINATION

22.1.1 Specific questions

Direct your questions according to the patient's complaint or in reference to foot problems you discover in the course of general evaluation. Inquire about surgical or traumatic events, particularly those involving the lower extremities, as well as any foot disorders.

If there is pain, ask the patient to point to it as clearly as possible with his finger. This provides only a partial guide to any diagnosis. Specify what triggers the pain: movement, contact, or footwear, for example. Determine whether pain is unilateral or bilateral, symmetrical or asymmetrical.

Ask about lifestyle:

- profession, normal physical activity, sports;
- usual type of shoes;
- recent change in footwear;
- risky physical activities (ballet, running, athletics, team sports involving pivoting, such as handball or basketball);
- any intensification of athletic training (fatigue, fractures);
- medications harmful to tendons or bones (certain antibiotics, such as quinolones, as well as corticosteroid use, for example).

22.1.2 Inspection

Visual inspection is very informative. Focus on these characteristics:

- color;
- moisture;
- swelling;
- hairiness;
- plantar hyperkeratosis
  (The sole of the foot can suffer cutaneous and subcutaneous thickening in areas subject to excessive demand; changes in skin thickness are an excellent way to gauge treatment progress.);
- vascular anomalies: varicosity, edema, induration;
- toe length and position;
- nail thickness, color, quality, possible ingrown toenail;
- shoe wear patterns indicative of posture and gait.

22.1.3 Standing examination

While mobility is the most important parameter in osteopathic examination, the foot is an exception; its static and structural features are important to observe. The foot is a distinctive singular architectural unit built around diverse elements whose form directly influences function. Any structural deformities can radically alter the functional mechanics of the foot and are clues to be taken into account.

Observe the outward appearance of the foot under load and when it is free. Differences noted in the two positions tell you about reduced compliance or movement abnormalities. Weight-bearing feet are classically examined using a podoscope, but this device is not essential.

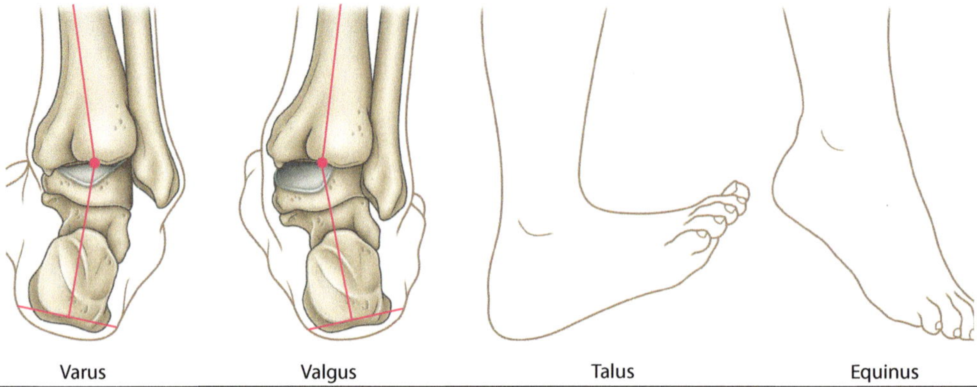

Fig. 22.1 Deformities of the hindfoot.

Hindfoot (Fig. 22.1)

In the frontal plane the calcaneal-Achilles tendon axis must be approximately perpendicular to the ground. Note any deviations of the hindfoot in valgus or in varus.

The normal axis of the hindfoot tends to have a slight valgus, not exceeding 5°. Any increase indicates flatfoot. Varus of the forefoot is always pathological and is mostly seen in the hollow of the high-arch foot. In the sagittal plane, note deformities in equinus or in vertical talus.

Longitudinal arches (Fig. 22.2)

The internal arch must sit above the ground in such a way that you can glide your finger underneath. Flatfoot, or pes planus, exists where there is reduced clearance. The opposite condition occurs in the high-arched foot, or pes cavus, where the external arch does not touch the ground.

Forefoot (Fig. 22.3)

Observe the forefoot in the frontal plane. If the medial border is elevated in relation to the lateral edge, the term is supinatus. If the external border is raised, the foot is in pronatus.

In the horizontal plane, the axis of the second metatarsal and the longitudinal axis of the calcaneus are normally in alignment. If the forefoot is twisted inward in relation to the rear foot, the term is adductus or metatarsus varus. If the forefoot is twisted outward in relation to the rear foot, the term is abductus or metatarsus valgus.

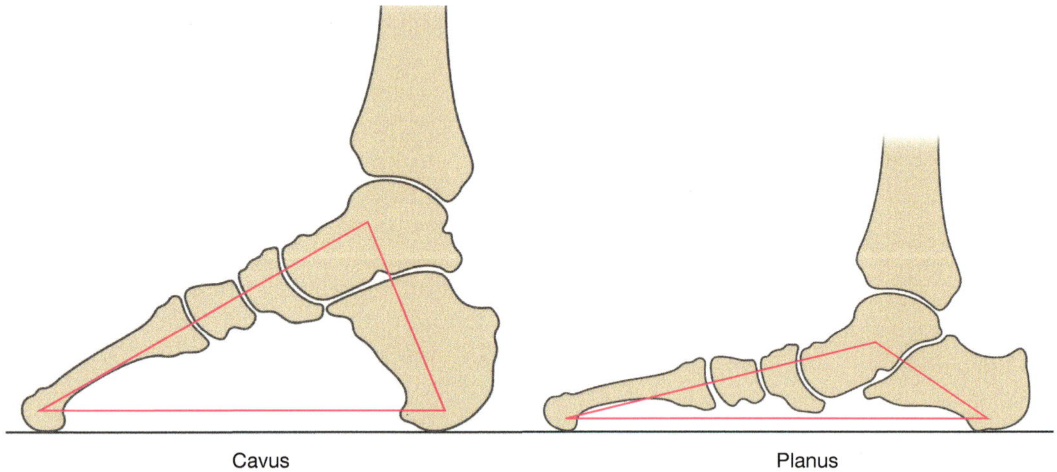

Fig. 22.2 Deformities of the longitudinal arches.

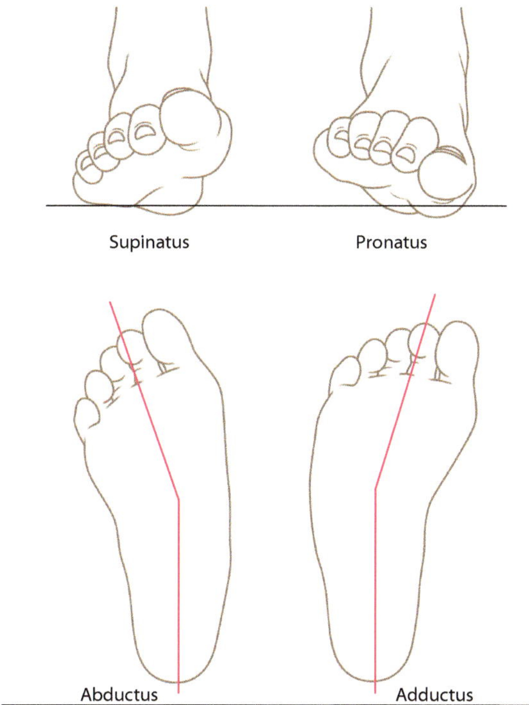

Fig. 22.3 Deformities of the forefoot.

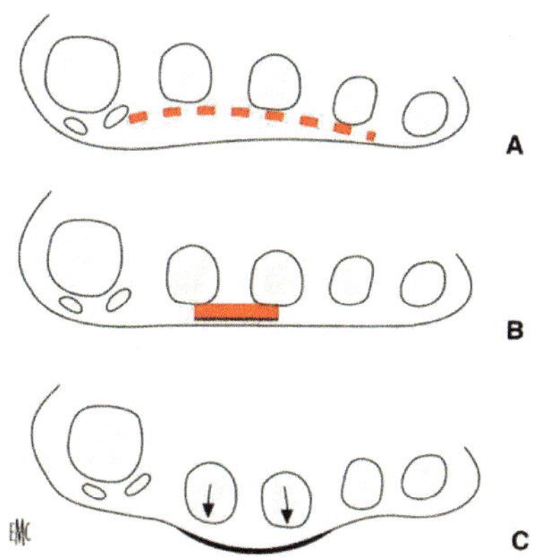

Fig. 22.4 Deformities of the transverse arch. (A) This is the classic conception of the "anterior arch" maintained by the oblique and transverse heads of the adductor hallucis. (B) Forefoot ground support is mainly through the intermediary of the metatarsal heads, particularly the second and third, which represent the fixed platform between medial and lateral balancing platforms. (C) The lowering of one or two metatarsal heads focuses pressures on a reduced bearing area that can show signs of strain. (Pierre Groulier, Georges Curvale, Alexandre Rochwerger, and Barbara Piclet. 1997. "Static metatarsalgias." EMC Musculoskeletal system 14-124-A-10. Paris: Elsevier. All rights reserved.)

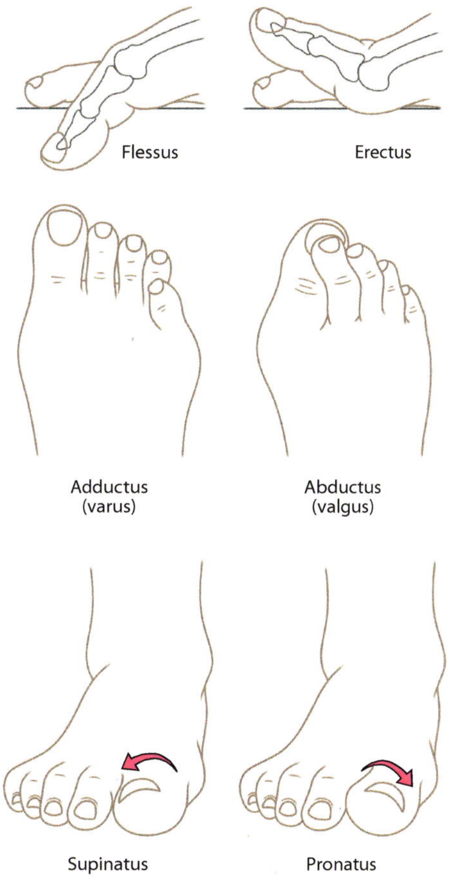

Fig. 22.5 Toe deformities.

Transverse arch (Fig. 22.4)

The transverse arch runs from side to side across the metatarsal heads. It cushions the forefoot and is only observable when weight is removed from the foot. Any exaggeration of the transverse arch constitutes a high-arched foot or cavus. Fallen arches are termed flatfoot. An inverted transverse arch is a convex forefoot or convexus.

Toes (Fig. 22.5)

In the sagittal plane, toes must rest flat on the ground. Toes that do not are termed claw toes. In the horizontal plane, the axis of each toe is normally an extension of the metatarsal axis. Inwardly deviated toes indicate varus; outwardly deviated toes indicate valgus.

Pediatric flatfoot

It is normal for the feet of newborns and infants to appear flat up until age three, when they normally grow out of it. In rare instances it persists, and the condition is often mistaken for rear-foot valgus, where the medial arch flattens. Pediatric flatfoot generally:

- is not painful, although it can cause fatigability on walking, unsightly gait, or abnormally worn-down shoes;
- normally resumes its curvature when body weight is removed or when the great toe is forcibly dorsiflexed;
- is flexible, because normally supporting ligaments are elongated, causing the talar head to displace inferomedially.

Flatfoot is precipitated by overweightness, hypotonia, rickets, exaggerated anteversion of the femoral neck, knock-knee, shortening of the sural triceps muscle, and so forth.

Sixty-five percent of infant static flatfoot cases evolve spontaneously, achieving complete correction between five and seven years; 30% remain asymptomatically flatfooted.

All valgus flatfeet benefit from good shoes with extra lateral support. Plantar orthotics can be worn to reinforce shoe action and to reassure parents when their children's discomfort persists beyond age five.

A painful flatfoot warrants an X-ray to rule out calcaneonavicular synostosis. This type of fusion is visible under three-dimensional radiography and can explain certain flatfeet discovered in infants or adolescents. Abnormal fusing between two bones hinders the smooth development of the hindfoot and impedes normal talar tilting and shifting around the block formed by the calcaneus and navicular.

22.2 FOOT AND TOE DEFORMITIES

22.2.1 Standard deformity terminology

Flatfoot (pes planus) (Fig. 22.6)

Flatfoot implies a collapse of the plantar arch. The talus is displaced medially and distally to the navicular. Added to this are mediotarsal eversion, abduction of the forefoot, and calcanael valgus. This scenario often associates with genu valgum (knock-knee).

When the foot remains flat through the course of growth and development, the child can find walking difficult, and shoes may show abnormal wear. While the flatfoot is rarely painful in itself, medial protuberance of the talus can rub against footwear and create discomfort.

A podoscope analyzes plantar form and imprint. Flatfoot is classified in three degrees (Fig. 22.7). A flatfoot produces a wide imprint. It overtakes both sides of the physiological axis of the foot that extends from the middle of the heel to the space between the second and third toes.

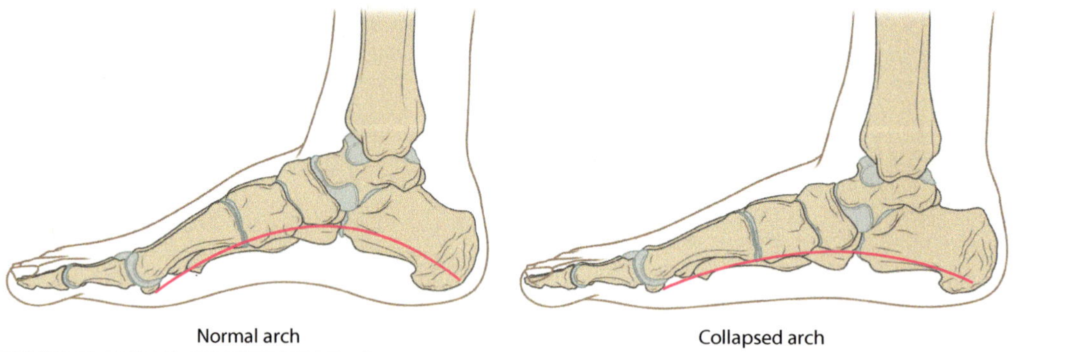

Fig. 22.6 Flatfoot.

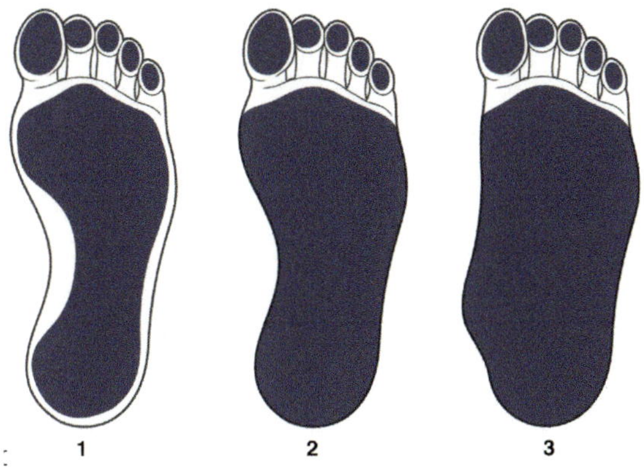

Fig. 22.7 Podoscopic aspect of flatfoot (After Lelièvre). 1. First degree; 2. Second degree; 3. Third degree. (A. A. Lopez and A. Goldcher. 2010. "History of the understanding of the biomechanics of the barefoot." EMC Podiatry 27-010-A-10: 1–15. Paris: Elsevier Masson. All rights reserved.)

Many adults have flat feet that are relatively well tolerated. The medial edge of the imprint is concave or straight. This impression is generally considered not to be as pathological as are feet whose medial border is convex (third degree).

In the majority of cases, standard treatment consists of shoe inserts or orthopedic footwear. From an osteopathic standpoint, it is imperative to check the axis of rotation of the lower extremity together with the mechanics of the hindfoot.

High instep (pes cavus) (Fig. 22.8)

The high-arched foot has an exaggerated plantar concavity. An abnormally high arch associates with a varus hindfoot. It presents with retraction of the plantar aponeurosis and shortened muscles. As the foot's intrinsic muscles weaken, the toes are drawn into claw-toe deformity. Initially the pads of the toes remain in contact with the ground, but eventually all contact is lost.

Podoscopic examination reveals an elevation difference between the talon and the metatarsals. This foot is able to flatten in standing, which is what distinguishes fixed high instep from flexible high instep (Fig. 22.9). Calcaneus hindfoot varus is constant, and the forefoot is often in adduction and varus.

The footprints depicted in Fig. 22.10 show the strip of lateral arch support at the lateral border of the foot tapering progressively from first degree. The band has disappeared entirely in the third-degree image. The anterior and posterior contacts become separate entirely, and the toes vanish.

Exaggerated anterior plantar contact manifests as the gradual onset of metatarsalgia. Pain in the ball of the foot is localized to the heads of the first and fifth metatarsals, where calluses tend to appear. Sometimes individual plantar calluses develop under each metatarsal head.

Be careful. The accentuation of the longitudinal arch of the foot is often due to a muscle imbalance. With a high instep, be sure to look for possible neurological anomalies or muscle fibroses in the calf. Be alert for spina bifida occulta at the level of the

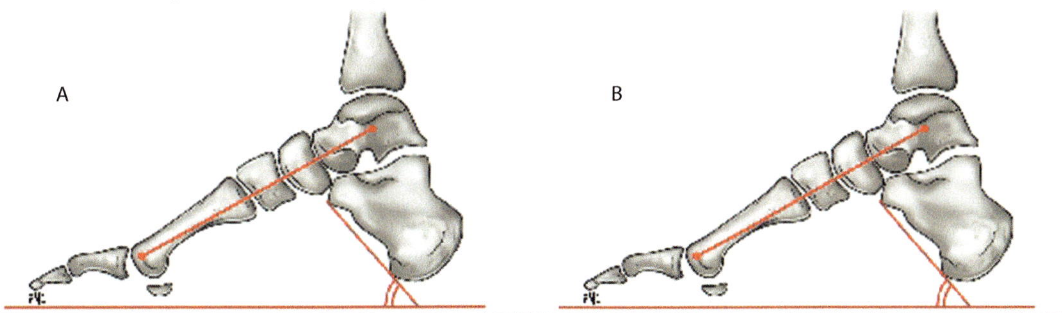

Fig. 22.8 Pes cavus. (A) Diagram of a direct anterior high instep characterized by a verticalization of the forefoot. The summit of the deformity is located in the cuneonavicular joint. (B) Posterior direct high instep by verticalization of calcaneus. (Georges Curvale and Alexandre Rochwerger. 2002. "Pieds creux." EMC Podiatry 27-060-A-20: 1–13. Paris: Elsevier Masson.)

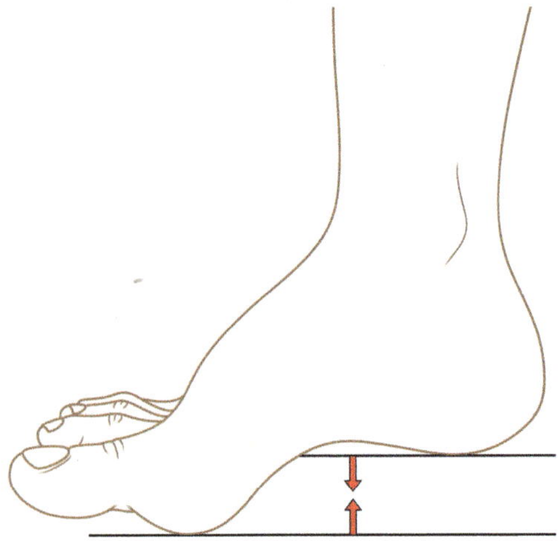

Fig. 22.9 Slope of the pes cavus. (J. Montagna, A. Chevrot, and J. M. Galmiche. 1986. "Static foot problems." EMC Medical radiology an imagery: musculoskeletal–neurological–maxillofacial 31-390-A-10.Paris: Elsevier Masson.

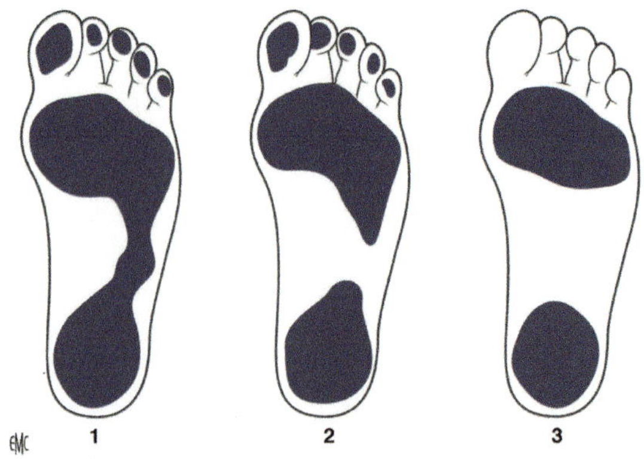

Fig. 22.10 Podoscopic impression of the pes cavus (After Lelièvre). (1) First degree; (2) Second degree; (3) Third degree. (A. A. Lopez and A. Goldcher. 2010. "History of the understanding of the biomechanics of the barefoot." EMC Podiatry 27-010-A-10: 1–15. Paris: Elsevier Masson.

lumbar spine. The high-arch foot is rare in infants. It is always considered abnormal. Refer the child to an infant orthopedist for a complete neuro-orthopedic workup.

Hallux valgus (Fig. 22.11)

Abnormal angulation of the great toe is the most common of foot problems. Hallux valgus is a complex deformity of the first toe characterized by:

- lateral deviation of the great toe that is great enough to overlap the second toe;
- rotation of the great toe, where its plantar surface faces outward with the nail facing inward;
- metatarsus varus in which the first metatarsal turns inward.

Once it appears, angulation is aggravated by muscle action:

- Inclination of the great toe alters the trajectory of the extensor and flexor tendons belonging to the big toe that forms the "rope of the arc."
- Muscle contraction accentuates the deviation, producing a progressive subluxation of the metatarsophalangeal joint.
- Elevation of the head of the first metatarsal causes it to rub against the shoe, leading to irritation or inflammation of the serous bursa beneath the bone. There is always risk of infection. Pressure from footwear can cause irritation of the subcutaneous collateral nerves, which worsens the pain.

Secondarily, the metatarsal head can dislocate from the sesamoid bones that are normally located on the plantar head of the first metatarsal. Painful arthritic changes can occur in the sesamoid and the metatarsal bones.

Hallux valgus can develop into osteoarthritis of the metatarsophalangeal joint. It also can lead to degradation of the neighboring toes, which become squeezed.

Metatarsalgia commonly afflicts the middle metatarsals, which are overloaded when the big toe loses its support function. Adolescent girls, in particular, can be vulnerable to bunion deformity due to a growth spurt of the foot as well as ill-fitting or overly pointy-toed shoes.

Sometimes metatarsus varus (intoeing) predisposes the foot to hallux valgus, as does the foot with an especially long great toe (Egyptian foot).

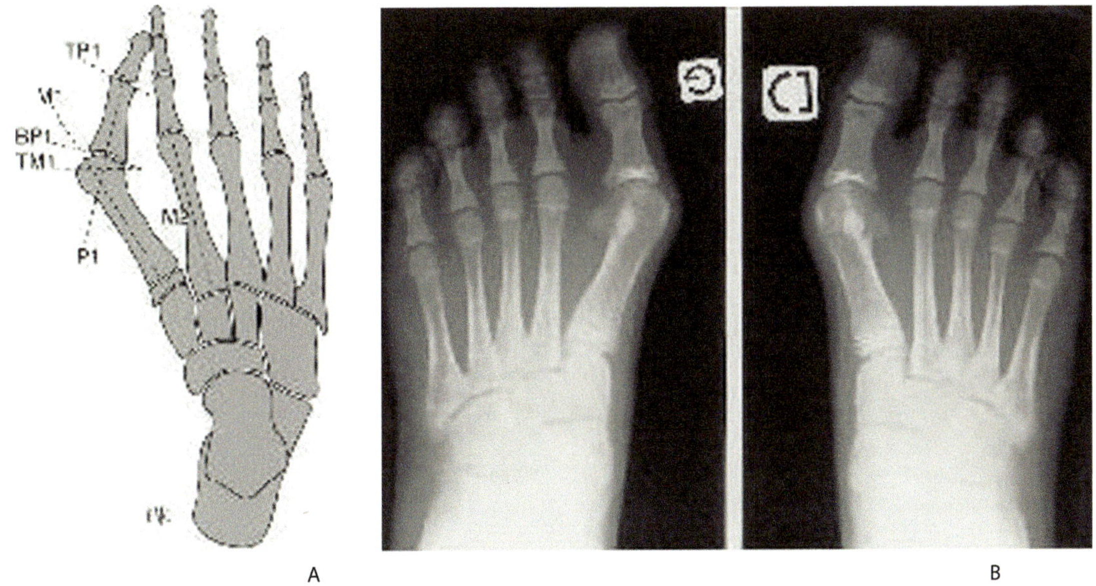

Fig. 22.11 Hallus valgus (HV). (A) Different elements of HV: Constants: P1/M1 angle greater than 20°; M1/M2 angle greater than 10°. Inconstants: valgus joint facet of M1(TM1/M1) less than 80°; metatarsophalangeal valgus joint (AMP (BP1/TM1), PI clinodactyly (TP1/BP1) greater than 10°). (B) Radiograph of an HV: Note the increased angles between P1 and M1, and M1 and M2, as well as the external subluxation of the external sesamoid. (Jean-Paul Metaizeau. 2000. "Congenital malpositions and malformations of the infant foot." EMC Musculoskeletal system 7 (1) 15-380-A-10: 1–13. Paris: Elsevier Masson.)

Other deformities of the great toe

Lateral crossover of the great toe

This anomaly is not to be confused with hallux valgus. The deviation is an angulation of the phalange itself and not the metatarsophalangeal joint. The second toe takes on a "gooseneck" shape on being compressed by the distal phalange of the big toe.

Hallux rigidus

This is a primary arthritis of the metatarsophalangeal joint of the great toe. It can begin as early as adolescence, when patients complain of stiffness and pain around the joint.

Lack of metatarsophalangeal dorsiflexion causes the phalange to lose contact with the ground, overloading neighboring metatarsals. As in all forms of arthritis, hallux rigidus impinges on the joint space—in this case the metatarsophalangeal junction. Osteophytes develop, and exostoses eventually form on the bone; surgery is often recommended at this stage.

Hallux varus

The great toe deviates medially.

Hallux flexus

The great toe is fixed in plantar flexion (hammertoe).

Deformities of the other toes

Claw toes (Fig. 22.12)

Claw toes are fairly common. They are often seen together with high arches brought on by muscle imbalances. You can find either distal or total claw toes. The consequence of this anomaly is exaggerated pressure on the toe tips and the formation of calluses on the

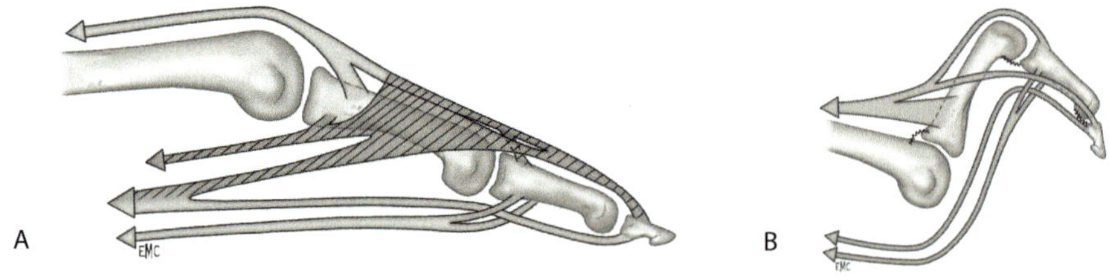

Fig. 22.12 Claw toes. (A) Normally, the skeletal muscles and lumbricals (shaded) stabilize the metatarsophalangeals, permitting the action of the long flexors and extensors. (B) Relative weakness of the interosseous and lombrical muscles causes a bending back of the first phalange toward the corresponding metatarsal, giving the toe a clawlike appearance that is initially flexible and reducible, becoming stiffened through muscular and capsular retractions. (Georges Curvale and Alexander Rochwerger. 2002. "Pieds creux." EMC Podiatry 27-060-A-20: 1–13. Paris: Elsevier Masson. All rights reserved.)

dorsal surfaces because of shoe pressure. Often all the outer toes are involved.

Hammer toe (Fig. 22.13)

This deformity features hyperextension of the metatarsophalangeal joint together with flexion of the first interphalangeal joint, causing it to bend and end up in dorsal conflict with the shoe. The second interphalangeal joint is fixed in extension; only the pad of the toe touches the ground. Hyperextension of the first phalange often results in subluxation followed by dislocation of the metatarsophalangeal joint.

Quintus varus (Fig. 22.14)

The fifth toe juts out, swerves inward, and overlaps the fourth toe. A bump forms at the toe. Bursitis can develop because of shoe pressure. Functional impairment and pain sometimes necessitates surgical correction with quintus varus.

22.3 PEDIATRIC FOOT PROBLEMS (TALIPES)

22.3.1 Congenital clubfoot

Deformation

Talipes equinovarus is one of the most common of congenital malformations of the foot. The foot appears to be rotated inward at the ankle. Virtually all newborns are routinely screened for it.

The deformity is complex:

- The heel of the foot is turned inward (varus).
- The forefoot is adducted.
- The foot points downward at the ankle (equinism) from retraction of the Achilles tendon.
- The middle section is twisted in inversion.

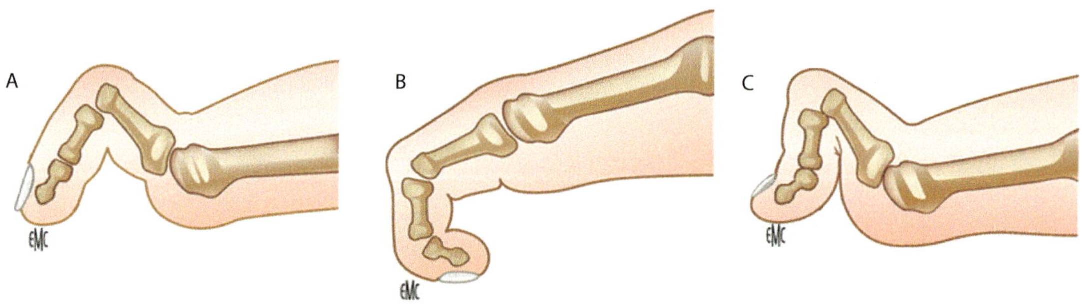

Fig. 22.13 Hammer toes. (A) Proximal claw; (B) Hammertoe (neutral metatarsophalangeal); (C) "Swan-neck" claw. (C. Ferrari-Portafaix, B. Piclet-Legre, and M. Helix-Giordanino. 2011. "Toes in toe claws: physiopathology, podological treatment, surgical treatment." EMC Podology 27-060-A-30: 1–12. Paris: Elsevier Masson. All rights reserved.)

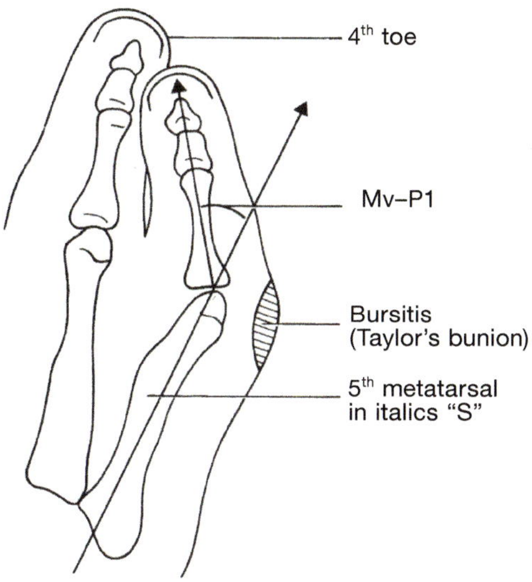

Fig. 22.14 Quintus varus. (A. Goldcher. 2012. Podology. Abrégés collection 6th edition. Paris: Elsevier Masson.)

There is a tendency to parallelism of the talar and calcaneal axis that run forward and downward on the oblique angle.

Examining the newborn's foot

If the foot seems fixed in inversion, hold the leg and gently touch the lateral border of the foot. If the foot is normal, the infant responds by dorsiflexion. If the foot is twisted in clubfoot, there is no response. If the infant fails to respond normally to this stimulation, gently flex the foot. In the normal baby you will be able to bring the foot against the tibia.

Evaluation and treatment

Left untreated, soft tissue retraction interferes with normal skeletal development, resulting in tarsal bone deformities that can become permanently misshapen. Treatment is best undertaken at birth (osteopathy, movement therapy, plaster splinting) if surgical intervention is to be avoided. With pediatric foot problems, some of our musculoligamentous and neural techniques can be added to more standard therapies.

22.3.2 Metatarsus varus

Metatarsus varus (intoeing) is a common deformity. The forefoot is lifted inward and upward, such that the victim walks on the outside of the foot. This adduction of the metatarsus is due to compression in utero. Because it is not a boney defect, stimulation of the lateral border of the feet with the fingers or a toothbrush is enough to see the toes fan out properly. In contrast to clubfoot, this abnormality is correctable.

22.3.3 Tarsal scaphoiditis (Kohler's disease)

Osteochondrosis of the navicular bone can affect children between the ages of 3 and 10. Tenderness on the medial border of the foot calls attention to it. Symptoms subside spontaneously after a few months, and the condition does not require surgery. X-rays show increased density and a flattening of the scaphoid (navicular) bone. Plantar support insoles can help to relieve the pain.

22.3.4 Sever's disease

Inflammation of the calcaneal growth plate occurs in the heels of growing children, typically between ages 6 and 15. It is common in adolescents who are physically active. The Achilles tendon is subject to overuse, excessive traction, direct microtrauma, and repetitive stress from shock waves generated when the heel hits the ground.

The disorder manifests as heel pain with no precise cause. Discomfort is aggravated by activity and subsides with rest. Pain is localized to the lateral posterior aspect of the heel and elicited by dorsiflexion of the foot. Walking on tiptoes is possible and pain-free, whereas heel walking is unbearable.

An X-ray is required to rule out a more serious condition. Irregular, condensed, or fragmented aspects of the ossification nucleus can show up in a normal child.

It is imperative that the child refrain from all sports for a period of time. He or she must also temporarily avoid any activity that involves a lot of heel movement, such as running or cycling. When the heel is used less for an interval of time, the effects of calcaneal inflammation subside.

22.4 ADULT FOOT PROBLEMS

22.4.1 Sprains

Sprains and their aftermath are a frequent cause for osteopathic consultation. Sprain involves a torn or partially torn ligament. There are three grades of ankle sprain:

- benign, which is a simple ligament overstretch where the ligament still provides joint stability;
- intermediate, which is a partial tear;
- serious, which is a complete ligament rupture.

By far the most common type of ankle sprains affect the lateral ligaments, whereas medial ligament injury is rare.

Lateral sprain

Lateral ankle sprain is cause by a violent "twist" to the lateral part of the ankle.

Patients often report having forcibly landed on the side of their foot. The initial pain is sudden and severe, localized to the outside of the foot. Functional instability is variable in lateral sprains. The ankle often swells and may develop bruising.

Sprained ankle diagnosis is made by locating the pain through palpation; the injured area is tender to the touch. In examining the ankle, look for pain located at fibers on the anterior lateral talar shelf. This is more common than injury near the fibular malleolus. For the intermediate fascicle, examine the lateral calcaneal insertion and the retromalleolar region to evaluate the posterior fascicle. Pain can also be triggered in unforced plantar varus flexion.

A possible bone fracture is indicated if you find tenderness at any of the following: posterior edge and tip of the lateral malleolus, base of the fifth metatarsal, the navicular bone, or the heel. (See Fig.22.15 "The Ottawa ankle rules.")

Determining the severity of a sprain is done clinically. Severe sprain involves intense pain and considerable swelling ("pigeon egg") followed by bruising on the internal surface of the heel. If the ankle is not swollen but just hurts, it is mildly sprained. Moderate sprain associates with some swelling.

Severe sprain can involve the anterior fascicle (simple), middle fascicle (double), and, more rarely, all three fascicles (triple). A tuning fork can be used to identify avulsion fractures.

Place the vibrating fork gently on the ligamentous insertions at the lateral malleolus. There will be diminished or absent sound over the fracture. An avulsion fracture is a microfracture of the malleolus, inferior to the ankle joint; it produces exquisite pain. A positive tuning fork test requires an X-ray.

All ankle sprains, even benign twists, deserve to be x-rayed (following the Ottawa ankle rules). Radiographs can eliminate malleolar fractures, as well as fractures of the distal tibia, talus, or calcaneus.

Ankle sprains commonly injure the following elements:

- fibular collateral ligament;
- fifth metatarsal/cuboid joint;
- distal talofibular joint;
- talonavicular joint;
- talocalcaneal joint;
- talomalleolar joints;
- distal part of the interosseous membrane
- peroneus longus and brevis.

These structures store traumatic energy and can disrupt foot mechanics for a long time. It is important to check them manually.

Ankle sprain diagnostics

Ankle sprain is the mask of all pathohological trauma to the hindfoot. This can be a diagnostic trap. Insufficient clinical examination can lead to an improper diagnosis of sprain for any significant trauma to the rear foot. The true damage may actually be something more serious, such as Achilles tendon rupture.

On the other hand, sprain frequently occurs together with traumatic lesions, such as osteochondral fracture of the talus, that go undetected. We have had the bizarre experience of patients arriving at our office diagnosed with a sprained ankle in the absence of any traumatic context!

Ottawa ankle rules (Fig. 22.15)

These recommendations were formulated in 1994 as guidelines to diagnose lateral ligament sprain and to help clinicians decide when to recommend radiography of the ankle and midfoot. Unnecessary X-rays can be avoided provided that:

- pain only exists along the lateral course and insertions of the lateral ankle ligament;
- there is no tenderness at other boney landmarks (the posterior edge or tip of the malleolus, base of the fifth metatarsal, the navicular, the heel, and so forth);
- the patient is able to bear weight taking more than four steps.

These guidelines have been validated in trials carried out on populations between 18 and 60 years of age. The patient must be clearly informed and brought back for a new exam in the days following.

Sprain and pediatrics

In children, the main differential diagnosis for sprain is the traumatic stretching of the lateral malleolar growth plate cartilage. The diagnosis is clinical. The pain will be located higher up on the malleolus. X-rays must be taken to rule out any epiphysary detachment. Severe ankle sprain in a child that occurs together with avulsion fracture of the malleolus or a lateral submalleolar accessory bone has a poor prognosis with high risk of repeated sprain.

Medial sprain

Medial ankle sprains merit great caution! With this type of trauma, look systematically for other diagnostics, because isolated medial sprain is rare.

Look for:

- fracture of the medial malleolus;
- fracture of the lateral malleolus;
- fracture of the fibula, sometimes at the neck;
- displacement of the tibialis posterior tendon. Pain at the posterior medial malleolar ridge, extra-articular

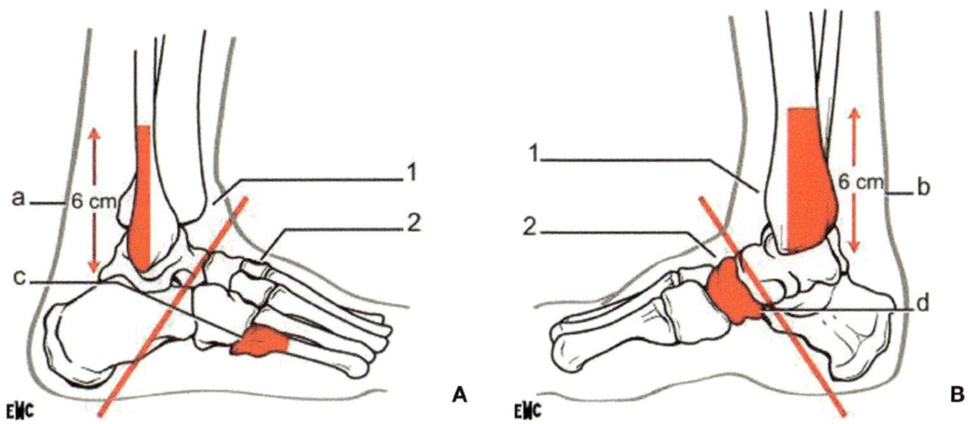

Fig. 22.15 The Ottawa ankle rules—lateral and medial view. Pain in the grey or coloured zone requires X-ray. A. Lateral view; B. Medial view; (a) posterior edge or tip of external malleolus; (b) posterior edge or tip of medial malleolus; (c) base of 5th metatarsal; (d) navicular; (1) malleolar zone; (2) midfoot.(B.Barrois, P.Ribinik, B.Davenne. Ankle sprains. EMC Physical rehabilitation kinesitherapy-medicine. 2002;8(2):1-8{Article 26 -250-D-10}. Paris: Elsevier Masson. All rights reserved.)

hematoma, or sometimes a small fleck of bone near the posterior medial malleolus reveals avulsion fracture.

Other rear-foot sprains

Because the mechanism of injury is inversion or eversion, ankle sprain concerns the whole foot. Here again clinical examination can direct you to other diagnostic locations:

- Subtalar joint sprain often associates with ankle sprain. Pain is found slightly lower, just in front of the tip of the lateral malleolus, in the depression formed by the sinus tarsi at the outside of the ankle.
- Sprain of the anterior fascicle of the distal tibiofibular ligaments involves pain located higher up than in lateral sprain, in the anterior lateral part of the ankle. Pain can be triggered by palpation or passively dorsiflexing the ankle in combination with lateral rotation of the foot around the axis of the leg. The talus tends to push the malleolus laterally, putting the ligament under tension.
- Midtarsal sprain (Chopart's joint) involves pain located on the outside top of the foot. Joint mobilization causes pain.
- Calcaneocuboid ligament sprain can occur in isolation.
- Tarsometatarsal sprain (Lisfranc) can range from a stable sprain to grossly unstable.

Foot fragility

The foot is delicate and far more vulnerable to sprain than the knee. In the long run, the aftermath of knee sprain carries far more nefarious consequences for the joint itself than does ankle sprain. Ankle sprains, however, are more destabilizing to the body's proprioceptive system.

One might even go so far as to say that the foot, because of its frailty, protects the knee. Conversely, the repercussions of ankle sprains are very deleterious to the knees.

22.4.2 Microcrystalline arthropathies

The following section is based on our own experiences as well as the work of professor Gérard Chales of the Rheumatology Department of South Hospital of Centre Hospitalier Universite at Rennes.

Gout and chondrocalcinosis are the most widespread of microcrystalline arthropathies. Some patients consult us absolutely convinced that they have a mechanical problem of the foot when, in fact, their pain is of another origin entirely.

Gout

This is a metabolic disease that lands in the joints. A person suffering from gout produces excessive amounts of uric acid that are stored in the blood. Elevated uric acid can be acute or chronic. Excessive uric acid reacts with sodium to form a salt called sodium urate, whose crystals deposit in various tissues such as the kidneys, joints, and ear cartilage. Ninety-five percent of cases affect men.

Clinically gout manifests as:

- pain that resurges at night, exacerbated by the very weight of bedclothes;
- local inflammation with areas of swelling, redness, and tenderness;
- general signs, such as nervousness, scant urine, a coated tongue, and sometimes slight fever, that occur to varying degrees.

Classically, arthritic gout affects foot joints, particularly the metatarsophalangeal joint of the big toe. Other joints such as the ankle, knee, or even the hand can be affected. Gout can land in the serous bursa, tendons and their sheathes, and the costal cartilages.

Salt crystals irritate and erode cartilage. Besides painful crisis, a number of latent forms can produce joint pain reminiscent of mechanical problems. In chronic gout, be careful with the kidney, as there is risk of stones and nephropathy that can lead to arterial hypertension and renal insufficiency.

A question of temperature

It is interesting to note that certain joints are more susceptible to gout than others due to temperature differences in the body. The lower the temperature the higher the risk of gout. Urate solubility rates are better at 37 °C than they are at 35 °C, the temperature of the big toe. Thus the most vulnerable joints are distal joints with the lowest body temperatures.

> **Gout.**
>
> Above all, diet:
> Cheese is to be banished at night. Salt, cold cuts, seafood, white wine, beer (even nonalcoholic), hard liquor, sodas, offal (animal intestines used for food), sorrel, and asparagus are all to be strictly avoided. Fruits and vegetables are recommended as is physical activity and weight loss.
>
> Avoid the application of cold:
> Advise patients against putting ice on a painful big toe. Even if pain goes away momentarily, it generally returns with a vengeance within a few hours. The application of clay or cabbage is more effective and easy enough to do.

Chondrocalcinosis

Painful cartilage calcification resembles gout. These deposits most commonly invade the knee, hip, and pubic symphysis, but they can produce referred pain in the foot. Radiographic imaging reveals calcium encrustations at joint cartilages. Calcium pyrophosphate crystals are also found in synovial fluid. Here again, latent forms can produce joint or musculotendinous pain that comes on with exertion, making you think it is mechanical in nature.

22.4.3 Neurological pain

Morton's neuroma (intermetatarsal syndrome)

This neuroma forms at the medial planter nerve, more precisely the second and third plantar digital nerves. Fibrous tissue thickens around nerves from mechanical irritation and rarely as part of a systemic illness or metabolic disorders.

A metatarsal tunnel lies between the metatarsal head and encloses digital nerves and vessels in company with the lumbrical tendon and its bursa. The inextensible canal is situated in a region vulnerable to frequent microtrauma and various morphological problems.

Digital nerves can be irritated directly by the repetitive strain of a shrunken or restricted passageway. Constrictive footwear can provoke neuroma in a matter of months or over a couple of years. Plantar fascia and ligaments thicken in response to the irritation. Sometimes nerve irritation occurs because of close contact with other structures in the intermetatarsal space, such as inflamed lumbrical bursa.

Morton's neuroma, also known as Morton's disease, involves stabbing pain at the anterior intermetatarsal space, most commonly the third. Numbness can occur in the corresponding toes, usually while walking, standing, or wearing certain shoes (shoe sign).

Pain is caused by plantar pressure in the intermetatarsal space, by the crowding of the metatarsal heads, or by extending the toes. Frequently some hypoesthesia affects the toes.

Many patients consult us for this type of metatarsalgia. Surgery can be avoided through peripheral nerve manipulation in combination with joint techniques presented in this text.

Tarsal tunnel syndrome

This entrapment condition is the counterpart to carpal tunnel syndrome. The tibial nerve becomes compressed as it travels through the tarsal tunnel to continue onto the bottom of the foot. Patients typically complain of burning pain and tingling in the foot radiating to the toes. This syndrome is rare but very amenable to joint and neural manipulation. Sometimes surgery is warranted.

22.4.4 Static metatarsalgia

Metatarsalgia is defined as pain beneath the metatarsal heads. This disorder is usually connected with abnormal constriction of the metatarsal bones. In the medical literature this is called static metatarsalgia. Other types of metatarsalgia can arise from such things as fatigue fracture or osteochondritis of the metatarsal head.

Static metatarsalgia is common in middle-aged women. It is connected to dysfunction of the big toe; instead of contacting the ground, the toe tends to overlap the neighboring toe. Symptoms are always linked to activity.

Static metatarsalgia has various causes: overload from obesity, abnormal morphology with an overly long or vertical metatarsal (high arch, equinisme), or fallen arch (flat or convex forefoot). They also can result from somatic dysfunctions affecting the mediotarsal cushioning system and the transverse arch.

22.4.5 Fatigue fracture

Fatigue fractures occur in bone that is subjected to repetitive stress. Boney changes result from excessive physical activity. These are not fractures, strictly speaking, but rather an osseous remodeling that ends up weakening bone. Nevertheless, without treatment this type of stress fracture can develop into true fracture.

Fatigue fractures can affect any bone, but the most commonly afflicted is the second metatarsal. Whatever the location, pain comes on gradually and is mechanical in nature, arising with exertion and vanishing at rest. Pain can be weak at the beginning and become progressively more intense until it becomes so extreme that sports activities are impossible. These fractures can interfere with daily life and make people lame.

Fatigue fractures are difficult to identify in radiography; nuclear bone scans detect them only when they have been chronic. Ankle pain that is not always precise or logical, but nevertheless chronic, is typical of fatigue fracture.

22.4.6 Rheumatoid arthritis

The foot and ankle are often targeted in the course of rheumatoid polyarthritis. Joint deformations can be severe and multiple. They can include flat feet, fallen arches, hallux valgus, claw toes, and metatarsophalangeal dislocations, all caused by destruction of the joint spaces. Metatarsalgias are common. The best recourse to avoid surgery is orthopedic footwear, but an operation is often unavoidable.

22.4.7 Algodystrophy

After the hand, the ankle and foot are next in line for algoneurodystrophy. The extremities are richly innervated and can be involved in the autonomic nervous system dysregulation that can happen in response to even minor trauma.

The condition occurs in two phases:

- the hot phase with painful foot edema
- the cold phase characterized by ankle stiffening

Diagnosis is based on clinical findings and possibly bone scan.

22.4.8 Vascular pain

In a patient with pre-existing vascular conditions or cardiovascular risk factors, all foot pain must raise suspicion of obliterating arteriopathy of the lower limbs. Many "sciatic" pains are in fact undiagnosed vascular pains.

When dealing with foot pain, even in the absence of edema or cyanosis, it is important to look for signs of arterial insufficiency. Take the pulse of the lower limb. Ask the patient about any possible intermittent claudication that might have caused them to suddenly stop walking because of pain. Such limping often occurs together with abolition of the peripheral pulse, cooling or color changes of the foot, and sometimes shortness of breath.

22.4.9 Referred pain

The foot and ankle can serve as witnesses to visceral dysfunction, something that is true of the entire osteoarticular system. As the distal extremity is subject to considerable load bearing, dysfunctions quickly become painful. We will see later in the book that referred visceral pains usually involve the intestinal and urogenital spheres.

Metatarsal contacts: Normal anterior arch ground contact is made predominantly with the first and fifth metatarsals. If the anterior arch becomes slightly flattened by the weight of the body, middle metatarsal contact is accentuated. This can lead to arch inversion, in which only the second, third, and fourth metatarsal heads in the rounded forefoot make any contact (Fig. 22.16).

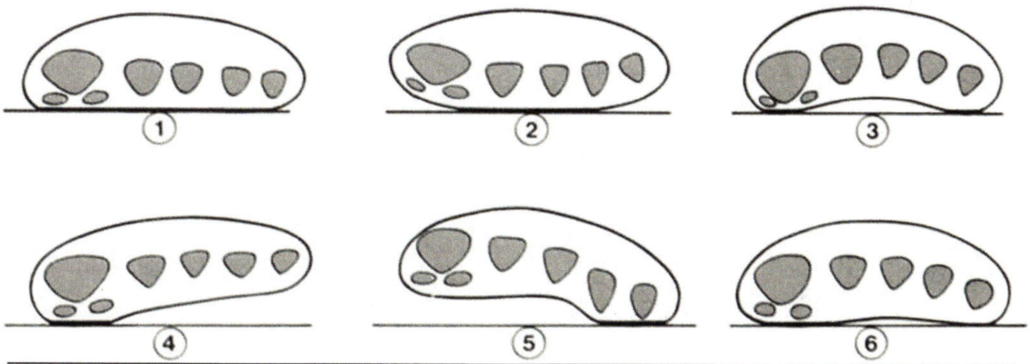

Fig. 22.16 Anterior arch of the foot.

The harmonious curve is shown in figure 6.

Hyper-contact can be:

- generalized to all the metatarsal heads—high instep or flatfoot (1 and 2);
- localized to the last metatarsals—first and second metatarsal heads (3) in the high transverse instep foot;
- localized to just one metatarsal:
  - the first head in pronation of the forefoot (4) in some athletes or in cases of the anterior internal hollow foot;
  - the fifth metatarsal head in supination of the forefoot (5) of traumatic or post-operative origin.

(J. Montagne, A. Chevrot, and J. J. Galmiche. 1986. "Static foot problems." EMC Medical radiology and imagery: musculoskeletal–neurological–maxilofacial 31-390-A-10 Paris: Elsevier Masson.)

Manipulation of the ankle and hindfoot

23

23.1 TIBIOFIBULAR JOINTS (FIG. 23.1)

23.1.1 Review

These joints must withstand considerable tension, especially when movement occurs outside the vertical axis of the leg. Their capsule is tensed and reinforced by the interosseous membrane, anterior and posterior ligaments, and muscles that are particularly connected to the capsule.

Interosseous membrane (Fig. 23.2)

This membrane connects the bodies of the fibula and tibia. Distally its oblique fibers have the same caudal and lateral orientation as the anterior tibiofibular ligament. Posteriorly they run in the same direction as the posterior tibiofibular ligament but terminate a little more proximally.

Tibiofibular ligaments (Fig. 23.2)

These fibrous bands extend caudally and laterally. While tough, they nevertheless permit small translation movements between the fibula and tibia.

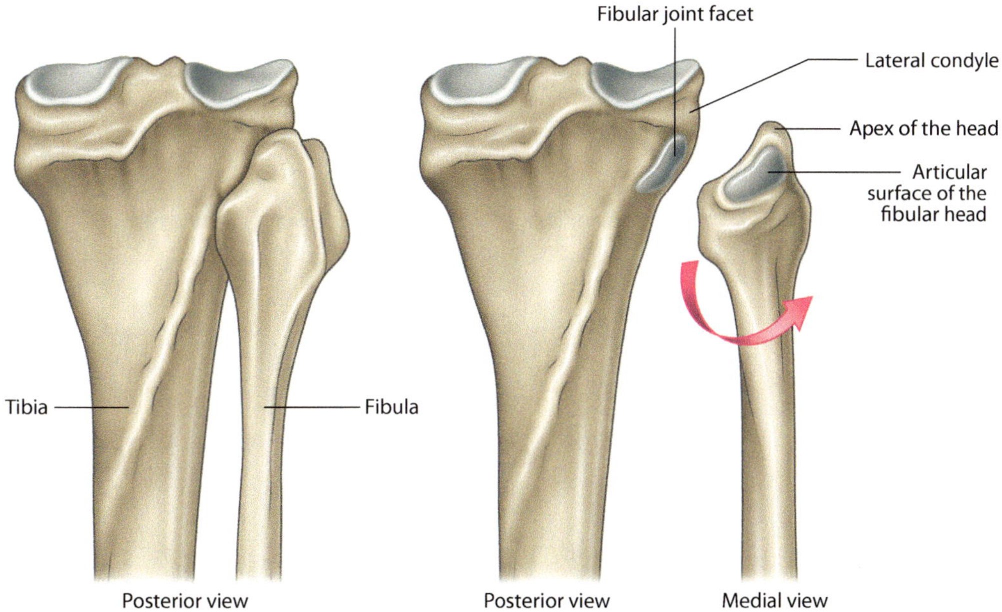

Fig. 23.1 Proximal tibiofibular joint.

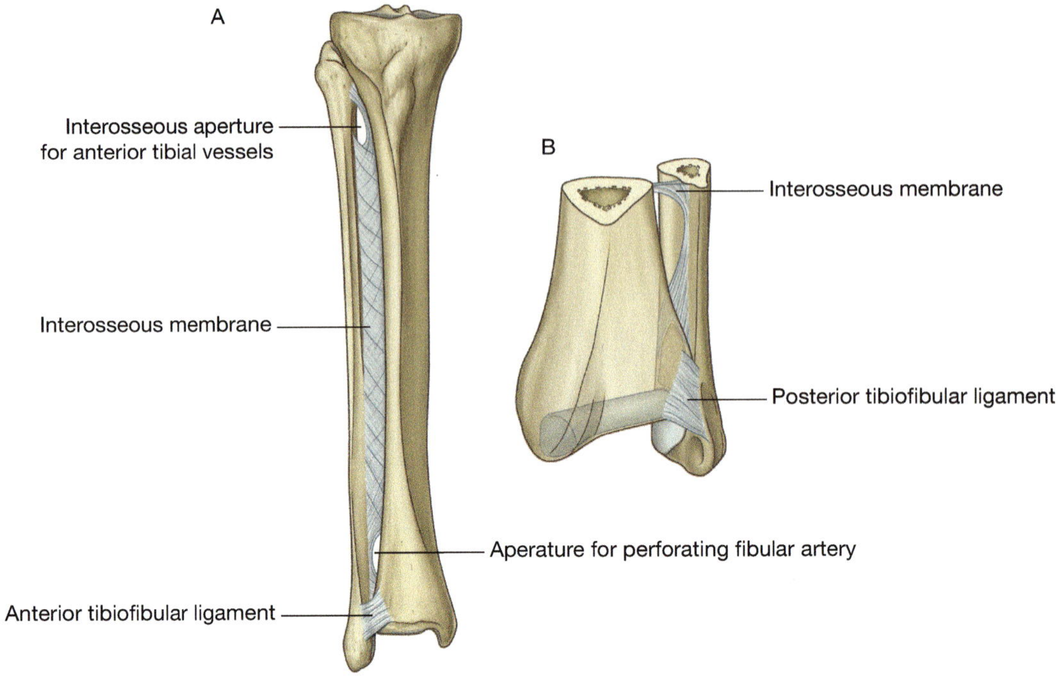

Fig. 23.2 Interosseous membrane and tibiofibular ligaments.

23.1.2 Techniques

Test in decubitus (Fig. 23.3)

The patient lies on his back, leg extended. You place your palms on the tibial and fibular malleoli. Shear the bones alternately in the sagittal plane. When you posteriorize the fibula with your palm, use your fingers to anteriorize the tibial malleolus. Perform this scissorlike movement in turns.

Apply the same technique to the interosseous membrane by placing your palms and fingers on the tibia and fibula as far as their caudal thirds. The membrane higher up is less involved in leg trauma. Make note of the areas of least mobility in order to release them.

Maneuver in decubitus

Shear the tibia and fibula several times. First, shear the malleoli in induction. Secondly, free the caudal part of the interosseous membrane. Induction must be done smoothly until you perceive a full tibiofibular movement.

Maneuver in procubitus (Fig.23.4)

We particularly like this technique, which allows you to take firm hold of the tibia and fibula. Grasp the malleoli between the index fingers and thumbs of your two hands. Traction the leg caudally. Maintain the lift while moving the fibula and tibia sagittally. Finish by applying traction-induction. Stabilize the patient's thigh with your knee so that the knee does not compensate for the traction.

Do the same technique focusing on the interosseous membrane. Follow the listening closely. Little by little you will see that the movement, which appeared to be quite sagittal at the start, has components of lateral flexion and rotation. The goal of this technique is to release small tissular constraints, which inhibit micromovements that are disturbing to the informational system.

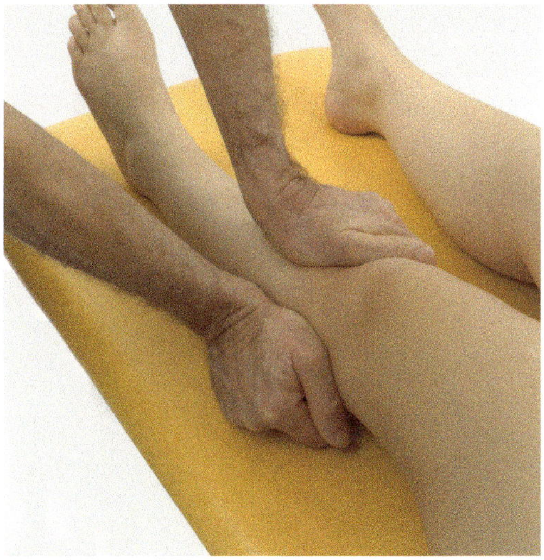

Fig. 23.3 Testing the proximal and distal tibiofibular joints.

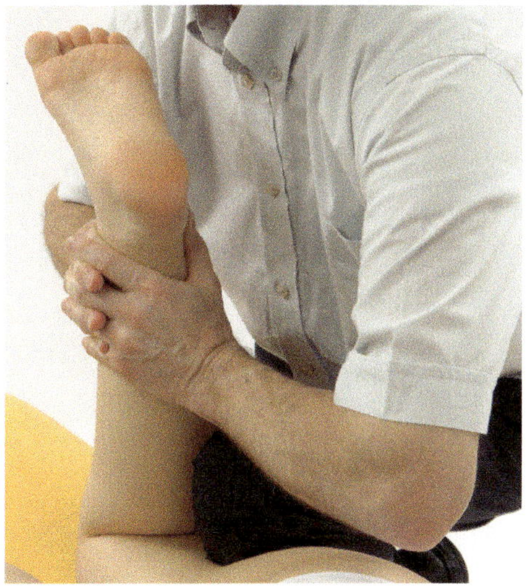

Fig. 23.4 Manipulation of the tibia and fibula in procubitus.

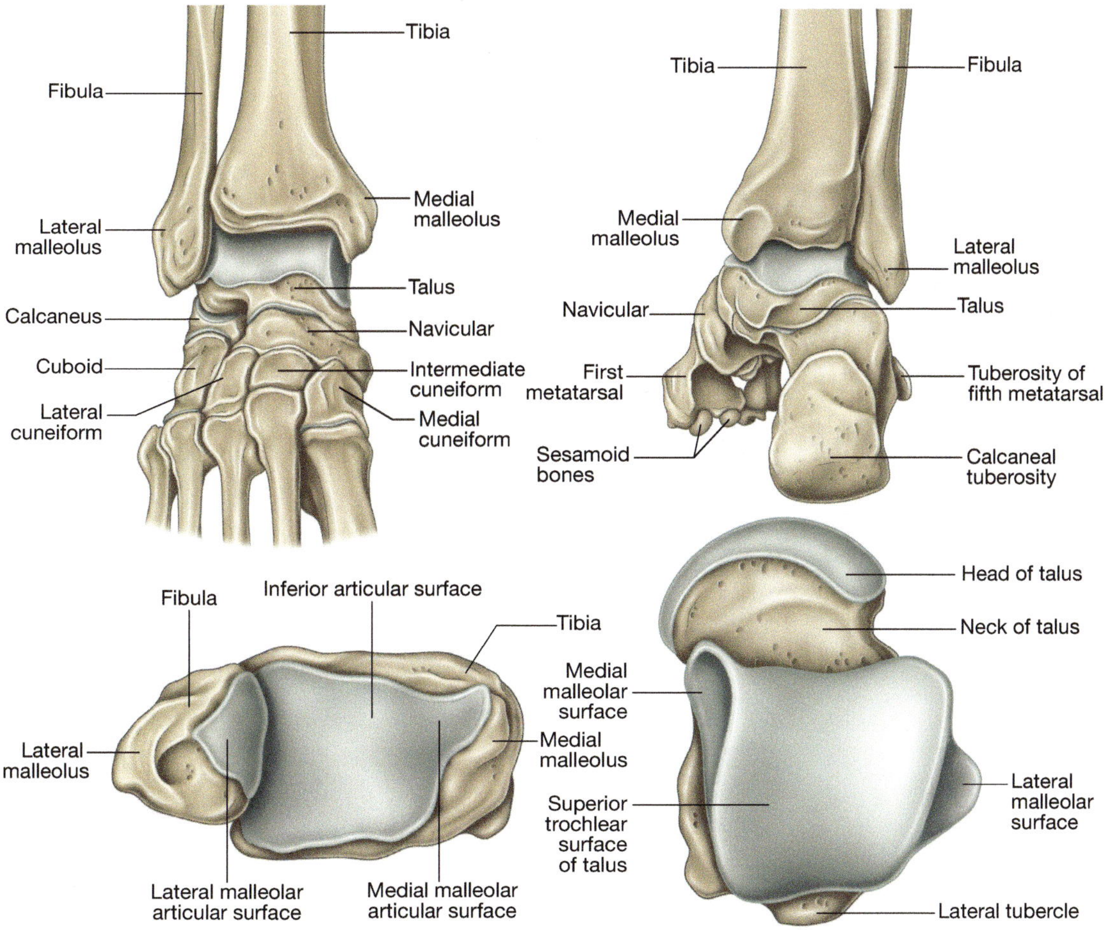

Fig. 23.5 Talomalleolar joint.

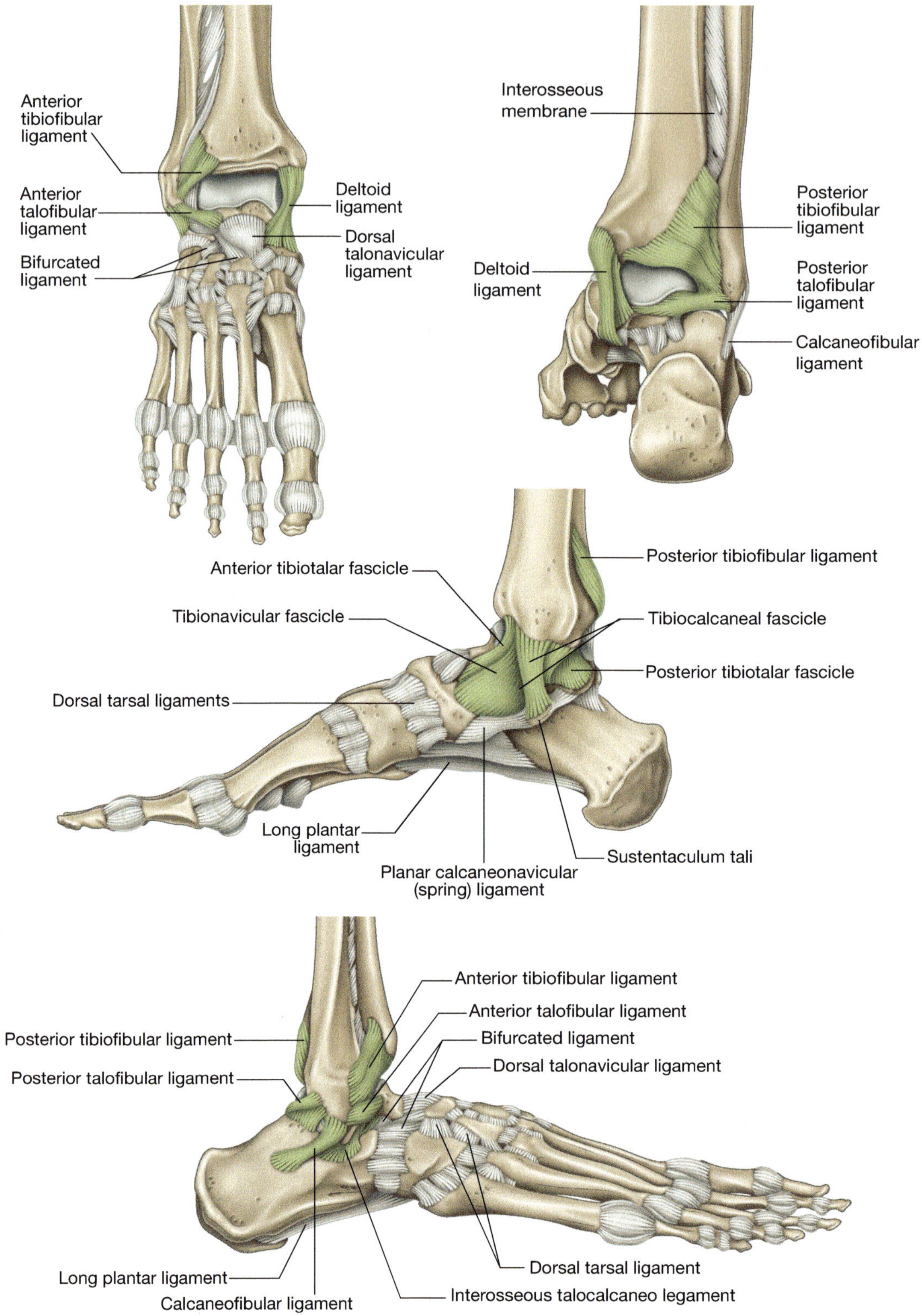

Fig. 23.6 Tibiotalar and talofibular ligaments.

23.2 TALOMALLEOLAR ARTICULATION (FIG. 23.5)

We focus primarily on reinforming the ligamentous proprioceptive system.

Apply the same traction technique following a more finely tuned listening. Traction-induction is applied more lightly and slowly. It is possible to find areas of microscarring due to repetitive sprain. These techniques are not very effective for general constitutional laxity. Nevertheless, subjects whose ankles are naturally lax are rather like a reed. Their ankles bend but do not break.

23.2.1 Review

The tibial and fibular malleoli articulate with the trochlea of the talus. Our techniques involve all the ligaments of this articulation, whether they are lateral, anterior, or posterior.

Trochlea of talus

This structure has three articular facets: one cranial and two lateral. The superior facet is wider in front than at the back and, remarkably, somewhat wider in the right foot (Testut 1896). The trochlea articulates with the caudal surface of the tibia and is flanked:

- laterally by the lateral malleolar facet;
- medially by a smaller medial malleolar facet.

The three talar surfaces articulate with the bimalleolar mortise of the ankle.

Ligaments (Fig. 23.6)

- The anterior tibiotalar ligament forms part of the deltoid or medial collateral ligament.
- The anterior talofibular ligament connects the fibula malleolus to the talus.
- The posterior talofibular ligament runs almost horizontally to connect the lateral malleolus to the posterior talar tubercle.

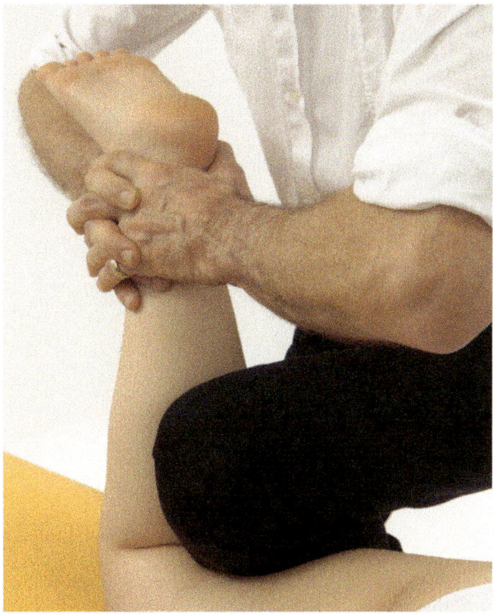

Fig. 23.7 Talomalleolar articulation test in procubitus.

23.2.2 Techniques

Test in procubitus (Fig. 23.7)

Following the same procedure as for the distal tibia and fibula, encircle the talus just below the malleoli. Maintain traction and mobilize the joint in the sagittal, frontal, and horizontal planes, looking for areas of reduced mobility.

Next, stimulate the mechanoreceptors of the various ligaments by allowing your hands to be directed by the listening. The body has an exceptional memory for trauma; listening will draw you precisely to the problematic zone.

Maneuver in procubitus (Fig. 23.8)

First, move the articular surfaces against one another to free any "jammed" joint fixations through joint surface polishing. Next, release the ligaments by allowing the listening to direct your hands, maintaining traction all the while.

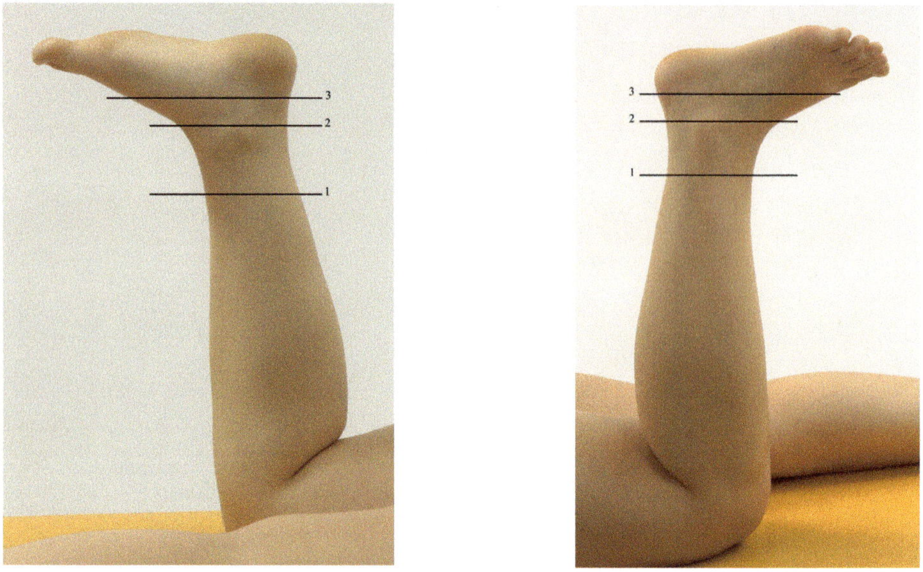

Fig. 23.8 Three manipulation levels of the ankle. (1) Distal tibiofibular; (2) Talomalleolar; (3) Malleolo-talocalcaneal.

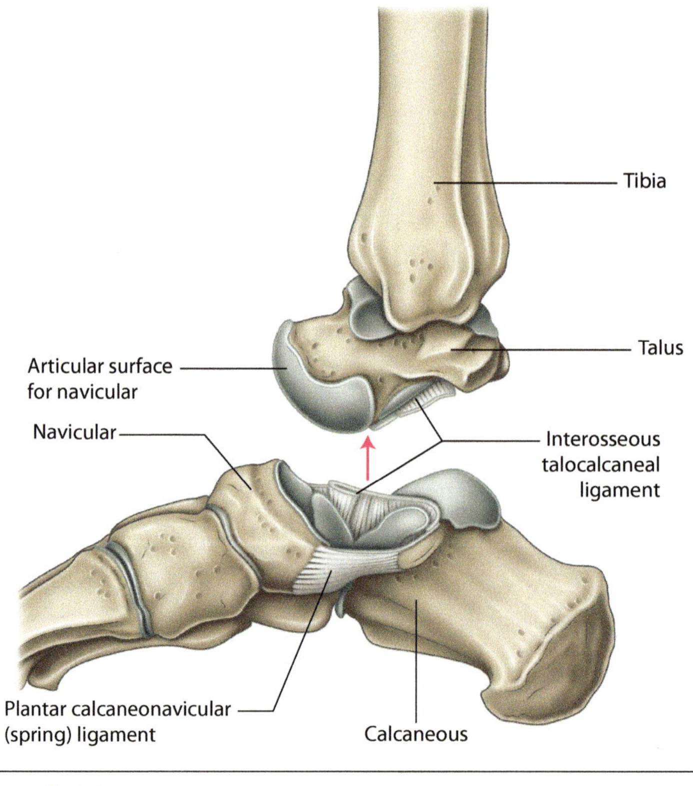

Fig. 23.9 Talocalcaneal joint.

23.3 MALLEOLO-TALOCALCANEAL ARTICULATION (FIG. 23.9)

It is difficult to differentiate the talocrural joint (composed of the distal malleolar clamp and the trochlea of the talus) from the talocalcaneal articulation, because their ligaments are intertwined.

23.3.1 Techniques

Test in procubitus

Both test and technique are performed in procubitus following exactly the same process as above. The only change this time is that the index fingers and thumbs contact the calcaneus alone.

Joints

With practice, you will be able to feel the three different articular levels: the malleolar clamp, the talomalleolar, and the talocalcaneal.

Ligaments (Fig. 23.10)

Medially

The collateral medial (or deltoid) ligament, together with its tibiocalcaneal portion, is easily identified because it joins the sustentaculum tali. It is quite false to think you can even nominally separate all the fibers of the medial collateral ligament; there are too many different fiber directions. On the other hand, it is important to locate properly and evaluate them so as not to miss even a small fixation.

Laterally

- Calcaneofibular ligament
- Interosseous talocalcaneal ligament
- Lateral talocalcaneal ligament

Maneuver in procubitus (Fig. 23.11)

Traction the leg as in the preceding techniques. Encircle the calcaneus just above the sustentaculum tali with your thumbs and index fingers. Begin by trying to individualize anterior, posterior, or lateral restrictions.

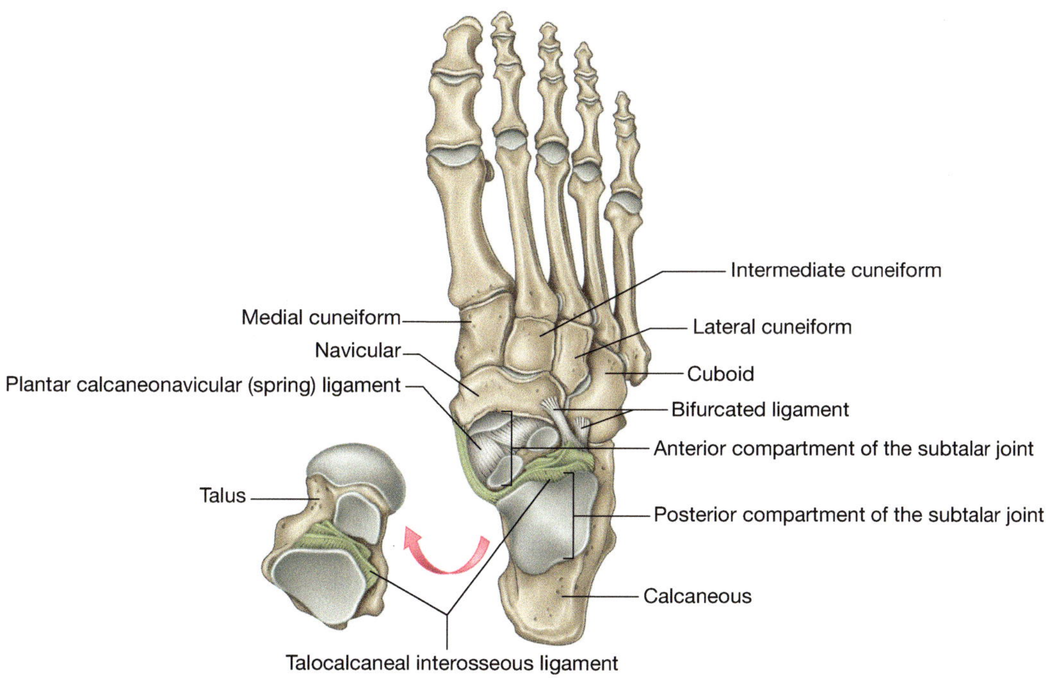

Fig. 23.10 Talocalcaneal ligaments.

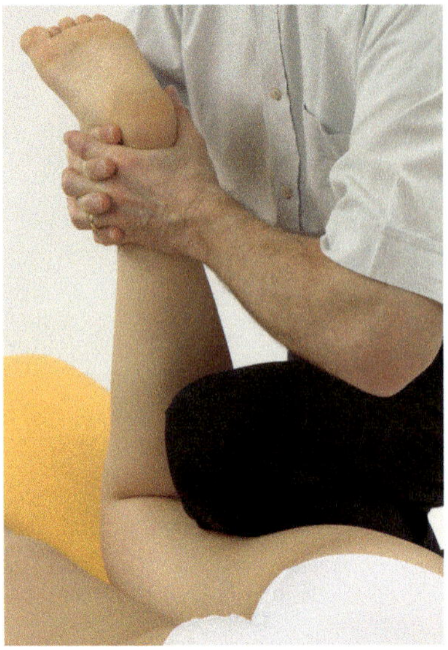

Fig. 23.11 Manipulation of the talocalcaneal joint in procubitus.

Stimulate the mechanoreceptors through traction-induction. Do not hesitate to emphasize the traction, even slightly overtaking the limit of induction.

23.4 TALONAVICULAR ARTICULATION (FIG. 23.12)

23.4.1 Review

A strong sheetlike ligament connects the talus to the navicular. As with the preceding ligaments, our techniques address the dorsal, plantar, anterior, and posterior ligaments.

23.4.2 Technique

In procubitus (Fig. 23.13)

Employ the same distal traction of the leg as above. Place one index finger and thumb on the neck of the talus and the other index finger and thumb on the navicular. Traction the foot joints accompanied by some rotation. In all of these ligament techniques we try to combine ligament work with intra-articular techniques to achieve a capsular and cartilage effect.

23.5 CALCANEOCUBOID ARTICULATION (FIG. 23.14)

23.5.1 Techniques

Following the same principle, place one index finger and one thumb on the cuboid and the other index finger and thumb on the calcaneus. Draw the cuboid away in traction-rotation and lateral flexion; at the end, perform an induction to release the ligament and the joint, which can both be jammed.

23.5.2 Bifurcated ligament (Fig. 23.15)

This ligament is very worthwhile to treat, because it joins the calcaneus to both the navicular and the cuboid. This dorsal ligament can be approached in either decubitus or procubitus.

Decubitus (Fig. 23.16)

The patient's foot rests on your thigh. Place one index finger and one thumb on the calcaneus, behind the cuboid and navicular. Draw the navicular and cuboid away with your other palm and fingers. Carry out several rotations in traction to mobilize the joint surfaces, completing the maneuver with traction-induction. You can fix the talus at the same time as the calcaneus to mobilize the transverse tarsal (Chopart's) joint space.

Procubitus (Fig. 23.17)

Place your knee on the back of the patient's thigh to traction the foot effectively.

Fix the calcaneus with the index finger and thumb of one hand, while your other hand performs joint mobilizations between the calcaneus, navicular, and cuboid. Finish with traction-induction.

These excellent techniques are particularly beneficial to sports enthusiasts (hikers, marathoners, basketball and football players). We frequently come upon fixations that are not yet symptomatic. Eventually decompensation occurs, bringing with it serious, sometimes incomprehensible, foot problems.

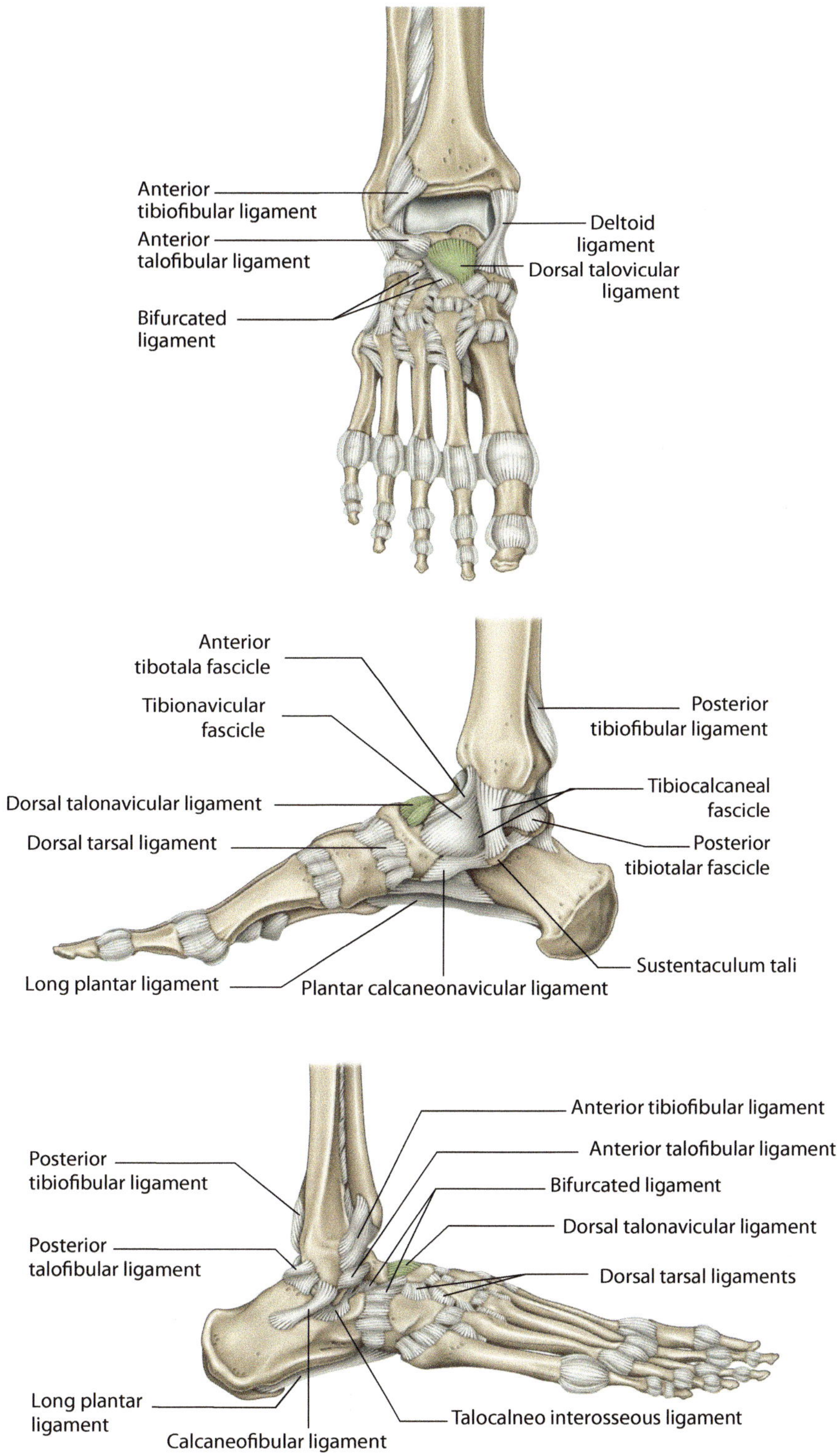

Fig. 23.12 Talonavicular joint.

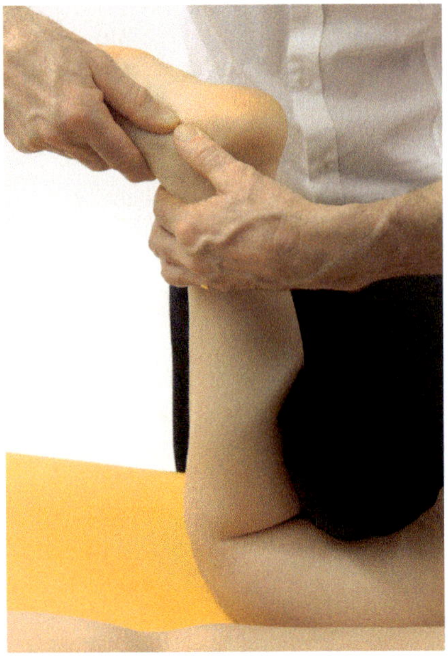

Fig. 23.13 Manipulation of the talonavicular ligaments.

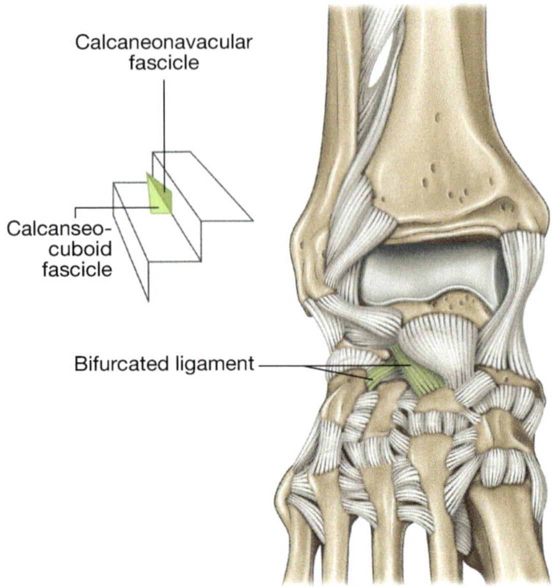

Fig. 23.15 Bifurcated ligament.

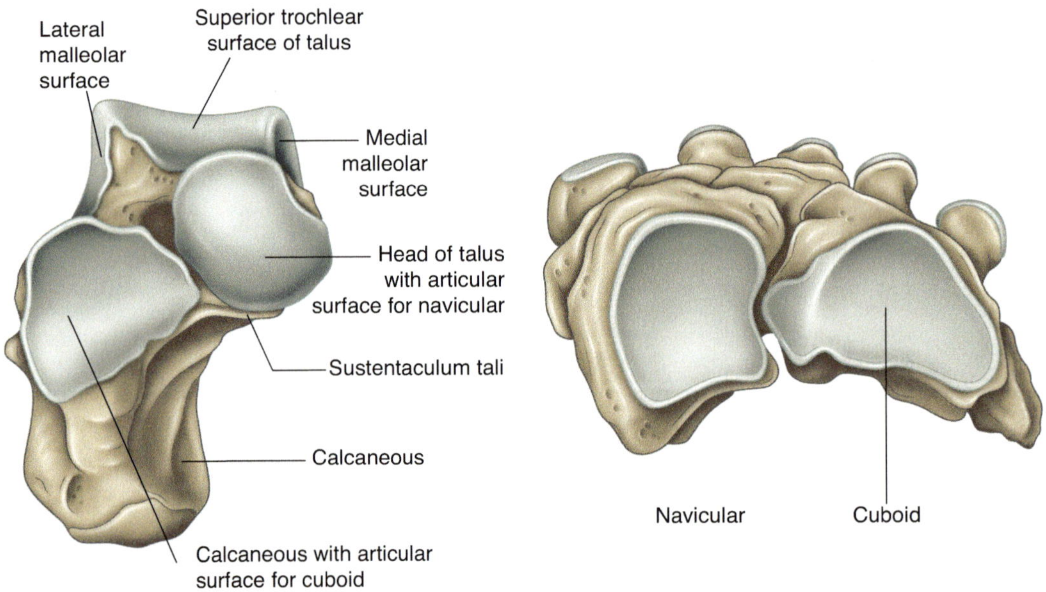

Fig. 23.14 Talonavicular and calcaneocuboid joints.

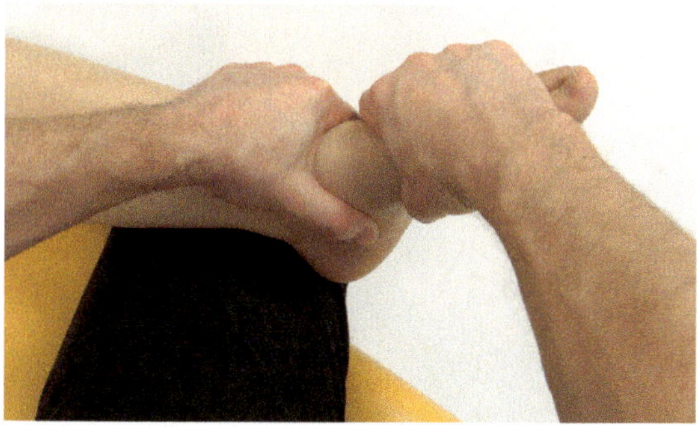

Fig. 23.16 Manipulation of the calcaneocuboid joint in decubitus.

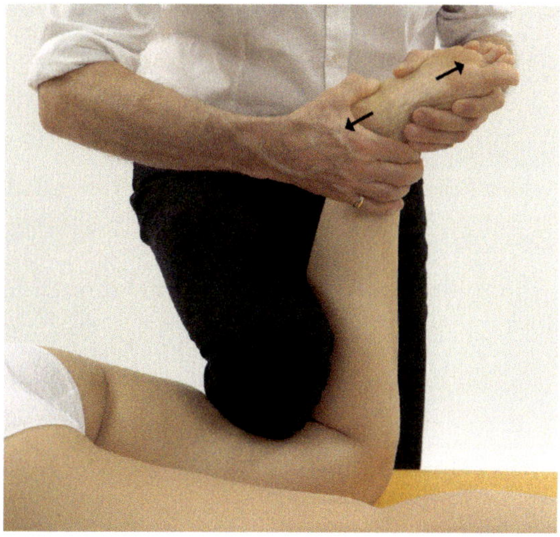

Fig. 23.17 Manipulation of the calaneocuboid joint in procubitus.

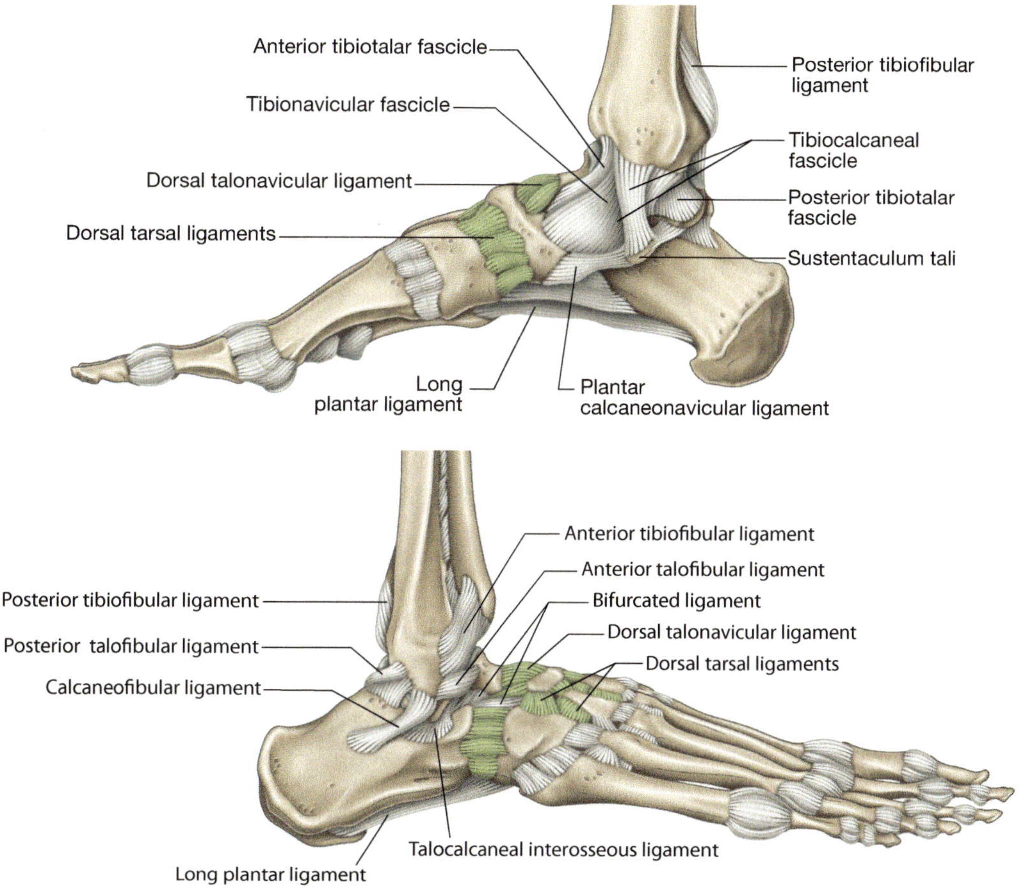

Fig. 23.18 Dorsal ligaments.

23.6 TREATING OTHER LIGAMENTS

23.6.1 Ligaments

Dorsal (Fig. 23.18)

Here we find cuneocuboid ligaments and intercuneiform ligaments.

Plantar ligaments

Recall how important the longitudinal arches are for allowing the foot to support the weight of the body in standing posture. Also recall the important cushioning effect of the torsion bar:

- the spring ligament, or calcaneonavicular ligament, located on the medial edge of the plantar surface, between the sustentaculum tali and the navicular;
- the plantar calcaneocuboid ligament.

23.6.2 Techniques

Dorsal ligaments in decubitus (Fig. 23.19)

The patient rests on his back with his foot on your thigh. Fix the cuboid and navicular between the thumb and index finger of one hand. With the index finger and thumb of your other hand, exert steady traction on the corresponding metatarsals. The movement implicates several joints at the same time: the junctions between the navicular, cuboid, cuneiforms, and the bases of the metatarsals.

You also can traction the cuneiforms directly, but the action is more difficult and less effective, especially on highly toned feet. Corrections are best made using induction incorporated into small movements of rotation and adduction-abduction.

Note: Maintain traction throughout the entire maneuver.

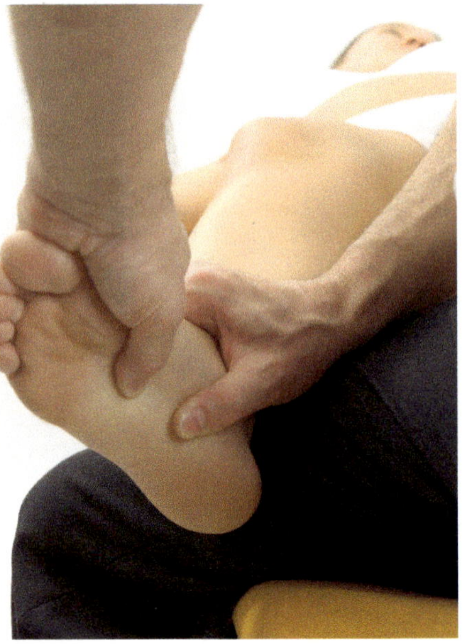

Fig. 23.19 Manipulation of the dorsal ligaments in decubitus.

Spring ligament (Fig. 23.20)

Search the medial underside of the foot for the spring ligament that connects the calcaneus to the navicular. It is located under the head of the talus, immediately in front of the sustentaculum tali.

Calcaneal ligament

Find this ligament by spreading the long plantar ligament laterally. In terms of manipulating the dorsal ligaments, systematically investigate the other plantar ligaments situated next to it, as we advise below.

Plantar ligaments (Fig. 23.21)

Any treatment of the dorsal ligaments usually involves the plantar calcaneonavicular, plantar calcaneocuboid, plantar cuneonavicular, interosseous coneocuboid, and intercuneiform ligaments. It is not a question of describing individual techniques for the estimated 114 ligaments of the foot (an approximate number), but we shall outline one routine that affects them all.

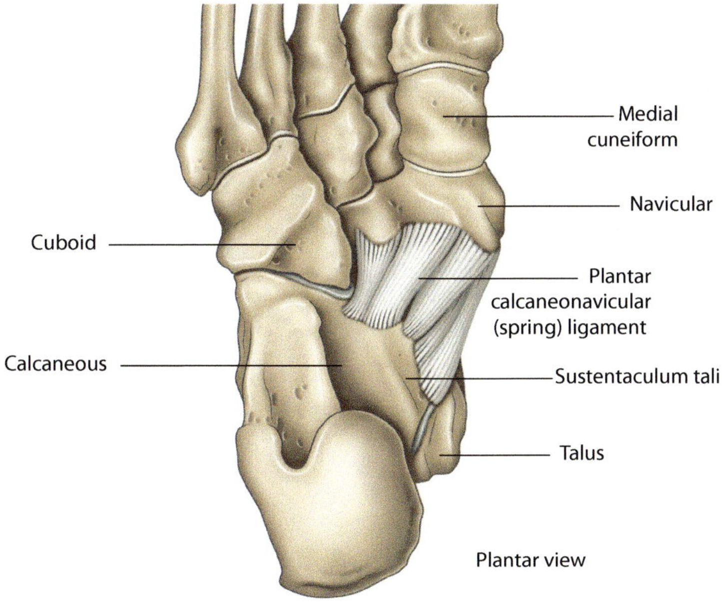

Fig. 23.20 Spring ligament.

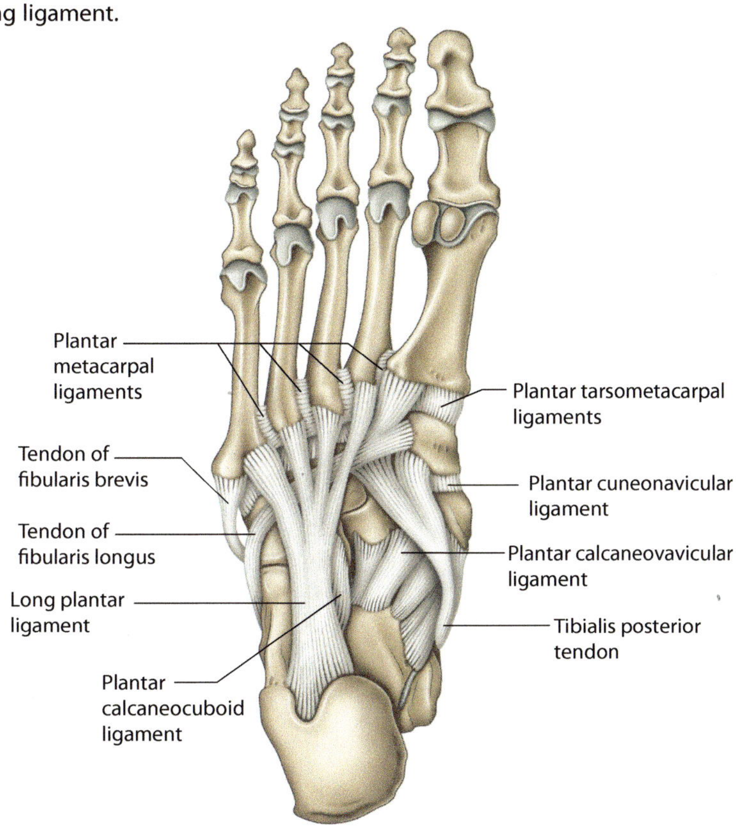

Fig. 23.21 Plantar calcaneocuboid ligament.

The routine

Begin by general listening to the entire body. A painful foot can certainly have other causes apart from local ligamentous fixation. If the foot is implicated in the listening, follow the principle that ligaments and muscle attachments are more important than bones themselves. It is recommended that you first mobilize the foot in a way that involves all the joints. This will permit you to:

- determine the location of the fixation globally;
- stimulate the local mechanoreceptors. This has the advantage of rendering the fixation more easily perceived, because proprioceptive stimulation often strengthens a restriction.

Perform a listening over the area of restriction. This will help to clarify the location, importance, and precise nature of the fixation. Local listening can be done by placing both hands simultaneously over the dorsal and plantar surfaces of the feet. This approach allows you to feel where the problems are located very quickly.

Once you have clearly felt the fixation and visualized its location, intensity, and how it figures in the foot mechanism, treat it with induction until a release is perceived.

In daily practice we regularly discover foot fixations. Certainly the most common are the result of eversion. The patient often speaks of "rolling the ankle" in the course of some everyday activity. It is very common to feel fixations of the fibula, talus, and fifth metatarsal joint.

Calibrating listening

If you are not confident in what you feel, you can certainly confirm your listening by engaging the tissues and joints a little more "mechanically." This in no way means a pure and simple joint mobilization. It is more about progressively and respectfully engaging the joint unit in the direction you perceive the listening to be.

Next, engage the foot in the direction opposite the perceived listening. See how easily the tissues move in each direction.

Normally, if your perception is correct, the tissues move easily in the direction of the listening but "bridle" and resist when you attempt to mobilize them in the opposite direction. It is good to measure and check your listening perceptions by validating or invalidating the movement parameters that you choose.

Treatment of the active stabilizers

24

24.1 ACTIVE STABILIZERS

Several muscles are involved in stabilizing the foot. Some of these muscles are directly linked to joint capsules. Active stabilizers can be divided according to location:

- the anterior group:
  - tibialis anterior;
  - extensor digitorum longus;
  - extensor hallucis longus.
- the lateral group:
  - fibularis longus;
  - fibularis brevis.
- the posterior group:
  - sural triceps made up of the soleus and the two gastrocnemius heads, including the tendon that serves as their calcaneal attachment, the Achilles tendon;
  - the inconsistent plantaris (It is not functionally as important as the other muscles.);
  - the flexors (Our preferred placement is in posterior medial division.).
- the posterior medial group (Insertions are posterior, tendons are medial.):
  - tibialis posterior;
  - flexor digitorum longus;
  - flexor hallucis longus.

We will begin with the lateral group, which is systematically and heavily impacted by sprain of the lateral compartment of the foot.

24.2 FIBULAR MUSCLES

These are the most important active stabilizers of the lateral foot, working in synergy with fibers of the fibular collateral ligament. Muscles can be thought of as the first bulwark against sprain. When their defense is breached, the ligaments are next to be overstretched or torn.

24.2.1 Review—fibularis brevis (Fig. 24.1)

Origin

- Fibula at the lateral surface

Course

- Distal, vertical

Termination

- Tuberosity of the fifth metatarsal. This highly strategic area is practically always involved in foot sprain.

Innervation

- Superficial fibular nerve (L5–S1)

Vascular supply

- Fibular artery

Actions

- Pronates the foot
- Assists in flexion of the foot

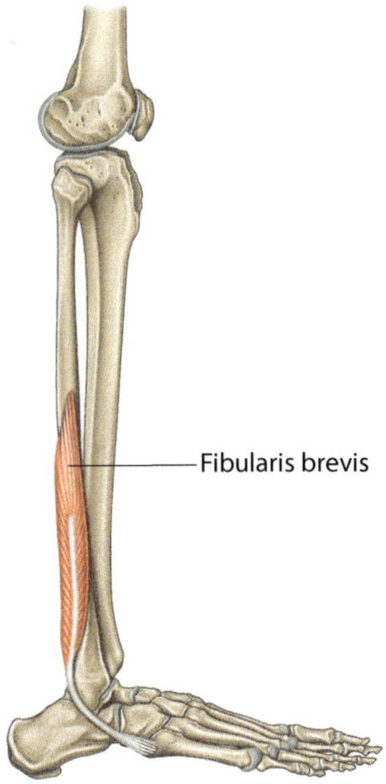

Fig. 24.1 Fibularis brevis muscle.

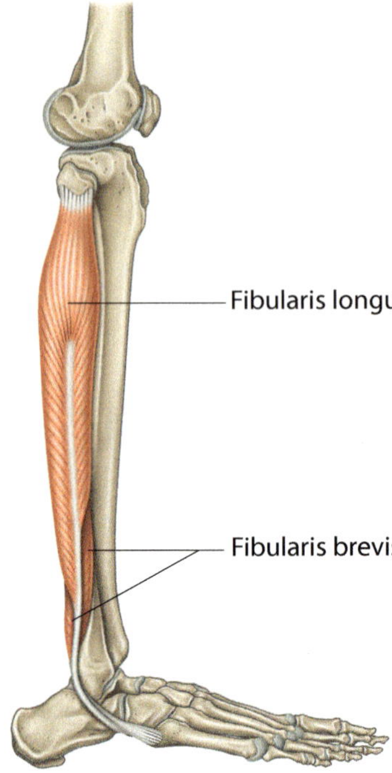

Fig. 24.2 Fibularis longus muscle.

24.2.2 Review—fibularis longus (Fig. 24.2)

Origin

- Capsule of the proximal tibiofibular joint
- Head of the fibula
- Cranial two-thirds of the fibula

Direction

- Vertical, distal

Termination

- First metatarsal
- Medial cuneiform
- Tendon, which runs ensheathed along a groove on the underside of cuboid to insert on the base of the first metatarsal

Innervation

- Superficial fibular nerve (L5–S1)

Vascularization

- Fibular artery

Actions

- Pronates the foot
- Plantar flexes the foot
- Tenses the transverse arch of the foot

24.2.3 Fibular retinacula (Fig. 24.3)

Two fibrous retaining bands overlay the fibularis tendons: a superior and an inferior retinaculum.

Superior retinaculum

This band extends from the lateral malleolus to the calcaneus, overlaying the tendons of the fibularis longus and brevis that run ensheathed in the malleolar groove. Both the retinaculum and the sheath are often injured in ankle sprain. Damage to the retinaculum not only impedes the normal course of these tendons but is also very disruptive to proprioception. When a retinaculum is left untreated, future sprains are likely due to inaccurate proprioceptive information.

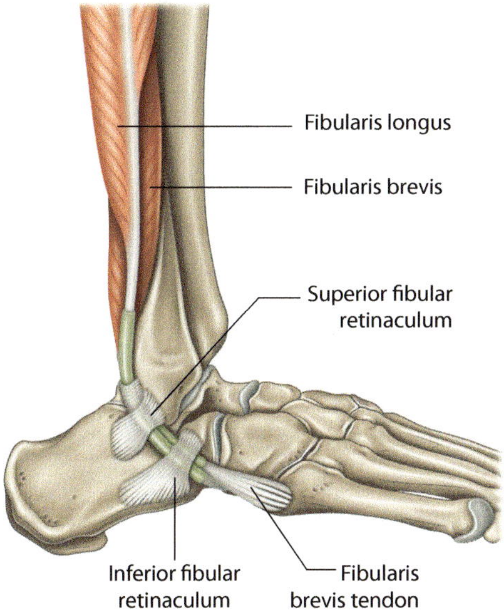

Fig. 24.3 Fibular retinacula.

Inferior retinaculum

This band overlays both fibularis tendons as they pass along the lateral malleolus of the foot. It is continuous with the extensor retinaculum at the lateral dorsal surface of the foot. It then inserts onto the lateral surface of the anterior part of the calcaneus. All lateral ankle sprains destabilize extensor muscle action and contribute to general instability of the lower limb.

Fibularis tendon dislocation

The tendons of the fibularis longus and brevis run behind the lateral malleolus and then divide as they continue toward the lateral edge and underside of the foot. The tendons may slip out of place in front of the fibular malleolus. This dislocation is rare and is often mistaken for lateral ankle sprain. The mechanism of injury, however, is altogether different.

Generally the tendon snaps out of position during sudden dorsal flexion. Forceful stretch of the peroneal muscles can also rip the sheath of the lateral retinaculum. Sometimes the dislocation is caused by the sudden active contraction of the fibular muscles attempting to defend the ankle against collision.

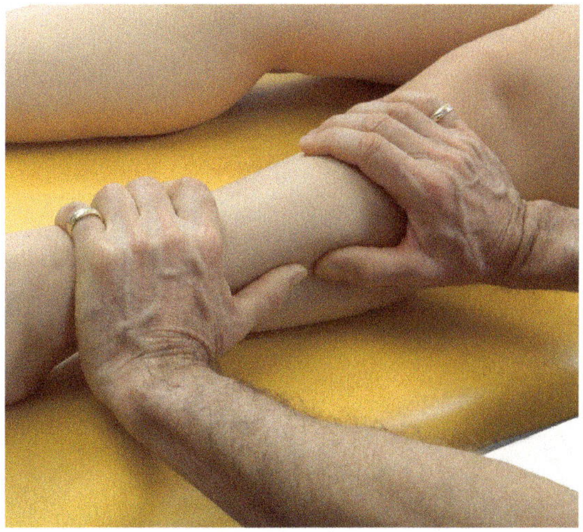

Fig. 24.4 Superficial fibular nerve manipulation.

Retromalleolar pain and edema are the usual symptoms. Patients often experience the tendons displacing out of their groove. The tendons usually snap back into place.

24.2.4 Techniques

Manipulations to the fibularis longus and brevis are common.

Pinpointing the lateral peroneal compartment of the leg

Look for the musculocutaneous junctions where the two muscle bodies meet. The patient rests supine, leg slightly flexed. Glide your thumb along the lateral fibular compartment until your thumb meets a small depression into which it suddenly falls. Usually this dip is precisely where the superficial nerve pierces the deep crural fascia.

Superficial peroneal nerve (Fig. 24.4)

Begin by freeing the nerve from its fascial depression by manipulating the immediately surrounding crural fascia by way of induction.

Musculotendinous junction (Fig. 24.5)

Perform a separation-induction technique at the fibularis longus and brevis. Starting at the cranial malleolus, glide your two thumbs up the leg until you feel the musculocutane-

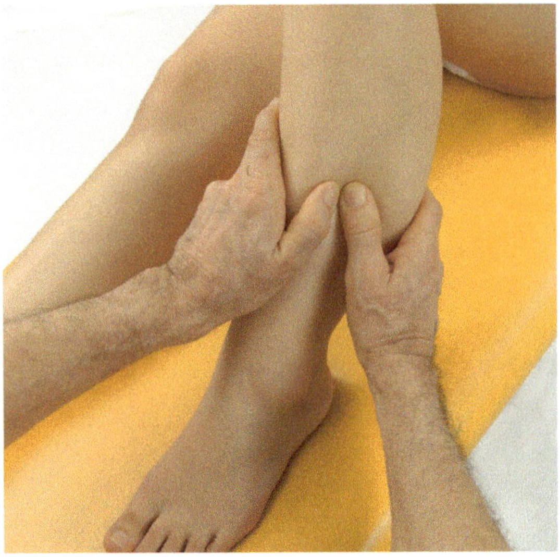

Fig. 24.5 Manipulation of the musculotendinous junction of the fibularis muscles.

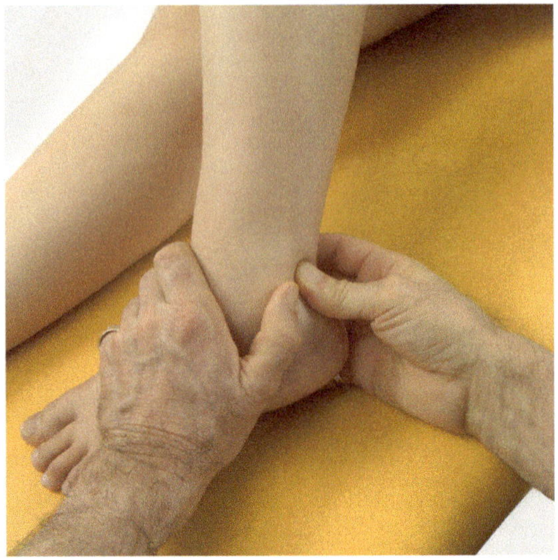

Fig. 24.6 Manipulation of the superior retinaculum.

ous junction. Spread your thumbs and maintain separation-induction for 12 seconds.

Retinacula in lateral decubitus (Figs. 24.6 and 24.7)

Work carefully, as retinacula are delicate and play a proprioception role in tendinous coordination and cohesion. As we know, they are routinely damaged in lateral ankle sprain, usually when the forefoot is somehow lodged and the leg continues moving.

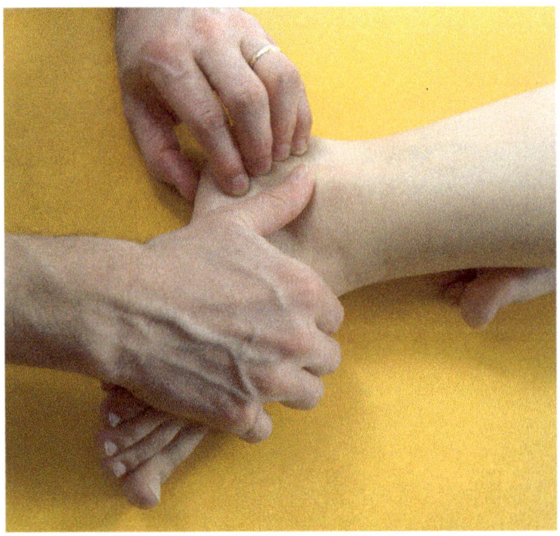

Fig. 24.7 Manipulation of fibular muscles and inferior retinaculum.

Adduct the leg to increase tension on the tendons passing under the retinacula. The patient lies on the side opposite the ankle in question. Explore the retinaculum with your finger pads, adding in small eversion and inversion movements of the foot. You can also place the retinaculum under tension by asking the patient to flex the foot a few times in order to evaluate how well the tendons glide under the retinacula.

24.3 SURAL TRICEPS

24.3.1 Soleus (Fig. 24.8)

While the muscle bodies of the gastrocnemius and soleus are of little interest, their proximal and distal insertions are worthwhile.

We have looked at the gastrocnemius and its close connection to the capsules in the knee chapter. We will now look at the soleus and then consider the Achilles tendon as it relates to the lateral fibular and posterior tibial muscles.

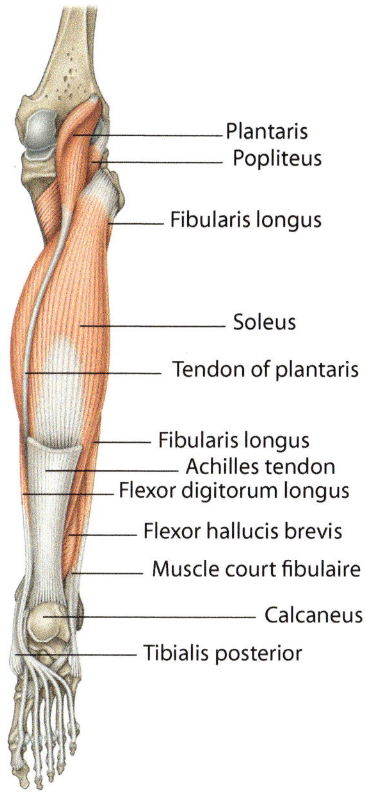

Fig. 24.8 Soleus muscle.

Origin

- The fibula–the head and proximal dorsal third
- The tendinous arch stretched between the fibular head and the tibia
- The proximal third of the tibia

Direction

- Proximally, vertical and slightly medial
- Distally, vertical

Termination

- Calcaneal tuberosity where it, together with the gastrocnemius, forms the Achilles tendon

Innervation

- Tibial nerve (S1–S2)

Vascularization

- Posterior fibular and tibial arteries, branches of the popliteal artery

Actions

- Plantar flexion
- Supination of the foot

24.3.2 Techniques

Our techniques are focused on the fibular attachment and tendinous arch.

Fibular attachment of soleus in decubitus (Fig. 24.9)

The patient lies with his leg flexed. Position yourself facing his leg. Push the gastrocnemius laterally with your thumb or index finger. Use your other thumb to contact the soleus where it attaches to the fibula. Search for indurated and sensitive fibers that you can release with spreading-induction.

Tendinous arch of soleus (Figs. 24.10 and 24.11)

Maintaining the gastrocnemius to the side, begin at the head of the fibula and direct your thumbs inward toward the proximal third of the tibia. It is not compression that counts but the transverse movement.

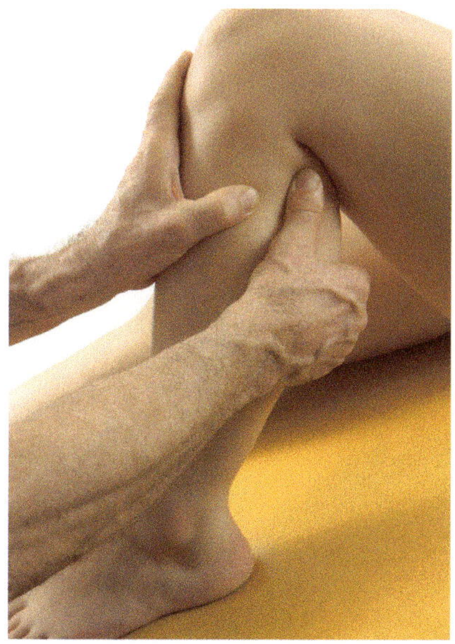

Fig. 24.9 Manipulation of soleus fibular attachment.

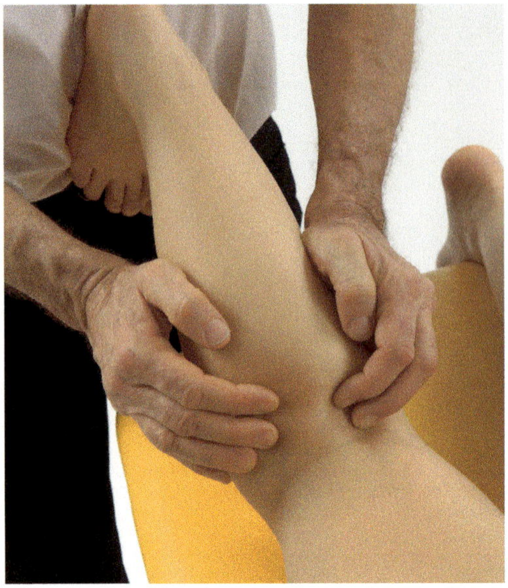

Fig. 24.10 Manipulation of tendinous arch of soleus muscle.

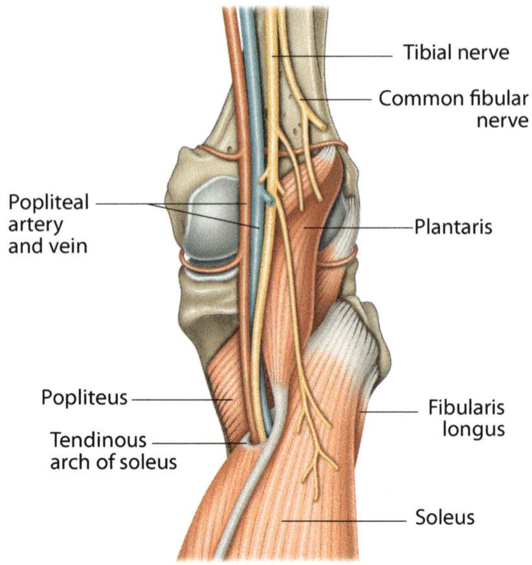

Fig. 24.11 Tendinous arch of soleus.

Precaution

Be careful in this region, as you are very near the fibular nerve, which does not appreciate compression. The patient will experience localized pain or numbness in the leg. If you feel a fine, fairly mobile thin cord, avoid it; it surely will be the fibular nerve.

Special note

Neurovascular structures run in front of the tendinous arch of the soleus. They are, from lateral to medial, the tibial nerve, the posterior tibial vein, and the posterior tibial artery branch of the popliteal artery.

Any retraction of the soleus tendinous arch can compress these elements. It is always a good idea, therefore, to compare the pulses of both posterior tibial arteries. If you feel one pulse is weaker, release the ipsilateral tendinous arch below the knee and see if the pulse improves.

Weakness of the posterior tibial pulse can come from a problem at the common external iliac, femoral, or popliteal vessels. It serves as an excellent witness pulse, allowing you to gauge the effectiveness of a particular vascular technique.

Posterior tibial vascular conflict (problem, insufficiency)

Sometimes patients consult for pain in the back of the leg. These discomforts are generally attributable to a torn muscle or its aftermath. As a rule, symptoms arise only during some physical activity such as walking or, less commonly, cycling. Vascular workups are usually negative because blood-flow tests are invariably done with the patient lying down, muting the effect of the insufficiency.

When symptoms come on rapidly with exertion, the posterior tibial artery is often involved. Symptoms that appear more gradually indicate a problem with the posterior tibial vein. These circulatory problems can be of traumatic or congenital origin. In rare instances they can be due to a general connective tissue disorder.

24.4 ACHILLES TENDON (FIG. 24.12)

Achilles tendon rupture and Achilles tendonitis can both occur with no great mechanical explanation. Tendons certainly can be overstretched by intense physical

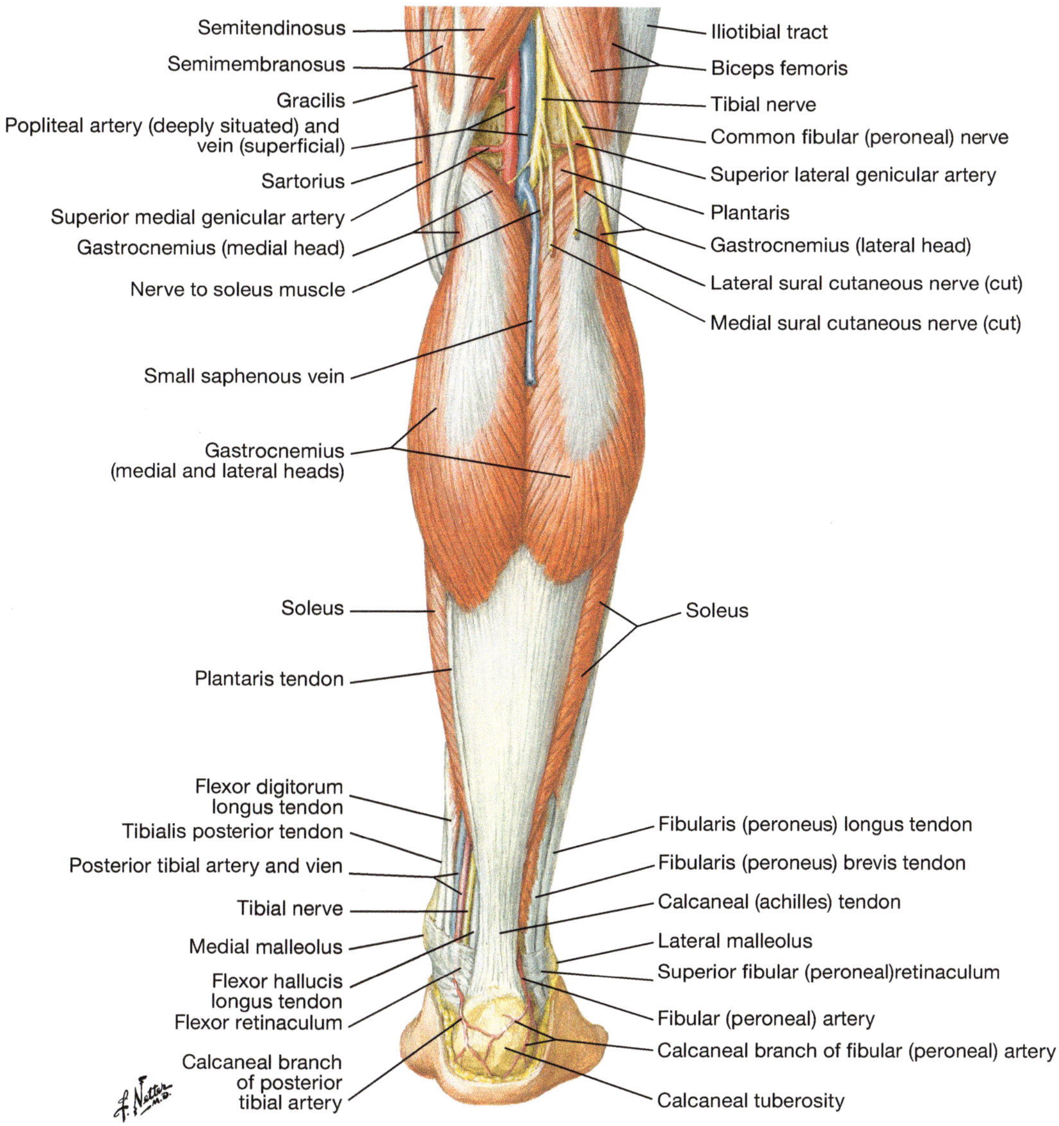

Fig. 24.12 Achilles tendon. (After Frank H. Netter. Atlas of human anatomy, 5th ed., plate 504. Used with permission of the editor.)

activities. It is good, therefore, to familiarize yourself with a few general principles pertaining to Achilles problems.

24.4.1 Bilateral Achilles pain

It is an established principle in manual therapy that when a patient complains of bilateral limb pain, the problem is more general than local. In such cases we tend to investigate possibilities along the lines of metabolism, hormones, toxicity, neuropathy, autoimmune disease, or inflammatory rheumatism disorders rather than mechanical causes.

Metabolic cause

Achilles pain can indicate latent gout or chondrocalcinosis. The affliction is more common in older adults who consume too much dairy, seafood, deli meats, chocolate, or salt. Treatment is first and foremost dietary. Men are especially prone to acute recurrences of gout and crystal deposition disease.

Discussion

We have had a number of instructive cases of gout where all biological markers were normal. It seems that in some instances the organism is able to rid itself of excessive uric acid buildup in the muscles, which explains why blood workups show nothing amiss.

One such patient, a urologist by profession as it so happened, consulted us for pain in the forefoot following a long walk. Unable to find any causal joint fixation, we suggested pseudogout as a possibility. Needless to say he did not believe us!

A pocket of fluid was evident behind his elbow. Puncture revealed the pouch to be filled with uric acid! In spite of this, he remained doubtful of our explanation. He altered his eating habits nevertheless and his problem abated.

Hormonal cause

This is most frequently a female problem, occurring at menopause or perimenopause, perhaps due to a lack of progesterone. We refer such patients for homeopathy or acupuncture.

Intoxication

Achilles problems affect patients taking antibiotics, beta blockers, high blood pressure medication, or cholesterol-lowering drugs. One of the first questions we ask a patient with musculotendinous complaints is, "Have you been taking medication regularly for a long time?" If we think their musculotendinous disorders are medication related, we advise them to have their doctor review their prescriptions.

24.4.2 Unilateral Achilles pain

Unilateral complaints can be of mechanical origin following some intensified activity, a vigorous walk, ill-fitting shoes, jumping, etc. Tendon pain can also be related to functional kidney disorders, very often pertaining to an overconsumption of meat and cheese.

Achilles tendon rupture diagnosis

Nearly 70% of torn Achilles tendons are diagnosed late. They are often treated as simple ankle sprains on first assessment.

Ruptures occur two finger widths above the calcaneus. Most cases of Achilles tendon ruptures involve a traumatic sports injury such as the forceful push-off of a jump entailing abrupt contraction of the sural triceps. Rupture is followed by an immediate sharp pain in the back of the ankle. The person feels as if he was lashed or kicked behind the ankle. Examination finds posterior pain above the heel.

Clinical diagnosis is simple and takes only seconds. The Brunet sign test is done with the patient lying facedown, feet hanging off the end of the table. The foot falls vertically at right angles to the leg on the side of the rupture. The healthy ankle maintains 15°–20° of plantar flexion provided by the sural triceps.

The Thompson test is done in the same position. When the tendon is intact, squeezing the ankle produces plantar flex. The test is positive when the ankle does not plantar flex when the calf is squeezed. This test is 100% reliable for Achilles tendon rupture. Other tests are somewhat less accurate.

A torn tendon can be masked by edema. Difficulty in pointing the toes is a nonspecific sign. Loss of active plantar flexion is not automatic as a diagnosis. This function can be provided by other tendons running along the lateral malleolus (tibialis posterior, peroneus longus and brevis, common and proper flexor tendons). Delayed dorsiflexion is often masked by pain.

24.4.3 Techniques

The tendon in decubitus or procubitus

Glide up from the calcaneus along the lateral and medial borders of the Achilles tendon. Very often the weakened tendon feels "lumpy." Our first goal is to even it out by performing a smoothing-induction technique around the tendon. Next, we use both thumbs to move the tendon transversely in order to restore its elasticity.

In all cases of painful Achilles, it is suggested that the patient avoid dairy, cold cuts, and red meat, especially in the evening when the organism has more difficulty eliminating due to inactivity and the horizontal position of the kidneys.

Achilles tendon and neighboring muscles

In decubitus (Fig.24.13)

The patient lies on his back, knee flexed. Facing the leg involved, use your thumb to move the fibularis tendons as if you want to separate them from the Achilles tendon. Follow up the leg as far as the musculotendinous junction. Proceed in the same way along the medial aspect, gently dividing the tendon from the flexor hallucis longus and tibialis posterior.

In chronic cases you often find adhesions between the tendon and muscle. Complete the treatment by maintaining separation-induction for 12 seconds.

In lateral decubitus (Fig. 24.14)

The patient lies on the side of the Achilles tendon in question; on the opposite side the leg is slightly flexed. In side-lying you can access the tendon higher up and go a little deeper. To reach the medial part of the tendon, for example, place your thumbs on the medial aspect and your fingers on the lateral part. Move the tendon generously from side to side.

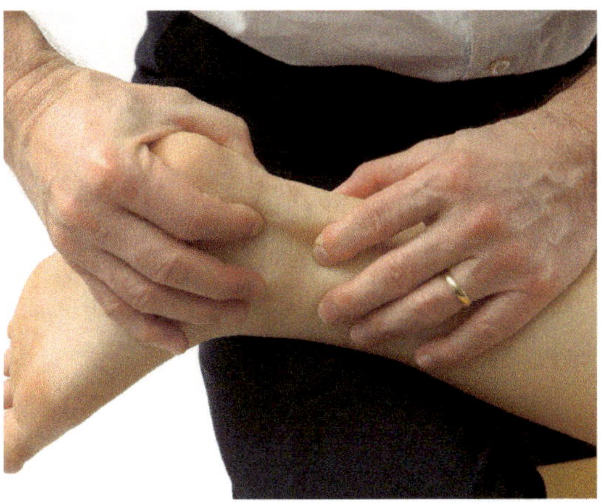

Fig. 24.13 Manipulation of the Achilles tendon.

24.5 TIBIALIS POSTERIOR (FIG. 24.15)

24.5.1 Review

Origin

- Tibiofibular interosseous membrane
- Tibia and fibula as far as the mid-calf

Direction and course

- It moves distally and turns medially at the distal part.
- The tendon passes in a groove behind the tibial malleolus, wrapped in a synovial sheath.
- It runs between the sustentaculum tali and the navicular.

Termination

The tibialis posterior tendon splits:

- The stronger medial tendon attaches to

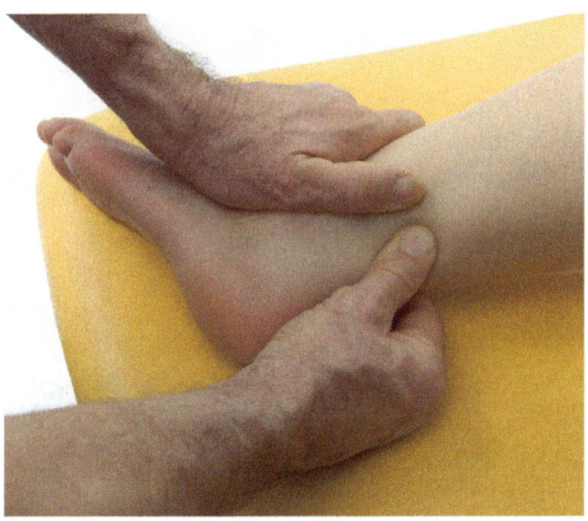

Fig. 24.14 Manipulation of Achilles tendon in relationship to neighboring muscles, in lateral decubitus.

the tuberosity of the navicular bone.
- The lateral tendon inserts on the three cuneiforms.

Innervation

- Tibial nerve (L4–L5)

Vascularization

- Posterior tibial artery (branch of the popliteal)

Actions

- Flexion and supination of the foot

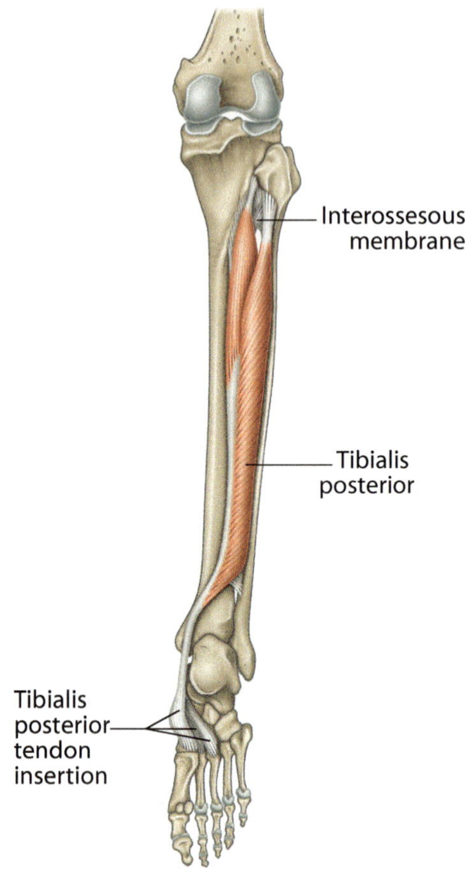

Fig. 24.15 Tibialis posterior muscle.

24.5.2 Techniques

Musculotendinous junction in procubitus (Fig. 24.16)

Starting at the tibial malleolus, follow up the tibialis posterior tendon (medial to the posterior tibial artery) as far as the muscle-tendon junction. Perform gliding-induction and separation-induction maneuvers at the junction.

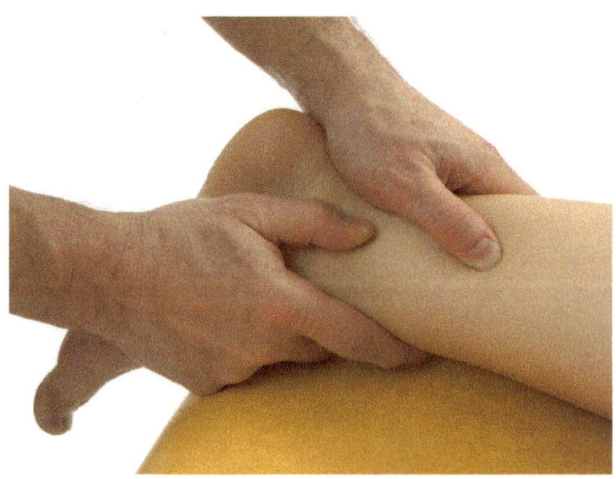

Fig. 24.16 Manipulation of musculotendinous junction of tibialis posterior.

Retromalleolar part

In procubitus (Fig. 24.17)

The patient lies facedown with his foot on your thigh. Place your thumbs on the most medial aspect of the tibial malleolus and glide the tendon transversely and longitudinally in its groove.

Next, mobilize the tibialis posterior in relation to the digitorum longus. Separate the two tendons up until the muscle-tendon junction.

In decubitus

The patient lies with his leg flexed. You place one thumb on the most medial aspect of the tibial malleolus and move the tendon transversely. Longitudinal gliding is rather difficult to perform in decubitus, so you can choose to do it in procubitus.

Plantar part in procubitus (Figs. 24.18 and 24.19)

The patient lies on the table, knee flexed, with your knee supporting his thigh. Be sure you are on the tibialis posterior tendon by asking the patient to flex and supinate his foot. Glide the tendon transversely in combination with small longitudinal movements.

Perform this mobilization either passively or actively. You can ask the patient to flex his tibialis posterior a few times, allowing you to fix the tendon at different points. Manipulate the tendon against the navicular tuberosity and the cuneiform bones by alternately fixing the lateral, intermediate, and medial cuneiforms during flexion. Be careful not to overcompress, as gliding is the effect we are after.

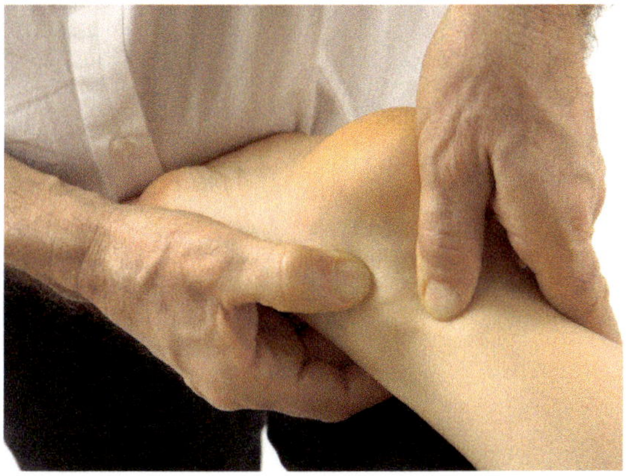

Fig. 24.17 Manipulation of retromalleolar part of tibialis posterior.

24.6 ANTERIOR GROUP

24.6.1 Review—tibialis anterior (Fig. 24.20)

Release this muscle when an ankle sprains in both inversion and eversion (dorsal flexion) at the same time. This happens when the distal foot is lodged against an obstacle or fixed on the ground while the leg keeps moving.

Origin

- Tibia, covering more than half its lateral surface
- Interosseous membrane
- Crural fascia

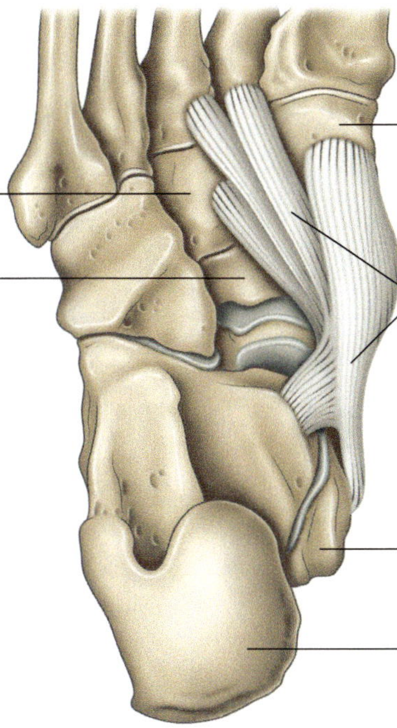

Fig. 24.18 Plantaris and tibialis posterior attachments.

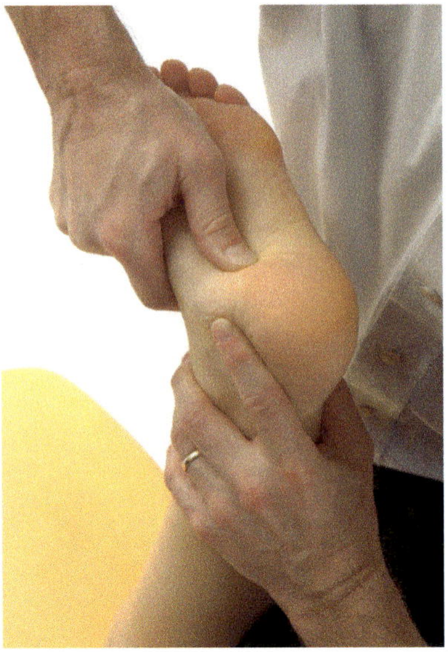

Fig. 24.19 Manipulation of the plantar part of tibialis posterior.

Direction and course

- It moves vertically, medially, and distally at its inferior end.
- The tendon passes under the superior and inferior extensor retinaculi that communicate with the inferior fibular retinacula.

Termination

- Medial cuneiform, beneath the plantar surface
- First metatarsal

Special note

With all tendons that glide on bone, a serous bursa surrounds the tendon.

Innervation

- Deep fibular nerve (L4–L5)

Vascularization

- Anterior tibial artery

Actions

- Dorsal flexion of the foot
- Supination of the foot

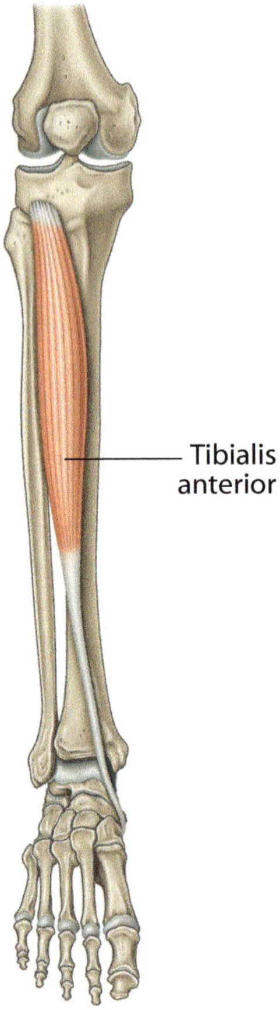

Fig. 24.20 Tibialis anterior muscle.

26.6.2 Review—extensor digitorum longus (Fig. 24.21)

Origin

- Tibia on the lateral condyle
- Fibula on the head and ventral border
- Crural fascia
- Interosseous membrane

Direction and course

- It runs vertically.
- Four tendons run beneath the extensor retinaculum in company with the tibialis anterior, each in its own synovial sheath.

Termination

- Distal phalanges of the second, third, fourth, and fifth toes

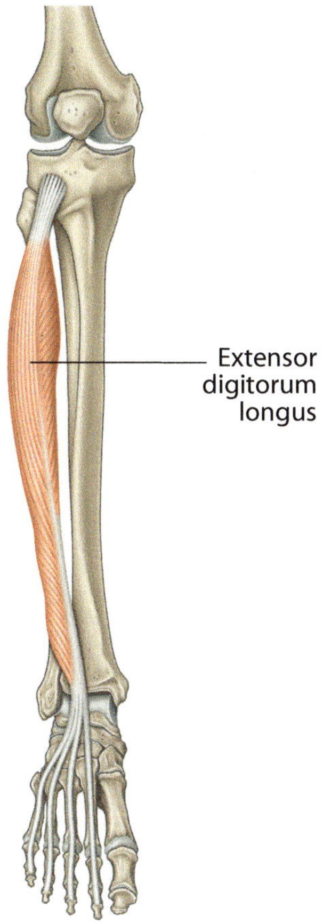

Fig. 24.21 Extensor digitorum longus muscle.

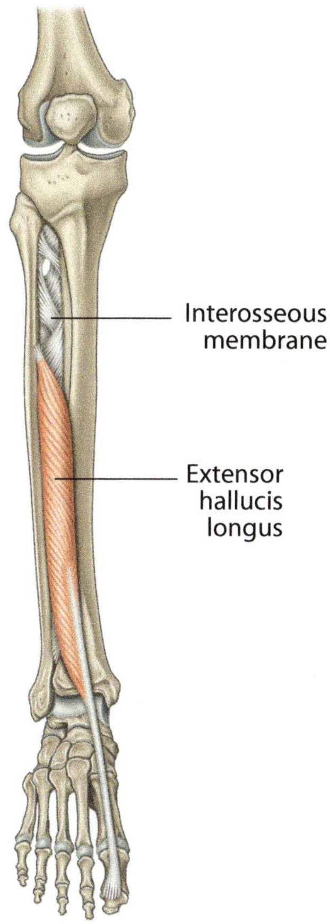

Fig. 24.22 Extensor hallucis longus muscle.

Innervation

- Deep fibular nerve (L5–S1)

Vascularization

- Anterior tibial artery

Actions

- Dorsal flexion of the foot and toes, working together with the tibialis anterior

24.6.3 Review—extensor hallucis longus (Fig. 24.22)

Origin

- Fibula on the medial surface
- Interosseous membrane

Direction and course

- It runs vertically and medially.
- The tendon glides under the superior and inferior extensor retinacula, running in its own synovial sheath.

Termination

- Hallux at its distal phalange

Innervation

- Deep fibular nerve (L4–S1)

Actions

- Creates dorsal flexion of the big toe and foot
- Assists with supination of the foot

24.6.4 Techniques

We have grouped the foot extensor together in the same section, as this makes sense in terms of treatment. Nevertheless there are some individual features worth emphasizing.

From lateral to medial they are arranged:

- extensor digitorum longus;
- extensor halluces;
- tibialis anterior.

We begin our manipulations at their distal parts and move progressively toward their proximal insertions.

Retinacula in decubitus (Figs. 24.23 and 24.24)

Sit at the end of the table with the patient's foot resting on your thigh. Gradually progress along the superior and inferior fibular retinacula until you reach the inferior and superior extensor retinacula. Glide the retinacula to discover any adhesions. Next, fix small areas overlaying the different tendons and ask the patient to perform a few dorsal flexions to increase the stretch. Frequently, only one tendon is restricted while the others glide easily. Proceed with small gliding- inductions.

Musculotendinous junction (Fig. 24.25)

This muscle-tendon junction is treated in the same position as above, with the patient's foot resting on the table, his leg a little more flexed. Glide one of your thumbs along the extensor tendons, starting just above the superior retinaculum. Pass first between the tibialis anterior and extensor digitorum longus. Then pass between the extensor digitorum longus and extensor hallucis longus.

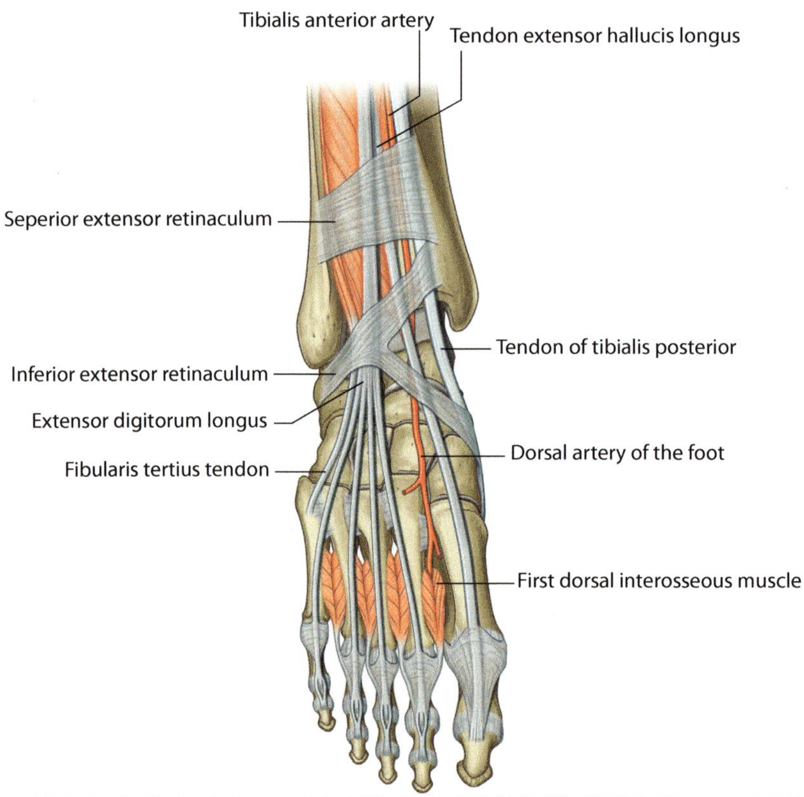

Fig. 24.23 Extensor retinacula.

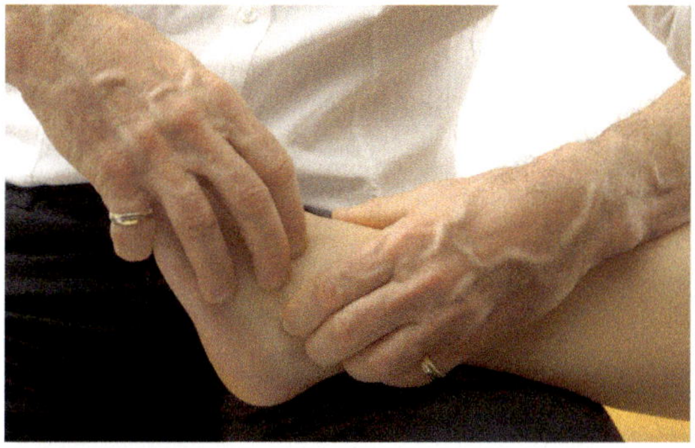

Fig. 24.24 Manipulation of extensor retinacula.

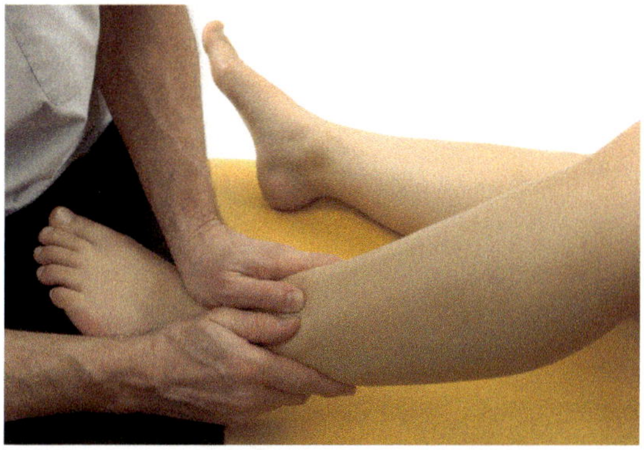

Fig. 24.25 Manipulation of musculotendinous junction of extensor muscles.

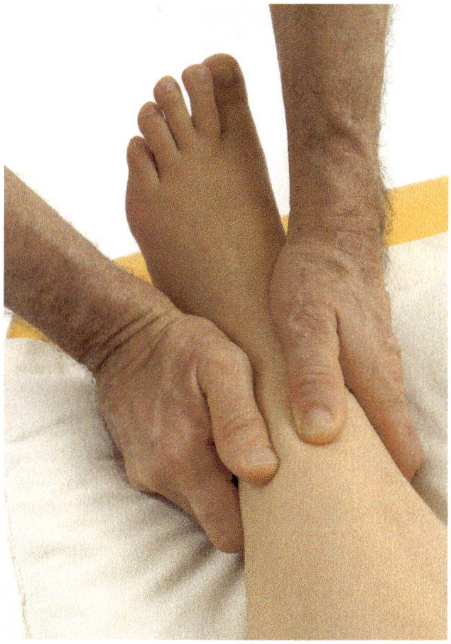

Fig. 24.26 Manipulation of interosseous membrane of extensor muscles.

Next, separate each muscle at the level of the musculotendinous junctions by maintaining separation-induction for several seconds.

This technique applies to people who participate in activities that demand intense muscle work, such as hiking, running, or jumping, and in the aftermath of tibia or fibula fracture. You can encounter musculo-aponeurotic constraints related to these musculotendinous junctions at the deep or superficial fibular nerves.

Proximal insertions

Interosseous membrane in decubitus (Fig. 24.26)

The three extensor muscles attach to the proximal part of the interosseous membrane. Manipulation of the distal tibiofibular junction has been described previously.

The patient rests on the table, leg outstretched, heel placed on a fairly flat cushion. Place one of your palms on the head of the fibula, the other on the neighboring tibia, and your fingers on the posterior leg. Carry out sagittal shearing movements. As you anteriorize the tibia, posteriorize the fibula and vice versa. Progress distally. When you find areas of reduced mobility, mobilize them by shearing-induction.

Fibular head: a special zone

Extensor digitorum longus fibers arise from the head of the fibula. Other muscle fibers merge with the tibialis anterior insertion on the lateral condyle of the tibia (Fig. 24.27).

The head of the fibula is a strategic zone that:

- offers an attachment for the:
  - fibular collateral ligament;
  - biceps femoris;
  - tibiofibular capsule;
  - fibularis longus;
  - soleus;
  - extensor digitorum longus (Fig. 24.21).
- relates to the fibular nerve;
- is very near the anterior tibial artery;

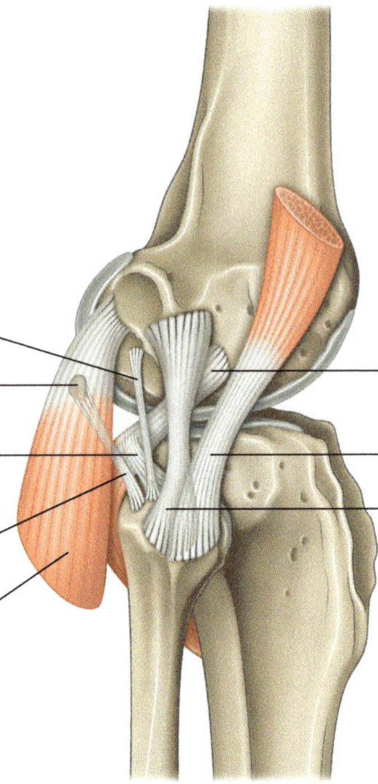

Fig. 24.27 Manipulation of interosseous membrane of extensor muscles.

- reflexogenically carries projections from the intestines and the bladder.

It is the "display case" of numerous fixations, sometimes causal or merely symptomatic, of ascending or descending imbalances.

Technique for the fibular head in decubitus (Fig. 24.28)

Search with your thumb along the tibial and fibular attachments of the extensor digitorum longus while your patient extends his toes. Note fixations of any other elements surrounding the fibular head. Treat the muscle insertions in sanding-induction. Also investigate the fibular attachments of the fibularis longus and biceps femoris.

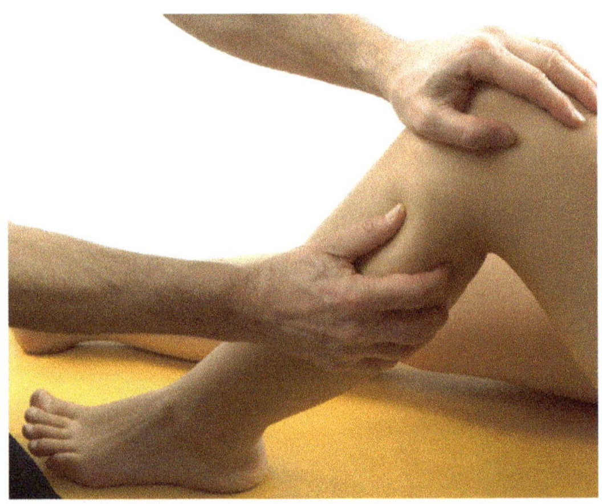

Fig. 24.28 Manipulation of the fibular head.

Treatment of the passive stabilizers

25

25.1 RETROMALLEOLAR GROOVES

It is possible to rapidly evaluate and treat all the tendons passing through the retromalleolar grooves. Fixations here are oftentimes numerous, to say nothing of their repercussions on the tendinous gliding systems.

25.1.1 Techniques

Topographical landmarks

Lateral retromalleolar grooves (Fig. 25.1)

From front to back we find the superior fibular retinaculum, fibularis brevis, and fibularis longus.

Medial retromalleolar grooves

From front to back we find the tibialis posterior, flexor digitorum longus, and flexor hallucis longus.

25.1.2 Achilles tendon

After inspecting and treating the retromalleolar grooves, move the Achilles tendon transversely with your thumbs. Next, follow along the medial and lateral borders, looking for any small, lumpy areas that you can then smooth out with induction.

Global test and technique in procubitus

The patient lies on the table, knee flexed. Begin by inspecting the retromalleolar

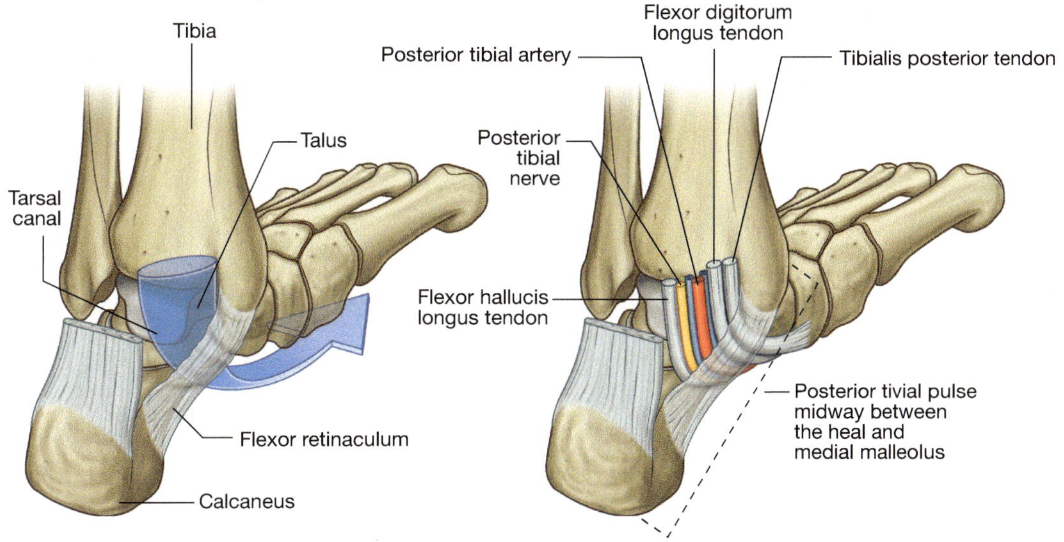

Fig. 25.1 Ankle joint (talocrural joint).

grooves individually. With experience you can assess them at the same time. Use your thumbs to glide the tendons longitudinally and transversely in the retromalleolar grooves to detect any possible fixations. Stretch the tendons directly and follow with stretch-induction. Combine flexion-extension and pronosupination of the foot to highlight the course of the tendons.

Technique in procubitus (Fig. 25.2)

Stand at the end of the table. The patient lies facedown with the plantar surface of his foot against your belly. This position leaves your hands free and allows you to create dorsal and plantar flexion movements with your body. Glide your thumbs meticulously along the retromalleolar grooves, both longitudinally and transversely.

First treat the restricted areas directly and follow up with induction. This manipulation is accompanied by flexion-extension of the ankle to amplify tendon tension. This excellent technique is not tiring and is a perfect way to inspect and treat all six tendons and their retinaculum at the same time.

Synovial sheaths

All flexor and extensor tendons cross the ankle joint. They are surrounded by synovial sheathes that pass beneath the retinacula and keep the tendons from being displaced. Treat these sheathes by stretching the tendons longitudinally or transversely, maintaining the stretch for 12 seconds.

25.2 FASCIA OF THE LEG AND FOOT

While a great many fascial techniques exist for the leg and foot, the fascia often spontaneously releases when you release muscles, ligaments, capsules, nerves, and arteries. There are, however, a few key points to be routinely checked and treated.

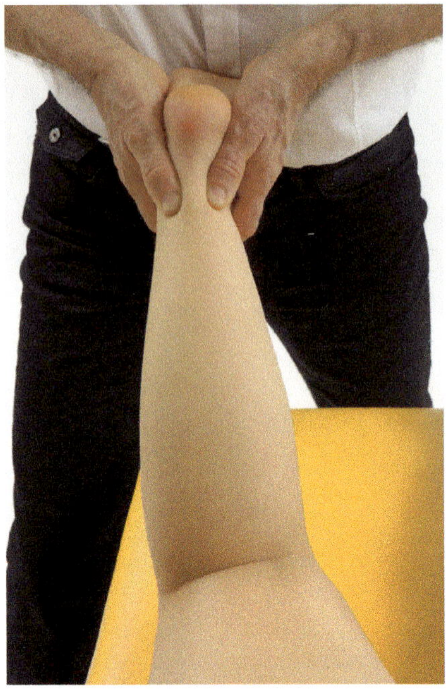

Fig. 25.2 Distal radioulnar articulation technique.

25.2.1 Review

Crural fascia

The deep fascia of the entire leg is continuous with the fascia lata through the intermediary of the popliteal fascia.

Iliotibial tract

We have described the iliotibial band in the hip and knee chapters. This thickening of the fascia lata, which inserts on the lateral tibial condyle on the infracondylar tubercle of Gerdy, is one of the first points to check.

Anterior lateral surface

Here we find the fibular muscles and their musculotendinous junction. The superficial fibular nerve pierces this depression in the leg. Manipulating this nerve releases the entire lateral surface of the crural fascia. Laterally the crural fascia is reinforced by the fibular retinaculum, whose manipulation is described above.

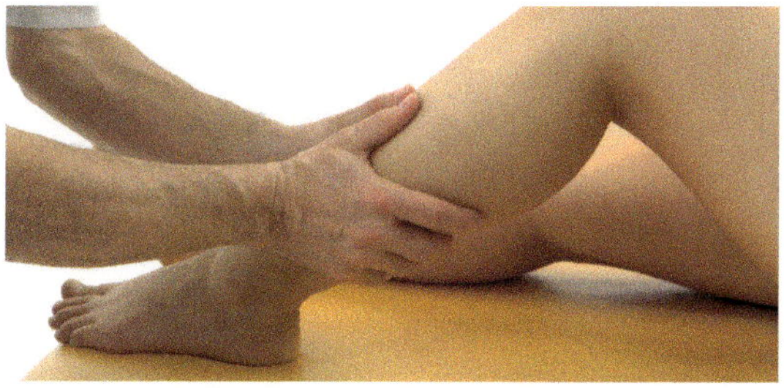

Fig. 25.3 Crural fascia technique.

Anterior medial surface

The crural fascia is also reinforced distally by the extensor retinaculum. It is important to follow the great saphenous vein up the leg to discover any fascial restrictions.

Dorsal surface

The fascia here is thinner than it is anteriorly. The best results in the leg are obtained in the area facing the tendinous arch of soleus. Perforating fibers of the sural cutaneous nerve cross the musculocutaneous junction of the gastrocnemius along this surface.

25.2.2 Technique in decubitus (Fig. 25.3)

Apply punctiform compression-induction and stretch-induction neural techniques on the main perforating sensory nerve threads as they pierce through fascial dips. Surround the crural fascia with both hands and manipulate it with clockwise and counterclockwise rotation-induction wherever you find fixations.

Special note

As we emphasized previously, these techniques are to be done at the end of a treatment session, with the aim of globally harmonizing tissues. Diagnosis is done by listening; treatment is done through induction; and re-evaluation is performed by a new listening. If the treatment is successful, the hand will quiet; there is no listening.

Treatment of the gliding apparatus

26

26.1 CHONDRAL POLISHING

26.1.1 Precision

The goal of polishing techniques is to smooth cartilage surfaces. The approach makes joints more functional by creating movement on the different subsystems that make up any given articulation.

While the word polishing may seem to be a misnomer, it accurately describes what our hands are doing as they "iron out" chondral surfaces. The gliding subsystem benefits the cartilage surface when we compress the joint cavity to act on the interface between fluid content and the joint surfaces.

Furthermore, chronic foot and ankle pain can destabilize all informational parameters of the foot. Synovial fluid and intra-articular pressure are part of information gathering. Cartilage gliding work affects joint position sense, even if cartilage itself is devoid of innervation.

26.1.2 Technique in procubitus

The patient lies facedown, knee flexed. You are situated on the same side as the foot to be treated. Place your hands one on top of the other over the plantar surface of the foot. To increase pressure transmitted to different cartilages, press your thorax against your hands. Creating movement with phases of compression-decompression mobilizes the foot alternately in flexion and extension, inversion and eversion.

Proceed slowly and softly. Without using force, simply feel for the sensation that your hands are "unwrinkling" the chondral surfaces. In chronic conditions, as with arthritis, you might perceive rough spots on the gliding surfaces that cause a "raspy" noise when mobilizing the joint.

Treatment of the osseous elements

27

The long bones of the leg are foremost in memorizing traumatic mechanical tensions. The intermediate part of the tibia remembers best at the ankle. With the fibula, the distal part is more involved. Mechanical tensions land proximally, mainly on the fibular head and the tibiofibular joint (Fig. 27.1). For whatever reason, intraosseous techniques are less effective for the fibula than for the tibia.

27.1 TECHNIQUES

27.1.1 Tibia in decubitus

The subject lies on his back, leg outstretched, heel resting on a small cushion (if the exam table is overly firm). Approach the bone either sagittally or transversely.

First method: sagittal (Fig. 27.2)

Stand beside the leg to be treated such that the weight of your body can fall over the palm of your hand. Starting from the distal tibia, exert sagittal pressure through your palms along the anterior border of the tibia. Stay somewhat on the bone to avoid irritating the sharp edge of the anterior surface.

The pressure is progressive and painless. Little by little you will feel elasticity variations through the bone. The tibia has an excellent memory for trauma, particularly fractures and knee or ankle sprains. In athletes, a direct kick to the tibia leaves an imprint.

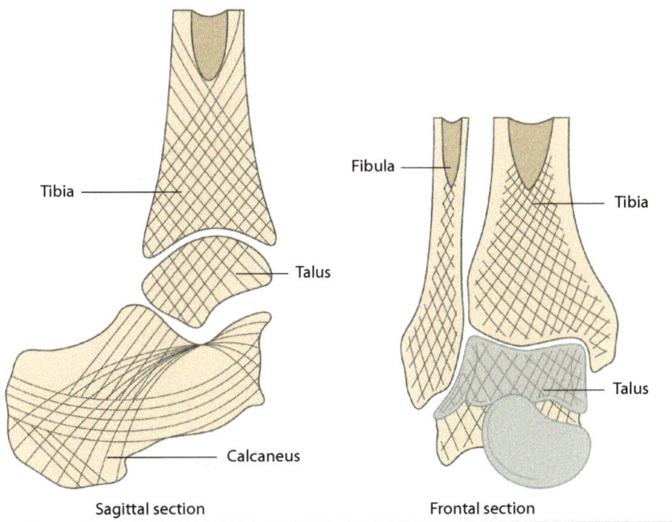

Fig. 27.1 Structures of the ankle.

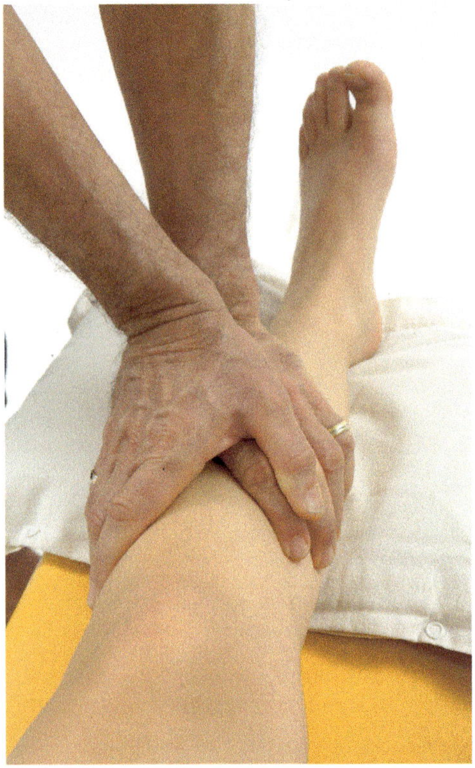

Fig. 27.2 Sagittal interosseous manipulation of the tibia.

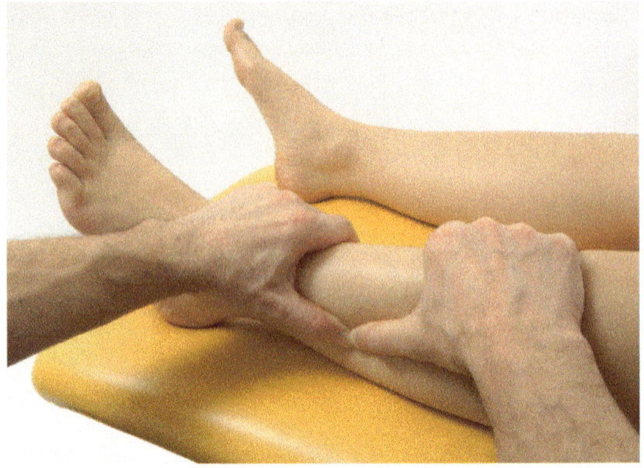

Fig. 27.3 Transversal interosseous manipulation of the tibia.

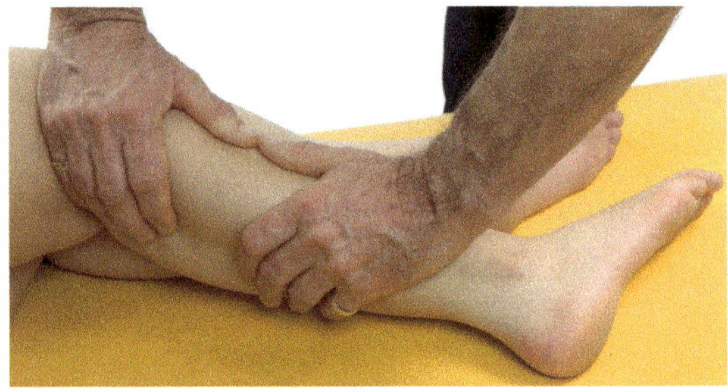

Fig. 27.4 Interosseous manipulation of the fibula.

With one hand on top of the other, apply force progressively, never uncomfortably, on the indurated part of the bone. The technique is done in induction. Practitioners are generally astonished at the degree to which elasticity can change through the course of treatment.

Second method: transversely (Fig. 27.3)

This time, situate yourself facing the leg in question. Place your fingers on the medial surface of the tibia and your thumbs on the outer leg. While one thumb pushes the lateral surface of the tibia medially, the fingers of your other hand draw the tibia laterally.

Practice this maneuver on the tibia and the fibula. The fibular muscles prevent you from making direct contact with the fibula. Their natural give can slightly distort your sense of osseous elasticity. With practice, however, you can easily tell the difference between boney and musculoligamentous elasticity.

27.1.2 Distal fibula in lateral decubitus (Fig. 27.4)

In our experience, almost every ankle sprain in the distal supramalleolar part of the fibula loses elasticity.

The patient lies on the side opposite the leg to be treated. You are facing the patient. Use your thumbs to apply gentle transversal compression to the fibula while maintaining a small measure of axial traction. Proceed as for the tibia.

Our goal is not merely the restoration of osseous elasticity but to facilitate bones in recovering their proprioceptive function.

Treatment of the forefoot and plantar region

28

28.1 TREATMENT OF THE PLANTAR REGION

This section focuses on musculoaponeurotic formations chosen for their importance to the informational system and for their frequency of injury. While other muscles and their aponeuroses are certainly worthy of interest depending on different foot lesions, our techniques simply are not efficacious in their treatment.

An example is large bands of thick connective tissue such as the plantar fascia. We do not deny their stabilizing and dynamic functions for the foot; rather, we find that these passive structures are mainly adaptable to broader myofascial chains.

28.1.1 Plantar fat

We have noted in previous chapters that fat plays a considerable role in cushioning the foot from pressure. Without it the balls of the foot would continually suffer injury. Fat is stabilized and supported by the plantar aponeurosis, which is compartmentalized by the medial and lateral septa and by the various muscles we studied in previous chapters.

Every nook and cranny of the plantar region should be investigated for anything that might destroy or displace this protective fatty layer. Fibrosis of any small, seemingly out-of-the-way part of the fat cushion can destabilize the informational system and cause its shock absorption abilities to deteriorate.

28.1.2 Dorsal foot muscles

There are basic differences between the muscles of the back of the foot and those on the arch. Plantar muscles operate under enormous mechanical constraint, up to six or seven times body weight, depending on body position or physical activity.

Manipulation of the dorsal muscles, which are fewer in number, produces very little general effect, except to the extent that they form part of the overall foot complex. It is nevertheless important to check for any adhesions or scars, because they disturb information generated from the feet.

Dorsal muscles help form the plantar arch by creating what is called the winch effect on the sole of the foot (Fig. 28.1). The plantar aponeurosis is tensed in toe extension. This has the effect of drawing the anterior and posterior plantar contacts closer, resulting in the plantar arch.

The metatarsophalangeal joints function like a winch whose crank is represented by the toes. This system functions equally well in passive and active toe extension.

This mechanism clearly shows that it is pointless to divide the foot into different compartments. The strength and dynamism of the foot depend on the ligamentous muscular and osseous systems. The 26 bones in each foot need to be considered. When you tell patients that out of 206 total skeletal bones 52 are in the feet, they are generally astounded.

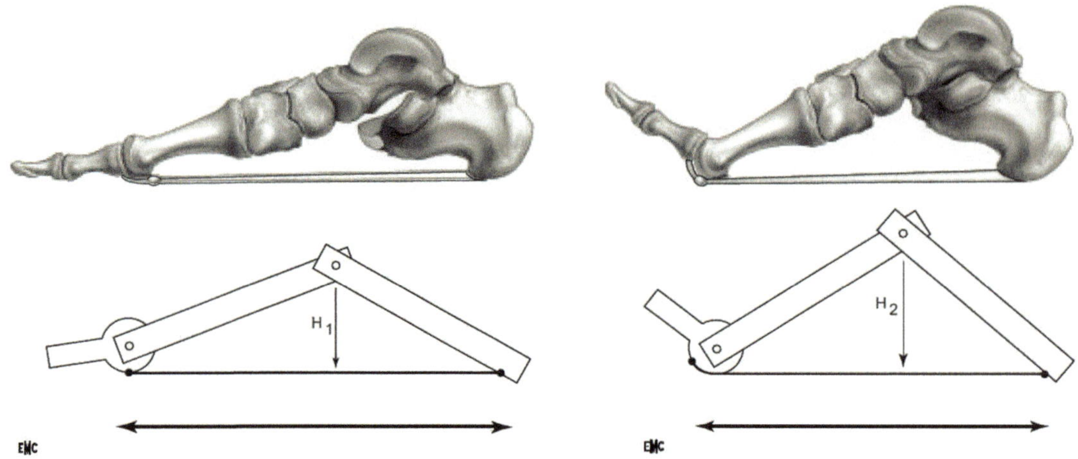

Fig. 28.1 Plantar arch windlass effect. When the great toe dorsiflexes, plantar elements are tensed, resulting in elevation of the internal arch and a shortening of the foot by way of the Hicks pulley mechanism. This effect is used clinically to assess reducibility of the flat foot. (N. Biga, D. Mouliès, and C. Mabit. 1999. "Static flat valgus foot [including congenital synostosis]." EMC Musculoskeletal system 14-110-A-10: 1–10. Paris: Elsevier Masson. All rights reserved.)

28.1.3 What of the 26 bones of the foot?

Numerous traditional osteopathic manuals describe excellent joint manipulations for the foot. We have little to add to this cadre. Their effects are undeniable in terms of the capsules, ligaments, and small muscles of the foot. The question is whether they work on joint fixations or whether genuine boney displacements even exist.

Apart from intraosseous techniques, osteopaths rarely treat bones themselves. For the most part our actions concern the soft tissues that attach to bones. Nevertheless, we have seen many patients in severe foot pain, in which genuine metatarsal and phalangeal microdisplacements were discovered.

You can sometimes feel very clearly when bones reposition themselves as they glide back into proper alignment. Musculoskeletal tensions are perhaps the first to cause and maintain this type of microgliding. By the time the small bone is out of place, however, repositioning it can release the neighboring soft tissues. Thus we must consider it both ways.

28.1.4 Key muscles of the plantar region

The plantar arch comprises numerous elements that allow the foot to bear considerable weight. We have devoted many years to determining the best way to stimulate the proprioceptive system to make foot pain go away. We have had the most success with the insertions of the following structures:

- fibularis longus;
- tibialis posterior;
- adductor hallucis;
- abductor hallucis;
- flexor hallucis brevis.

28.1.5 Fibularis longus

Review: tendinous groove of the cuboid (Fig. 28.2)

A fibrous sulcus houses the fibularis longus tendon, which continues under the foot to attach to the tuberosity of the first metatarsal and medial cuneiform.

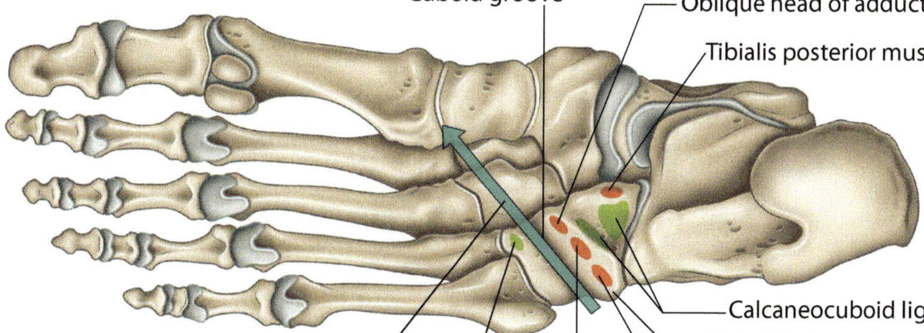

Fig. 28.2 Tendinous groove of cuboid.

Technique in procubitus (Fig. 28.3)

The patient lies facedown, knee flexed. Place one of your thumbs on the fibular trochlea of the calcaneus and the other on the fibrous peroneal groove of the cuboid. Stretch the tendon by moving the foot in pronation/supination. Next, use your thumb to release any hardened areas you encounter on the fibrous cuboid canal. Finally, work the attachments of the first metatarsal and medial cuneiform. To feel the tendon clearly, ask the patient to pronate the foot several times.

28.1.6 Tibialis posterior

Review: navicular tuberosity

The main tibialis posterior tendon inserts into the navicular tuberosity. The plantar portions insert onto the three cuneiform bones (Fig. 28.4).

Technique in procubitus

The patient lies facedown, knee flexed. Place one thumb between the sustenaculum tali and the navicular tuberosity while the other thumb also contacts the navicular. Effect a compression-induction on any roughened areas where there is reduced gliding. Proceed in the same fashion for the cuneiform attachments.

28.1.7 Adductor hallucis (Fig. 28.5)

Review

The adductor has two different insertions and plays a key role in supporting the medial arch. The adductor hallucis arises by two heads, an oblique and a transverse.

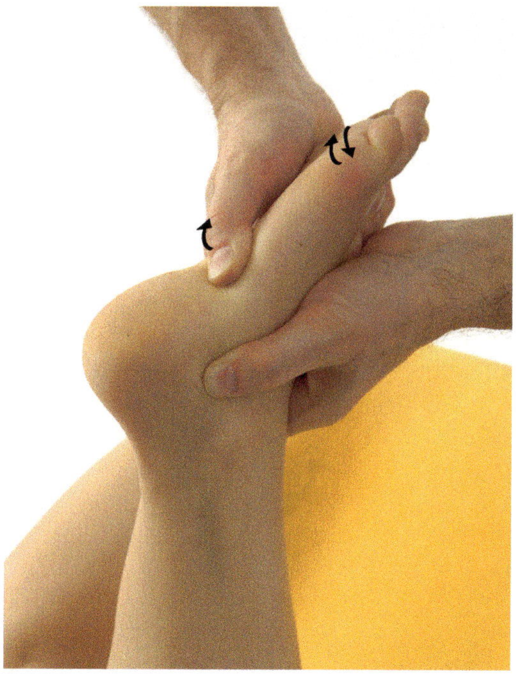

Fig. 28.3 Fibularis longus technique at the plantar arch.

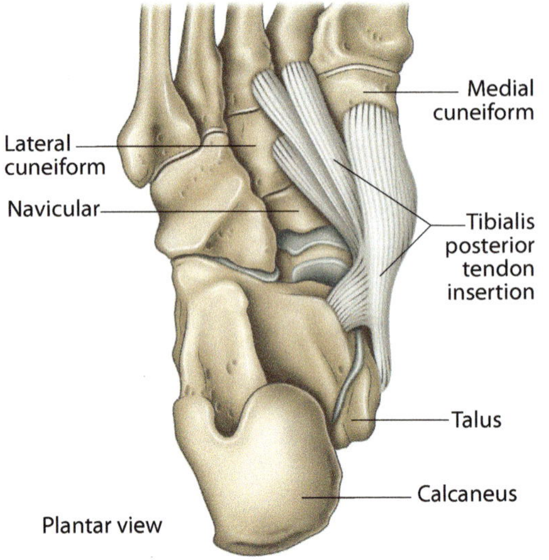

Fig. 28.4 Distal attachments of the tibialis posterior.

Oblique head

The oblique head attaches on:

- the cuboid;
- the lateral cuneiform;
- the second and third metatarsals (sometimes the fourth).

It often exchanges fibers with the calcaneocuboid ligament, fibularis longus, and flexor hallucis brevis. The oblique head defends the ankle against sprain. It is a plantar arch tensor and adducts the great toe.

Transverse head

The transverse head arises from the third, fourth, and fifth metatarsophalangeal joints and the deep transverse ligament. The two heads converge at the lateral sesamoid bone of the great toe. Note that the medial sesamoid of the first metatarsal serves as an attachment for the adductor hallucis and flexor hallucis brevis.

Technique in procubitus (Fig. 28.6)

The patient lies facedown, knee flexed. Hollow out the plantar arch by folding the foot with one hand, bringing the medial and lateral borders of the feet together. Your other thumb searches out the insertions of the adductor hallucis on the plantar surface of the cuboid and lateral cuneiform. It also searches out the bases of the second and third metatarsals. Work the tendons with induction.

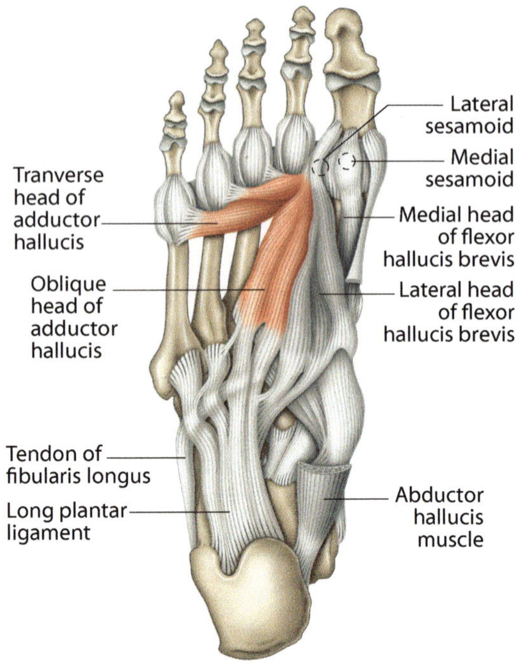

Fig. 28.5 Adductor hallucis.

Next, move the thumb in the direction of the distal extremities of the third, fourth, and fifth metatarsals. Work the insertions in induction. Finally, manipulate the terminal insertion on the lateral sesamoid bone of the great toe, located directly beneath the lateral aspect of head of the first metatarsal.

28.1.8 Abductor hallucis (Fig. 28.7)

Review

The abductor hallucis muscle inserts onto:

- the calcaneal tuberosity;
- the flexor retinaculum;
- the plantar aponeurosis.

The abductor hallucis forms the tendinous arch that attaches to the medial sesamoid

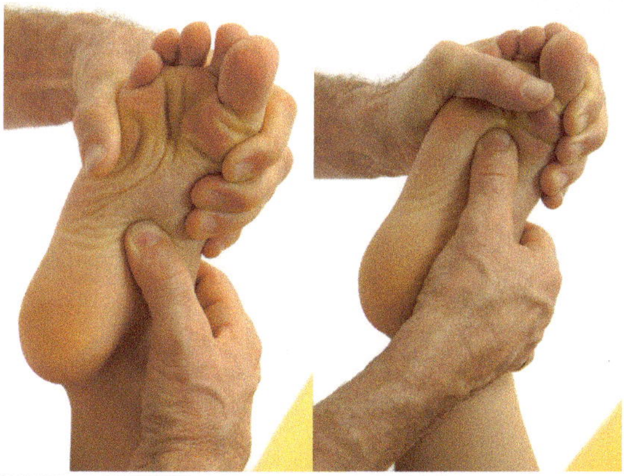

Fig. 28.6 Manipulation of adductor hallucis.

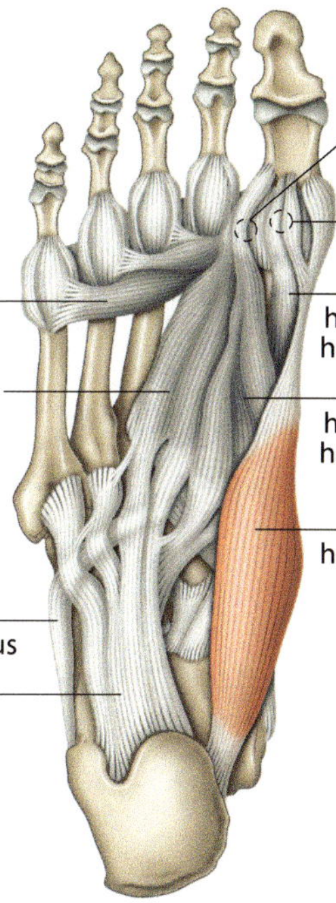

Fig. 28.7 Aductor hallucis.

bone and to the base of the first proximal phalange. It merges with the flexor hallucis brevis into a common tendon.

Note that the following insert onto the sesamoids of the first metatarsal:

- adductor hallucis;
- abductor hallucis;
- flexor hallucis brevis.

This makes it a key element in arch support and foot proprioception.

Technique in procubitus (Fig. 28.8)

The patient lies facedown, knee flexed. Place one of your thumbs on the calcaneal tuberosity (medial part of the calcaneus) and the other on the medial sesamoid of the first metatarsal. Stretch the two insertions distally, diminishing the plantar arch concavity. Work the muscle in induction.

28.1.9 Flexor hallucis brevis (Fig. 28.9)

Review

The flexor hallucis brevis inserts onto:

- the medial cuneiform;
- the long plantar ligament;
- the tibialis posterior tendon.

It terminates by two portions:

- The medial head:
  - abductor hallucis;
  - medial sesamoid of the first metatarsal;
  - first proximal phalange.
- The lateral head:
  - adductor hallucis;
  - lateral sesamoid;
  - Ffirst proximal phalange.

Runners (particularly sprinters) and ballet dancers are prone to injuring this muscle. The flexor hallucis brevis flexes the great toe, enabling dancers to stand on pointe.

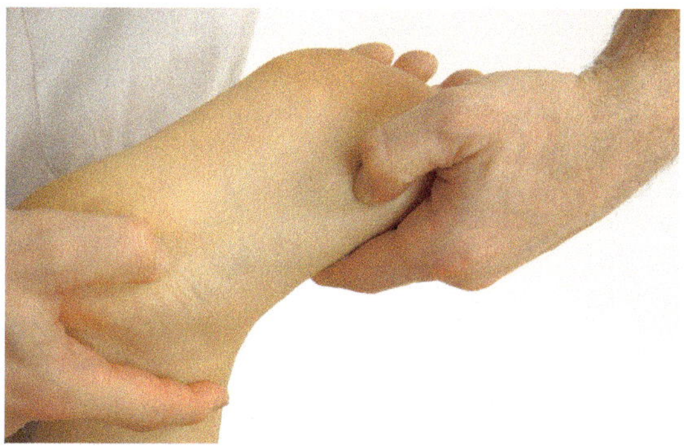

Fig. 28.8 Manipulation of abductor hallucis.

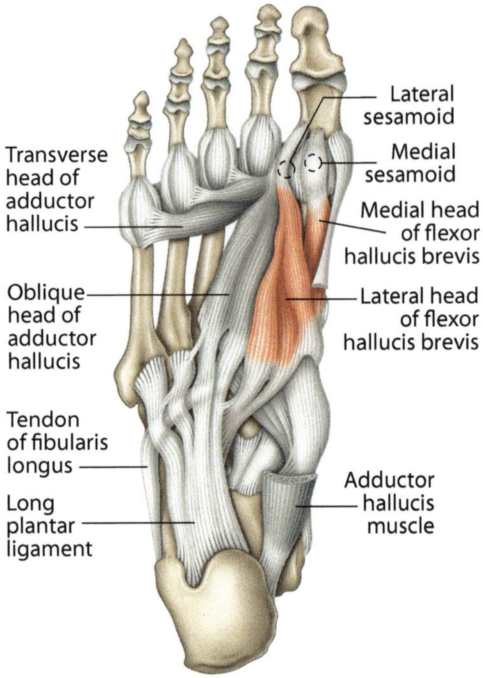

Fig. 28.9 Adductor hallucis.

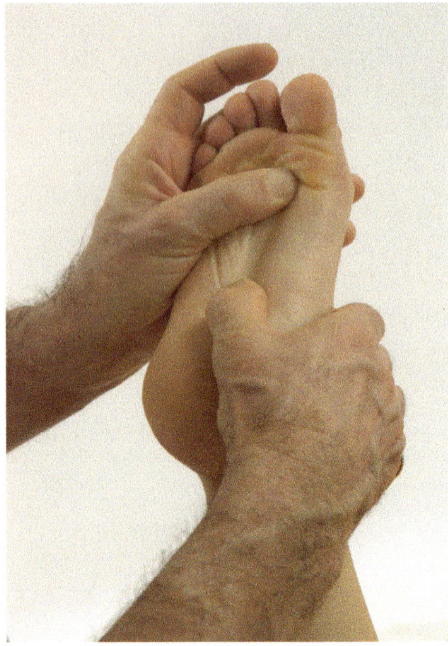

Fig. 28.10 Manipulation of flexor hallucis brevis.

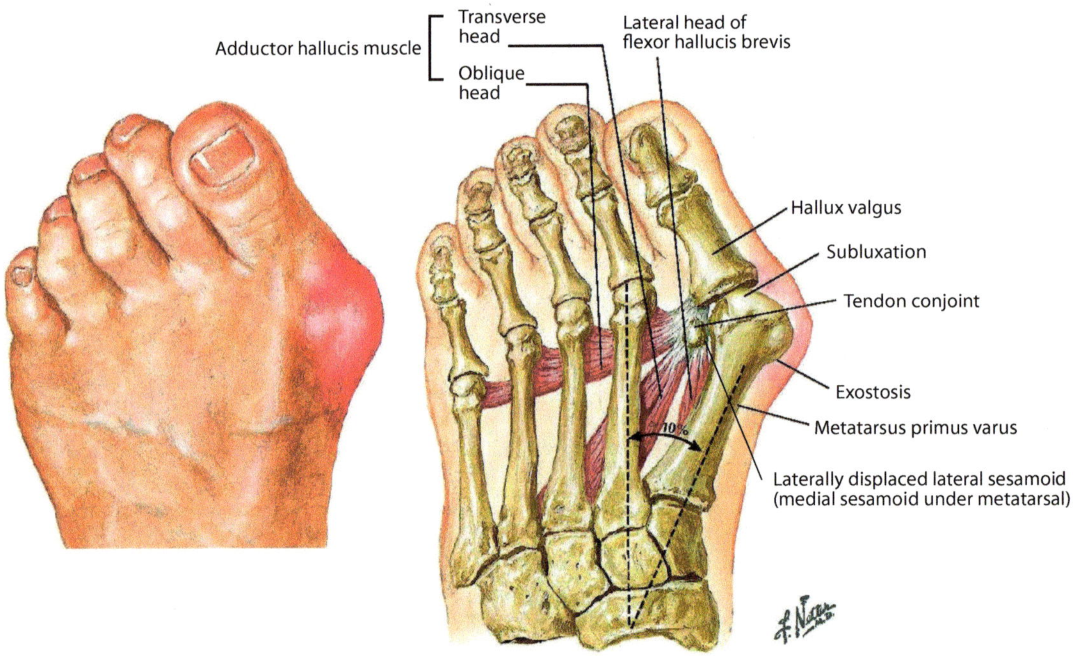

Fig. 28.11 Advanced hallux valgus. (After Walter Greene, ed., Netter's Orthopaedics, 44. Used with permission of the editor.)

Technique in procubitus (Fig. 28.10)

The patient lies facedown, knee flexed. Place one of your thumbs on the medial cuneiform just in front of the navicular. Position your other thumb on the lateral and medial sesamoids of the first metatarsal. Glide the insertions medially and laterally while rotating the foot with small amounts of abduction and adduction of the cuneiform, first metatarsal, and proximal phalangeal axis.

28.2 TREATMENT OF THE HALLUX VALGUS (FIG. 28.11)

28.2.1 Review

The hallux veers laterally; the metatarsal deviates medially. This condition is often accompanied by subluxation of the metatarsophalangeal joint. Bunions can be congenital or acquired. They are much more common in women and are sometimes aggravated by menopause.

Pain can be excruciating, especially when associated with bursal inflammation. When the deviation makes it difficult to find shoes, and walking discomfort becomes severe, surgery is the main recourse.

28.2.2 Treatment

What can be done?

Let us be clear at the outset. Our action has no effect on the deviation angle, but it can significantly reduce pain. Hallux valgus raises intra-articular pressure. Changes in metatarsophalangeal joint pressure have synovial, cartilaginous, and neurovascular consequences.

Release neural tensions first

Nerves of the first metatarsophalangeal joint are:

- the deep fibular nerve;
- the medial dorsal nerve;
- the superficial fibular nerve.

Techniques

Deep fibular and medial dorsal cutaneous nerves in decubitus (Fig. 28.12)

The patient lies facedown, the foot resting either on your thigh or on the table. Place one finger on the medial border of the first metatarsal and glide along the dorsal aponeurosis of the foot until you come to a depression. Feel in this dip for a small fascial ring; this indicates the location of the deep fibular and medial dorsal cutaneous nerves. First, release the nerves by "enlarging" the depression and fascial collar. Next, perform a light compression-induction on the two nerves themselves.

Superficial fibular nerve

Release the lateral compartment of the leg. Refer to the earlier chapter pertaining to the musculotendinous junction of the fibularis longus and brevis through which the nerve passes. The superficial fibular nerve pierces the deep fascia of the leg and branches into the medial dorsal cutaneous nerve.

Metatarsophalangeal traction-induction (Fig. 28.13)

Once the nerves have been released, progressively traction the metatarsophalangeal distally. Once under traction, be careful to rotate and laterally flex only the joint, carefully following the direction of the listening, to avoid the risk of creating excruciating pain. After a few rounds you will feel the gradual return of pain-free metatarsophalangeal mobility.

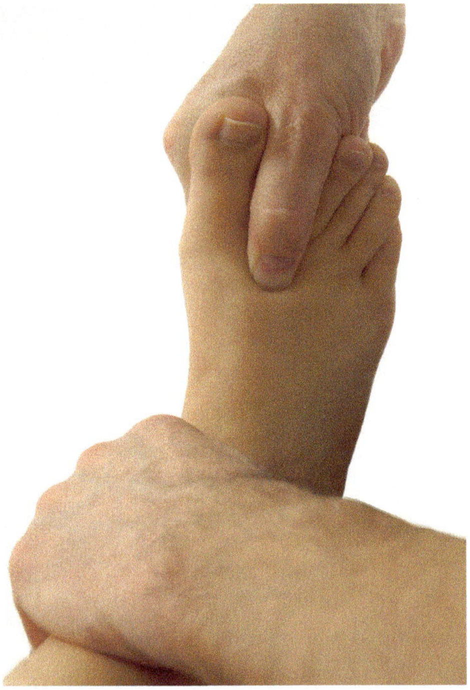

Fig. 28.12 Manipulation of the deep fibular nerves.

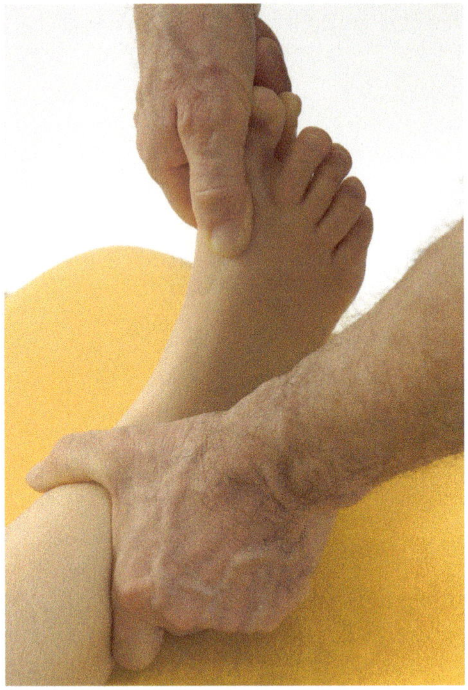

Fig. 28.13 Metatarsophalangeal traction-induction.

Neural manipulations

29

The nerves of the foot can be assembled into three groups:

- nerves of the anterior surface;
- nerves of the posterior surface;
- nerves of the plantar region.

29.1 NERVES OF THE ANTERIOR SURFACE OF THE FOOT (FIG. 29.1)

29.1.1 Leg

Superficial fibular nerve

We have studied the superficial fibular nerve located between the long and short fibular muscles at their musculotendinous junction. There is often a small depression where the nerve pierces the crural fascia between the muscles. The nerve is often surrounded by a fascial ring.

Saphenous nerve

We considered the saphenous nerve at the knee as it passes through the adductor (Hunter's) canal. It runs down the tibial side of the leg following the lateral surface of the great saphenous vein, where it is known as a "satellite."

Technique in decubitus

Trace your thumb down the lateral surface of the great saphenous vein. Apply small stretch-induction movements wherever you find sensitive points along the saphenous nerve.

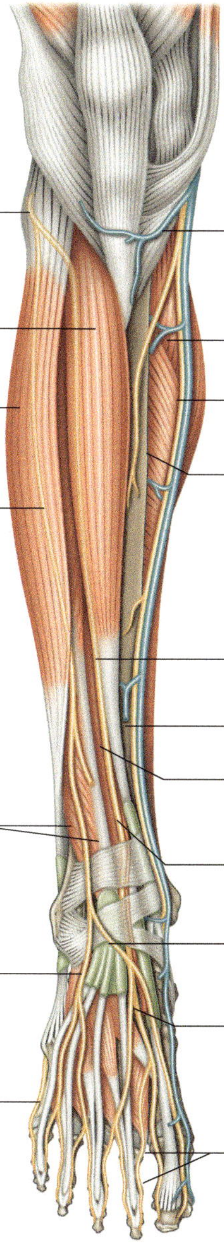

Fig. 29.1 Nerves of the anterior foot surface.

29.1.2 Foot

The anterior foot is rich in cutaneous nerve fibers that can be evaluated by gliding them up and down or side to side.

Saphenous nerve

Landmarks

Locate this nerve in front of the tibial malleolus. This is a key region for manipulating the saphenous nerve, which runs first along the lateral surface of the saphenous vein and then overlaps it.

> **Clinical note**
>
> The saphenous nerve ends before reaching the column of the first ray. This nerve is important because it happens to be a branch of the femoral nerve arising from the lumbar plexus, while all other branches to the foot come from the sciatic nerve arising from the sacral plexus.

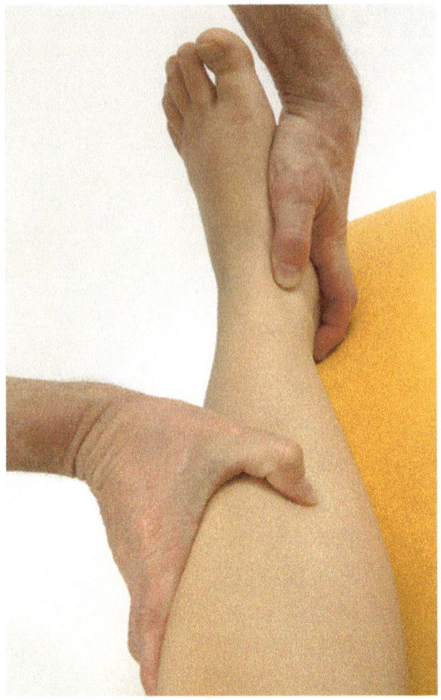

Fig. 29.2 Manipulation of the saphenous nerve at the instep and leg.

Technique in decubitus (Fig. 29.2)

Position yourself laterally to the foot in question. Use one hand to mobilize the foot several times in plantar flexion. Place the thumb of your other hand just below the painful or fixed part of the saphenous nerve. While moving the foot, directly glide the nerve distally and then in induction. The medial instep of the foot relates to the bladder and intestine, because of the saphenous connection to the femoral nerve.

Medial and intermediate dorsal cutaneous and nerves

Location

These branches of the superficial fibular nerve can be irritated by overly tight shoes, socks, or stockings that provoke acute neuralgia, particularly at the medial dorsal branch. The patient believes he might have sprained his ankle, but this is not usually the case.

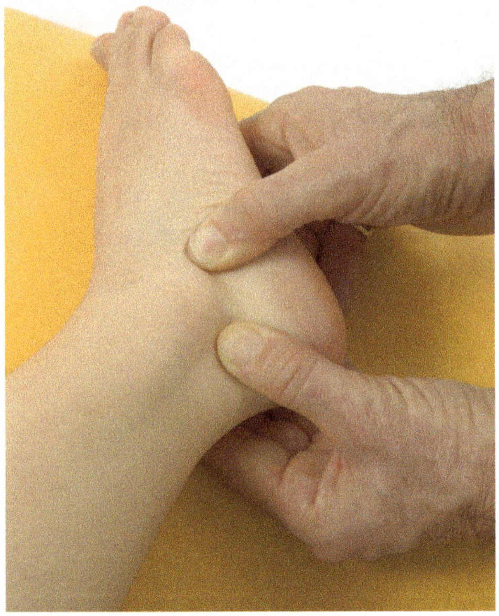

Fig. 29.3 Manipulation of the lateral dorsal cutaneous nerve.

Technique in decubitus

Position yourself beside the foot concerned. Place your thumb just below the painful parts of the nerve. Glide the nerve distally while simultaneously flexing the foot with your other hand.

Lateral dorsal cutaneous nerve

Location

The lateral dorsal cutaneous nerve is a continuation of the sural nerve that wraps around the fibular malleolus and courses to the fourth and fifth metatarsals. This nerve is of interest because it is located next to the fibular collateral ligaments. It is often sensitive and becomes indurated in the aftermath of ankle sprain. When the foot is blue following sprain, you can be sure this nerve has been injured.

Technique in lateral decubitus (Fig. 29.3)

The patient lies on the side opposite the lateral dorsal cutaneous nerve to be treated. You are situated behind him. Glide one finger under the distal end of the fibular malleolus, staying in contact with the bone. Glide your finger from front to back in search of a small indurated and sensitive nerve fiber that you can treat with induction.

Cutaneous manipulations

General principle

Cutaneous treatment involves tractioning the skin that overlays deep or cutaneous nerve branches. This rule applies to the foot in general, but three zones are of particular interest:

- beneath the fibular malleolus, where the lateral dorsal cutaneous runs;
- in front to the instep, for the dorsal cutaneous branch;
- between the first and second toes, to affect the deep fibular nerve that forms an anastomosis with the medial dorsal cutaneous nerve (description of this technique to follow).

Cutaneous technique for the deep fibular nerve performed in decubitus

The patient lies on the table, leg outstretched or slightly flexed. Stabilize the foot by placing one hand over the malleoli. Glide your other thumb or index finger between the first and second toes on the dorsal surface. Your thumb or index finger will come to a stop over a small fascial depression created by fibers of the dorsal fascia of the foot. The deep fibular nerve (Fig. 29.4) is surrounded here by a fascial bridge that is open distally.

First, lift the fascial bridge with your thumb or index finger and spread it open. This fascia is often compressed by shoes alone. The resulting dorsal foot pain makes no sense to patients who are searching in vain for a possible trauma that might have caused such painful neuralgia.

Next, treat the fascial bridge with compression-induction using a very light touch on the nerve.

> **Clinical note**
>
> There is often a relationship between intestinal problems and medial dorsal foot sensitivity. This correlation can be explained in part because the saphenous nerve branches from the femoral nerve that arises from the lumbar plexus.

29.2 NERVES OF THE POSTERIOR SURFACE OF THE FOOT

Treating the area behind the fibular malleolus is extremely beneficial. While several medial calcaneal branches run along the medial malleolus, these filaments, which derive from the tibial nerve, respond less to our techniques.

29.2.1 Retromalleolar fibular zone

Landmark (Fig. 29.5)

We pinpoint the lateral dorsal cutaneous nerve at the anterior lateral foot; we find it again just behind the fibular malleolus. If you

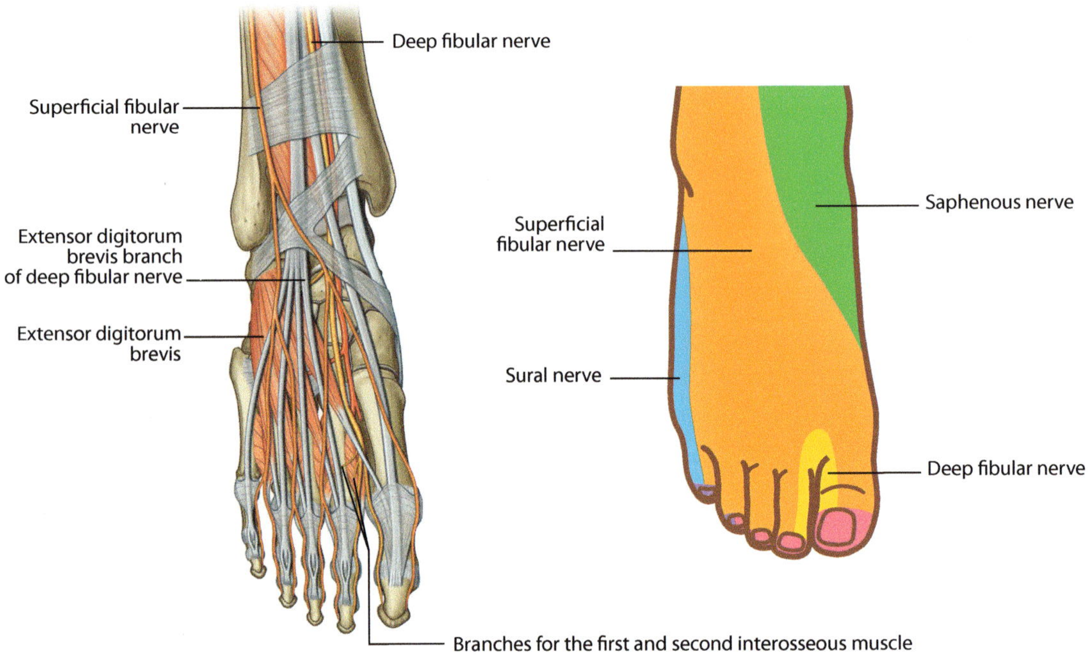

Fig. 29.4 Deep fibular nerve.

follow this nerve proximally you meet the sural nerve, which is its parent.

Technique in procubitus

The patient lies facedown on the table, his foot either just off the table or supported by a cushion. Glide your thumb behind the fibular malleolus and direct it toward the musculotendinous triceps junction.

You will easily feel the medial sural cutaneous nerve positioned against the lateral part of the Achilles tendon. Here you will find the anastomosis located between the medial sural cutaneous nerve and the fibular communicating nerves where they merge to form the sural nerve. This is a valuable area to release in combination with urogenital or intestinal treatment.

29.2.2 Retromalleolar tibial zone

Location (Fig. 29.6)

The posterior tibial nerve has significant influence on the foot. This nerve, by way of

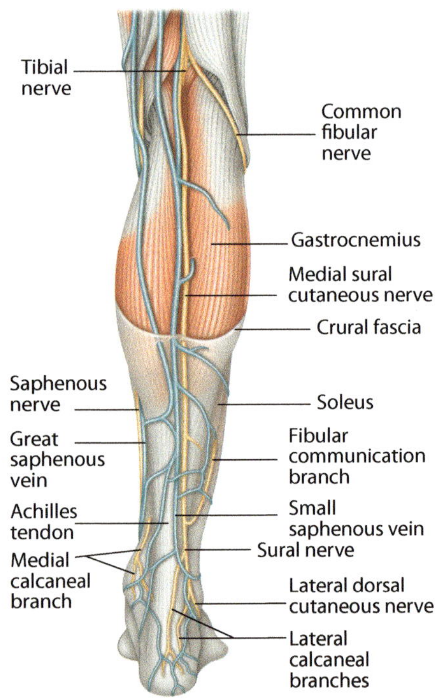

Fig. 29.5 Retrofibular posterior nerves.

Vascular manipulations

30

The foot receives its blood supply from two principal arteries, the anterior and posterior tibial vessels. The most effective arterial manipulations are performed on the large trunks, where the stretch-sensitive mechanoreceptors are most readily activated.

30.1 ANTERIOR TIBIAL ARTERY

30.1.1 Witness pulse: dorsal artery of the foot

The continuation of the anterior tibial artery (Fig. 30.1) on the dorsal surface of the

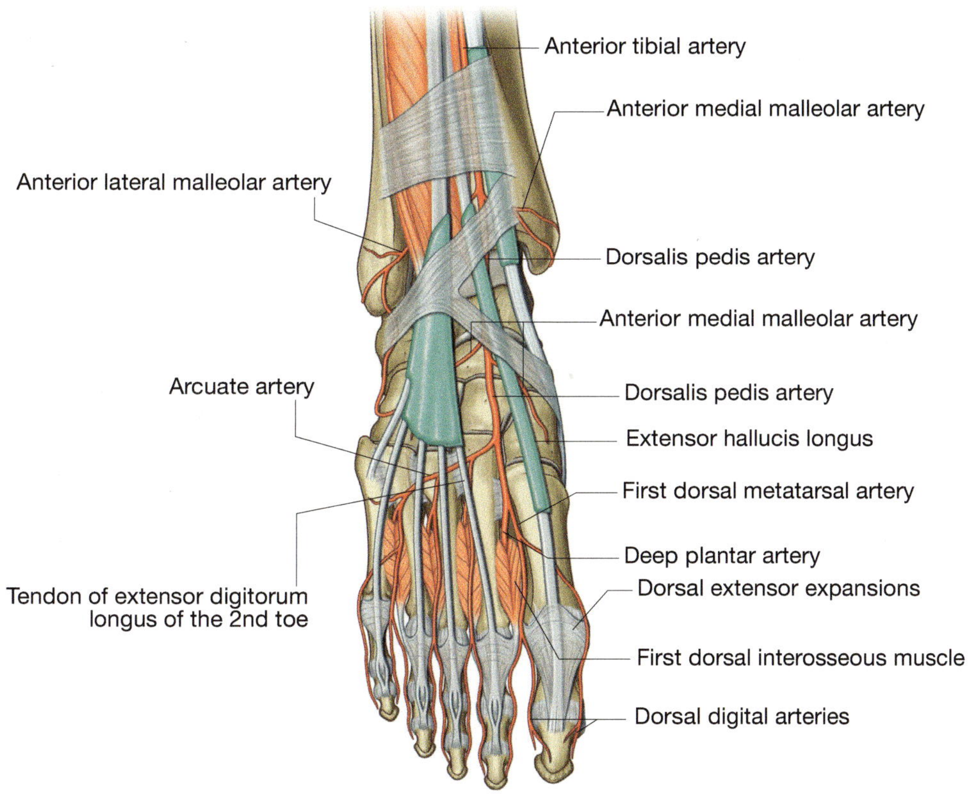

Fig. 30.1 Dorsal artery of the foot.

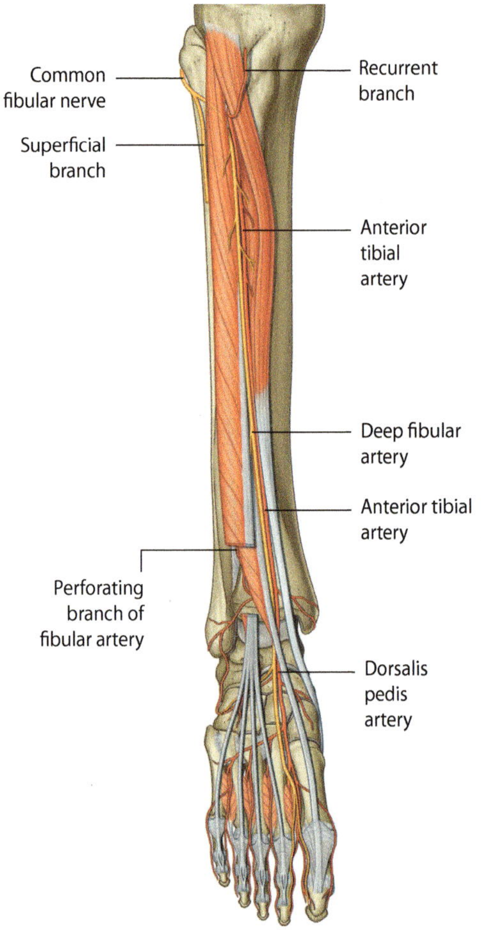

Fig. 30.2 Dorsal anterior tibial arteries of the foot.

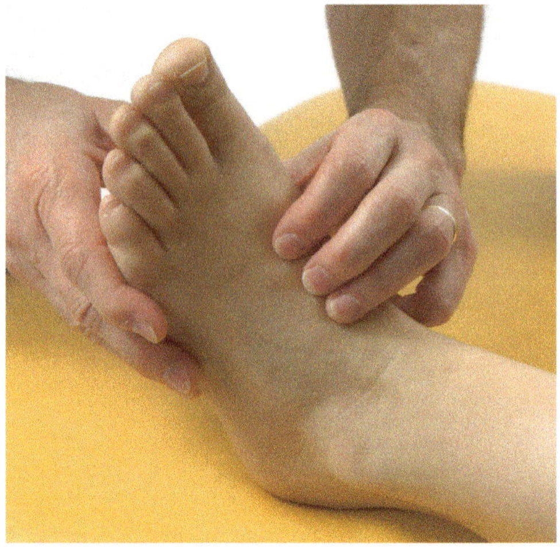

Fig. 30.3 Witness pulse of the dorsalis pedis artery.

foot is called the dorsalis pedis artery (Fig. 30.2). The pulse can be palpated on the back of the foot between the extensor hallucis and extensor digitorum muscles (Fig. 30.3).

Place two or three fingers delicately and very flat on the back of the foot, perpendicular to the course of the artery. Do not apply any pressure in order to sense the pulsations.

30.1.2 Technique

At the origin

Location

The anterior tibial artery reaches the anterior compartment of the leg through the proximal part of the interosseous space. In the anterior compartment it descends along the interosseous membrane, which is covered by the extensor muscles. It is not directly palpable at this juncture. It passes through an aperture in the upper border of the membrane called Hyrtle's fibrous tibial vessel canal (Tustut 1896). Here you can generally feel the pulse using a very light contact between the tibialis anterior and extensor digitorum, a little below the tibial prominence.

Technique (Fig. 30.4)

Once you have located the pulse, use your thumbs to perform spreading-induction maneuvers on either side of the pulsation. Focus on gently separating the tibialis anterior from the extensor digitorum.

Variation (Fig. 30.5)

You can check the effectiveness of your maneuver while manipulating the artery at its origin in the upper leg. Do this at the same time you are feeling variations in the witness pulse at the dorsalis pedis artery on the top of the foot.

Implications

The anterior tibial artery furnishes the major nourishing branches that supply the

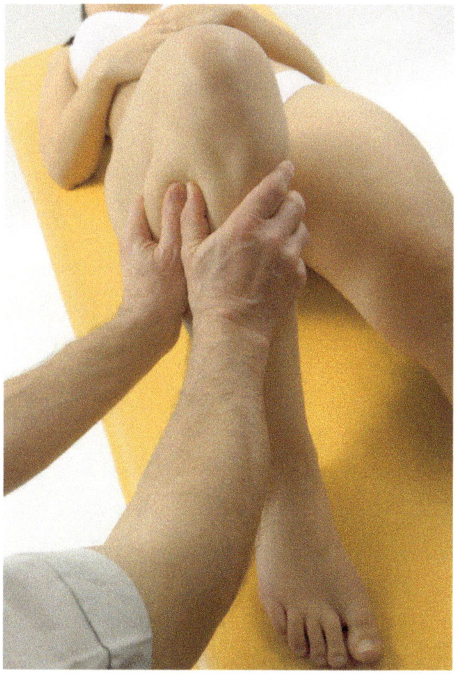

Fig. 30.4 Manipulation of the anterior tibial artery at its origin.

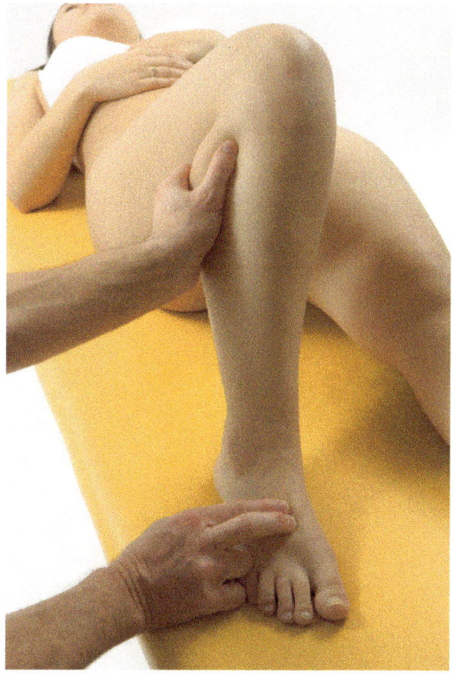

Fig. 30.5 Manipulation of the anterior tibial artery at its origin (variation).

lateral collateral ligament of the ankle joint. Function in the artery, as well as in veins and lymphatic channels, can be disturbed for a long time after trauma. In cases of significant residual ankle edema, notably in the aftermath of sprain, check the pulse of this artery at the Hyrtle canal. Any diminution indicates abnormal tension on the arterial pedicle.

If the pulse is weak, manipulate the artery at the leg. You will often find that swelling at the ankle clearly diminishes in the hours following the manipulation, even if you never touched the ankle itself. Always remember that good arterial circulation is essential to optimal scar healing and ligamentous reconstruction.

At the instep

Pinpointing the pulse

The best place to feel the anterior tibial pulse at the instep is either above the superior extensor retinaculum or below the inferior extensor retinaculum. The pulse is more difficult to feel here than at its posterior tibial counterpart.

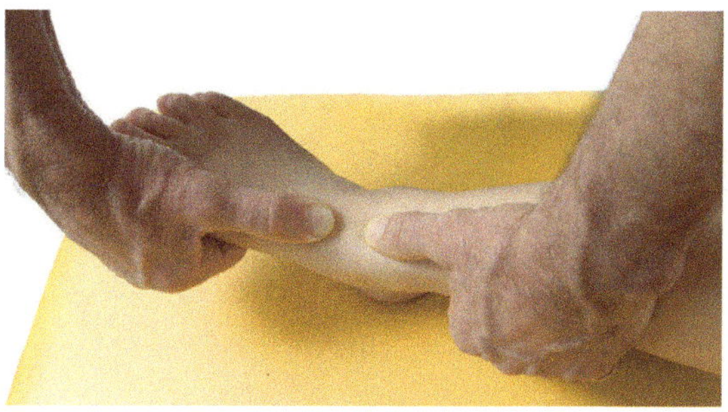

Fig. 30.6 Manipulation of the anterior tibial artery at the instep.

The anterior tibial artery is located:

- medially in relation to the extensor digitorum;
- laterally in relationship to the tibialis anterior and the deep fibular nerve.

It is easier to feel the artery if you first ask the patient to dorsiflex his foot. Place your index and middle fingers between the tibialis anterior and the extensor hallucis longus, and then ask the patient to relax his foot.

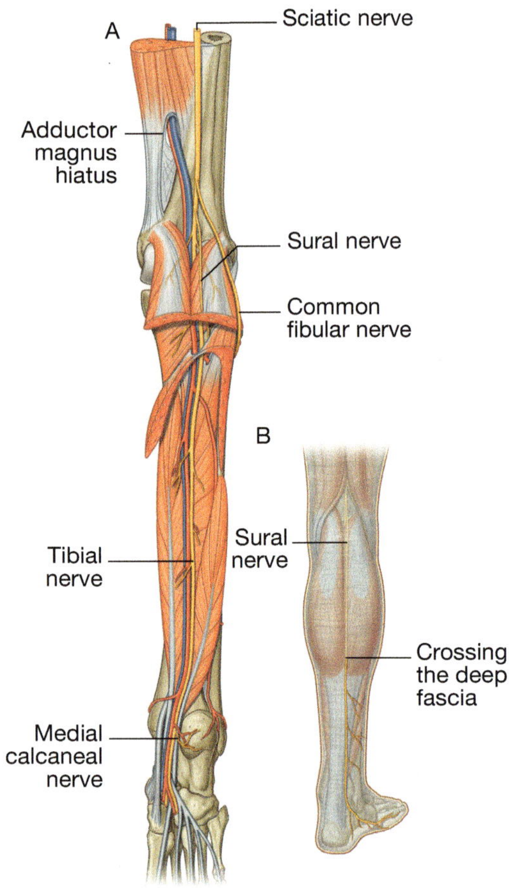

Fig. 30.7 Posterior tibial artery.

Technique (Fig. 30.6)

Choose two points of contact on the artery on either side of the extensor retinacula. Perform a stretch-induction of the anterior tibial artery. Maintain the stretch for 12 seconds. Next, stretch the dorsal metatarsal arteries through traction-induction of each toe. As with the nerves, use very light compression and emphasize elongation.

30.2 POSTERIOR TIBIAL ARTERY

This artery serves as a witness to vascular manipulation of the lesser pelvis, hip, knee, and foot. As noted previously, this pulse is easier to perceive than the anterior tibial

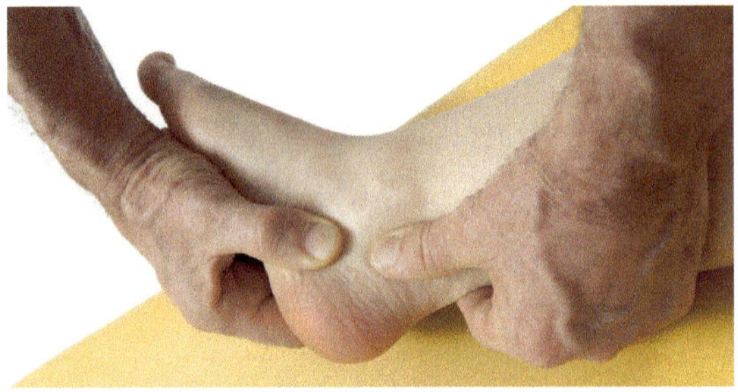

Fig. 30.8 Manipulation of the posterior tibial artery in lateral decubitus.

pulse. Manipulation of the posterior tibial artery has more widespread impact than does working the anterior tibial vessel.

30.2.1 Landmarks (Fig. 30.7)

The posterior tibial artery is located behind the medial malleolus. Ask the patient to flex his toes so that you can more easily feel the muscle. Place your thumb immediately behind the muscle.

30.2.2 Technique in lateral decubitus (Fig. 30.8)

The patient lies on the side opposite the artery to be manipulated, leg somewhat flexed. Place yourself either behind or in front of your patient. After locating the pulse, place one finger proximally and the other distally to create and maintain distal traction. Repeat this technique five or six times and then proceed with traction-induction of the artery.

Clinical note

In the case of either the posterior or anterior tibial arteries, always compare both sides. This allows you to discover a possible weak side or to confirm whether or not you have improved circulation by your maneuver. You can sometimes stretch the medial plantar artery, but this is rarely done. Manipulating the posterior tibial artery is usually enough to reestablish good general plantar circulation.

31 The emotional foot

Below are lists of attitudes, behaviors, and psychological tendencies we have found in observing hundreds of patients who experienced frequent ankle sprains. As with every joint, there are exceptions to these general propensities. A person cannot be put into a box, and there are always nuances. Still, a certain dominating tendency is there. The way a person contacts the ground is revealing.

Here is what we have noticed.

31.1 FEET FIRMLY PLANTED, POSITIONED IN LATERAL ROTATION

The well-planted person stands with his feet flat and open to the ground, legs slightly apart. You have a sense that the weight of his body is well supported and balanced on two feet.

This stance may express these characteristics:

- pragmatism;
- reality;
- the desire to make things happen;
- stability;
- action;
- energy;
- momentum toward the other;
- mission;
- future;
- roots;
- being a part of one's own territory;
- reactivity;
- spontaneity;
- desire to dominate.

31.2 FEET LESS GROUNDED, POSITIONED IN MEDIAL ROTATION

This stance may express these characteristics:

- instability;
- passivity;
- timidity;
- lack of pragmatism;
- poor sense of territory;
- absence of roots;
- lack of conviction;
- dreaminess;
- rejection of reality;
- the imaginary;
- fantasy;
- hesitation;
- withdrawal;
- reflection;
- fear of going over hurdles.

Conclusion

The techniques presented in this book are easy to perform and can be readily incorporated into clinical practice. Even so, their effectiveness demands nothing short of precision!

The anatomical education of the hand requires much perseverance and patience. Daily learning is the key to progress. Every patient enhances the development of our practice by either pushing our limits or filling in certain knowledge gaps. This is how any therapist improves.

The manual therapist's mind must cultivate the ability to connect theoretical knowledge with what the hand feels. As Professor Delmas (1981) wrote, "Learning anatomy is not limited to the study of cadavers, but must be integrated with an understanding of how it functions in the living."

The lower extremity is of capital importance to any therapist interested in human mechanics. It is the starting point of countless imbalances. A fresh approach often leads to advancement in patient care.

Bipedalism requires mechanical and neurological strategies involving all three joints of the lower extremity. Each has its own specifications:

- The hip finds stability in conjugating structural sturdiness with powerful muscles.
- The knee is the realm of the sensorimotor program, whereby it makes up for relative structural instability with unparalleled proprioceptivity and muscle responsiveness.
- The foot is an architectural complex whose deformability confers strength and flexibility to the unit.

We have also seen that beyond the classic biomechanical duality of mobility and stability, the lower extremity possesses an invisible quality: shock absorption. Cushioning relies in large measure on the viscoelasticity of supporting tissues. Our techniques have a very good effect on this parameter.

"For a joint to fulfill its contract, which is to say provide a normal function for an entire lifetime, it must keep to the supreme law of overall balance between its elements" (Ficat and Ficat 1987).

This quote could have come from Andrew Taylor Still, the founder of osteopathy. Instead it derives from a pair of orthopedic surgeons named Ficat and Ficat, whose frame of reference is certainly quite different from our own. Nevertheless, their thinking rather perfectly describes the intention of this book, which is to help normalize the joint in the context of the whole body.

We also gladly consider the joints in the context of a person's existence—their whole "way of being."

Bibliography

Arnoczky, S. P., Warren R. F. 1982. "Microvasculature of the human meniscus." *Am J Sports Med* 2 (10): 90–95.

Barral, J. P., and A. Croibier. 2004. *Manipulations des nerfs périphériques.* Paris: Elsevier Masson.

Barral, J. P., and A. Croibier. 2009. *Manipulations vasculaires viscérales.* Paris: Elsevier Masson.

Barral, J. P., and A. Croibier. 2011. *Nouvelle approche manipulative: Membre supérieur.* Paris: Elsevier Masson.

Barral, J. P., J. P. Mathieu, and P. Mercier. 1992. *Diagnostic articulaire vertébral.* 2nd ed. Aix-en-Provence, France: Cido & De Verlaque [F].

Beaufils, P., and R. Verdonk. 2010. *The meniscus.* Berlin: Springer-Verlag.

Bénichou, J., and M. Libotte. 2002. *Le livre du pied et de la marche.* Paris: Odile Jacob.

Blackwood, C. B., T. J. Yuen, B.J. Sangeorzan, and W.R. Ledoux. 2005. "The midtarsal joint locking mechanism." *Foot Ankle Int* 26 (12): 1074–1080.

Blaha, J. D., and E. Wojtys. 2006. "Motion and Stability of the Normal Knee." In *Insall & Scott Surgery of the Knee* 4th ed., edited by W. Norman Scott, M.D., 227–239. Philadelphia: Churchill Livingstone.

Castaing, J. 1977. *Anatomie fonctionnelle de l'appareil locomoteur: Fascicule 4—La hanche.* Paris: Vigot.

Cazeau, C. 2006. "Faut-il s'intéresser à la bipédie? Analyse anatomique et biomécanique dans diverses classes animales. Utilité pour la recherche de la phylogénie humaine." *Maîtrise Orthopédique* no.155. www.maitrise-orthop.com/viewPage.do?id=664.

Chiron, P. 2001. "Technique et indications de l'arthroscopie de hanche." *Cahiers d'enseignement de la SOFCOT* 2001. 78: 33–50.

Croibier, A. 1991. *Trou obturateur énigme ostéopathique.* Mémoire Collégiale Académique.

Croibier, A. 2005. *Diagnostic ostéopathique général.* Paris: Elsevier Masson.

Davies, P. C. W. 1996. *Les forces de la nature.* Paris: Flammarion.

De Doncker, E., and C. Kowalski. 1976. *Cinésiologie et rééducation du pied.* Paris: Elsevier Masson.

De Rosnay, J. 1975. *Le Macroscope: vers une vision globale.* Paris: Editions du Seuil Collection Points Essais.

Delmas, A. 1958. "L'acquisition de la station érigée." In *Les processus de l'Hominisation,* 9–36. Colloques internationaux CNRS.

Dolto, B. "Pelvis plaque tournante entre le tronc et les jambes." *Ann Méd Phys* 337–345, 1967, 406 –415, 1968.

Dolto, B. 1976. *Le corps entre les mains.* Paris: Hermann.

Dufour M., and M. Pillu. 2006. *Biomécanique fonctionnelle: Membres-Tête-Tronc. Rappels anatomiques, stabilités, mobilités, contraintes.* Issy-les-Moulineaux, France: Elsevier Masson.

Dye, S.F. 2008. "The envelope of function." In *The Crucial Principles Care of the Knee*, edited by J. A. Feagin and J. A. Steadman, 51–57. Philadelphia: J. R. Lippincott, Williams & Wilkins.

Ethier, C. R., and C. A. Simmons. 2007. *Introductory Biomechanics: From Cells to Organisms.* New York: Cambridge University Press.

Ficat, P., and C. Ficat. 1987. *Pathologie mécanique de la hanche.* Paris: Elsevier Masson.

Fick, R. 1911. *Handbuch der Anatomie und mechanik der gelenke unter berücksichtigung der bewegenden muskeln.* Dritter Teil: Spezielle gelenke-und Muskelmechanik. Lena (Allemagne): Verlag von Gustav Fischer.

Fox, E. L., and D. K. Mathews. 1984. *Bases physiologiques de l'activité physique.* Traduit et adapté par F. Peronnet. Decarie et Vigot.

Freeman, M. A., and B. Wyke. 1967. "The innervation of the ankle joint: An anatomical and histological study in the cat." *Acta Anat* 68: 321–333.

Fryette, H. H. 1983. *Principes des techniques ostéopathiques.* Bruxelles: SBO-RTM.

Gillot, V. 1995. "Veines plantaires et pompe veineuse." *Phlébologie* 48: 49–70.

Giraudet, G. 1976. *Biomécanique Humaine appliquée à la rééducation.* Paris: Elsevier Masson, Paris.

Goldcher, A. 2007. *Podologie* 5th ed. Paris: Elsevier Masson.

Greenwald, A. S. 1974. "Joint congruence, a dynamic concept." *In The hip: Proceedings of the second open scientific meeting of the hip society*, edited by W. H. Harris, 3–21.

Hendrix, G. 1934. "Pathologie des déformations statiques des voûtes du pied." *Bul Soc Belge Orth* 6 (3).

Hogervorst, T., and R. A. Brand. 1998. "Current Concepts Review: Mechanoreceptors in Joint Function." *J Bone Joint Surg Am* 80: 1365–1378.

Hoppenfeld, S. 2004. *Examen clinique des membres et du rachis.* Paris: Elsevier Masson.

Jerosch, J., M. Prymka, and W. H. Castro. 1996. "Proprioception of the knee joints with a lesion of the medial meniscus." *Acta Orthop Belg* 62: 41–45.

Kapandji, A. I. 1987. "La biomécanique 'Patate.' " *Ann Chir Main* 6 (3): 260–263.

Kapandji, A. I. 2009. *Anatomie Fonctionnelle Volume II: Membre Inférieur* 6th ed. Paris: Maloine.

Kapandji, A. I. 2011. *Qu'est-ce que la biomécanique?* Montpellier: Sauramps Médical.

Kim, Y., and H. Azuma. 1995. "The nerve endings of the acetabular labrum." *Clin Orthop* 320: 176–181.

Klein, P., and P. Sommerfeld. 2008. *Biomécanique des membres inférieurs. Bases et concepts, bassin, membres inférieurs.* Issy-les-Moulineaux: Elsevier Masson (F).

Kranich, E. M. 2006. *L'Homme et son corps: Anthropologie anatomique, physiologique et psychologique.* Triades.

Leliévre, J. 1981. *Pathologié du pied.* Paris: Elsevier Masson.

Le Minor, J. M. 2011. "Caractéristiques morphologiques évolutives du pied humain au sein des primates." In *Le pied* edited by G. Morvan et al., 17–43. Montpellier: Sauramps.

Lephart, S. M., D. M. Pinciviero, and S. L. Rozzi. 1998. "Proprioception of the ankle and knee." *Sports Medicine* 25: 149–155.

Liebschner, M. A. K., and T. S. Keller. "Hydraulic strengthening affects the stiffness and strength of cortical bone."

Annals of Biomedical Engineering 33 (1): 26–38.

MacConaill, M. A., and J. V. Basmajian. 1977. *Muscles and Movements: A basis for human kinesiology.* New revised edition. New York: Krieger Publishing Co.

Maestro, M., J. J. Rivet, and B. Ferré. 2011. *Le pied comment ça marche?* Montpellier: Sauramps Médical.

Misery, L. 2000. *La peau neuronale ou les nerfs à fleur de peau: Collection Vivre et Comprendre.* Ellipses Marketing.

Moore, K. L., and A. F. Dalley. 2001. *Anatomie médicale: Aspects fondamentaux et applications cliniques.* Paris: De Boeck.

Morin, E. 2005. *Introduction à la pensée complexe.* Paris: Editions du Seuil Collection Points Essais.

Netter, F. 2003. *Atlas of Human Anatomy* 3rd ed. Teterboro, N.J.: Icon Learning System.

Olivier, G. 1965. *Anatomie anthropologique.* Paris: Vigotis.

Olivier, G. 1965. *L'évolution et l'Homme.* Paris: Payot.

Olivier, G. 1978. *Homme ou singe.* Paris: Vuibert.

Paturet, G. 1951. *Traité d'anatomie humaine.* Paris: Elsevier Masson.

Piveteau, J. 1973. *Origine et destinée de l'Homme.* Paris: Elsevier Masson.

Rabischong, P. 2011. "Anatomie compréhensive du pied dans la locomotion." In *Le pied,* edited by G. Morvan et al., 45–57. Montpellier: Sauramps.

Rabischong, P. 2011. "Anatomie compréhensive du pied dans la locomotion. " In *Le pied,* edited by G. Morvan et al., Société d'Imagerie Musculo-Squelettique, 45–58. Montpellier: Sauramps.

Richards, G. 1986. "Free hands or enslaved feet? A note on the implications of ground-dwelling bipedalism." *J Hum Evol* 15: 143–150.

Rohen, J. W., and Ch. Yokochi. 1985. *Anatomie Humaine: Atlas photographique de l'Anatomie systématique et topographique Tome 1.* Paris: Vigot.

Rohen, J. W., and Ch. Yokochi. 1985. *Anatomie Humaine: Atlas photographique de l'Anatomie systématique et topographique Tome 2.* Paris: Vigot.

Schuenke, M., E. Schulte, and U. Schumacher. 2010. *Thieme Atlas of Anatomy: General Anatomy and Musculoskeletal System.* Stuttgart and New York: Thieme.

Still, A. T. 1992. *Osteopathy, Research and Practice.* Seattle: Eastland Press.

Testut, L. 1896. *Traité d'Anatomie Humaine.* Paris: Doin.

Testut, L., and A. Latarjet. 1948. *Traité d'Anatomie Humaine* 9th éd. revue et corrigée. Paris: Doin.

Testut, L., and O. Jacob. 1935. *Anatomie topographique.* Paris: Doin.

Valois, H. V. 1944. *La place de l'homme dans l'échelle des êtres.* Paris: CDU.

Von Bertalanffy, l. 1973. *Théorie Générale des Systèmes.* Paris: Dunod.

Wyke, B. 1972. "Articular neurology: a review." *Physiotherapy* 58: 94–99.